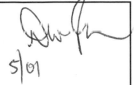

The Sunfood Diet Success System

36 Lessons In Health Transformation

David Wolfe
www.davidwolfe.com

Published by
Maul Brothers Publishing
San Diego, California

The Sunfood Diet Success System
By David Wolfe

This book contains little-known truths regarding the human body's amazing secrets.

A Note To The Reader:
Each lesson in this book contains facts, concepts, and ideas which build upon the lessons before it. Therefore, on the first time through, we urge the reader to avoid skipping around. The reading will surely prove most fruitful if you begin at the Table Of Contents and read straight through. It is our desire that a thousand years hence the contents of this book will be as up-to-date as at this moment. A lifestyle based on the cosmic laws is always in order and never becomes obsolete.

Unless otherwise noted, all poems are the author's work.

Disclaimer:
This book is sold for information purposes only. Neither the author nor the publisher will be held accountable for the use or misuse of the information contained in this book. This book is not intended as medical advice because the author and publisher of this work do not recommend the use of cooked foods or medicines to alleviate health challenges. Because there is always some risk involved, the author, publisher, and/or distributors of this book are not responsible for any adverse detoxification effects or consequences resulting from the use of any suggestions or procedures described hereafter.

ISBN #0-9653533-6-2
First Edition: April 1, 1999
Second Edition: January 1, 2000
Third Edition: October 1, 2000
Outside Cover Art: Ken Seaney, Ground Zero Graphic Design
Inside Cover Art: Dafna Mordecai, raw-foodist and professional artist
(Limited edition prints of the inside covers are available from Nature's 1st Law)
Interior Color Art: DiLuce Graphics
Total Book Design and Text Layout: David Wolfe
Copyright © 2000 Arlin, Wolfe

**Printed in North America on Recycled Paper by
Maul Brothers Publishing
P.O. Box 900202, San Diego, CA 92190 U.S.A.
Call or write for a FREE catalog: 1-800-205-2350**

What People Are Saying About
The Sunfood Diet Success System

"The philosophy and teachings of **The Sunfood Diet Success System** are terrific. The foundational law is the key understanding of this book: 'one thing does lead to another.' David Wolfe, in a beautifully authentic way, plants the awareness of the power of a live-food diet and healthy thinking that is transforming to each individual and to the very planet itself. I will be highly recommending this book to all at the Tree Of Life Rejuvenation Center." — Gabriel Cousens M.D. (H) author of **Conscious Eating** and **Spiritual Nutrition And The Rainbow Diet**

"This breakthrough book not only demonstrates a profound under-standing of Nature's physical laws of health-building, but also masterful-ly integrates the under-recognized motivational, mental, and emotional components needed to create overall success in life. A unique contribu-tion to the field and I highly recommend it to all success seekers." — Viktoras Kulvinskas MS, author of **Survival Into The 21st Century**

"Just as a fragrant tropical mango, glistening in the Sun, is an open invitation to eat it, reading **The Sunfood Diet Success System** is an open invitation to live it. Written by one who clearly does, this book is an inspiring synthesis of life-proven success technologies and the author's understanding of Nature's unchanging laws." — Eliot Jay Rosen, author of Los Angeles Times bestselling book **Experiencing The Soul**

"David Wolfe has emerged as the most important voice in the raw-food movement. This book is destined to be the new 'Bible' of the movement, perfect for both the beginner and the veteran raw fooder. The ancient Essenes lived to an average age of over 100 eating precisely the way this book advocates." — Rev. Dr. Abba Nazariah, worldwide head of the Essene Church Of Christ

"Never before have I come across a book which covers the entire spectrum of issues related to raw-food eating so honestly, concisely, and practically. This book will bring success because it covers every conceivable topic you are likely to encounter on your path to vibrant health and personal/spiritual development. If you only purchase one book this year, make it this one. Quite simply it will transform you and your life forever. This book is priceless." — Karen Knowler, coordinator of The FRESH Network, London, England

"Three cheers for 'The Sunfood Diet' — Raw! Raw! Raw! and for David Wolfe, an enlightened proponent of live food, who includes in his teaching the spirit of compassion by advocating the vegan lifestyle." — Light, founder of Gentle World

"David Wolfe has synergized a first class methodology for transitioning to and attaining limitless health and success on every level. With unyielding courage and compassion, David has removed the veils, pitfalls, and obstacles which keep us from achieving our full potential. He shares the simple, yet profound, truth of eating naturally. Put this book to work for you right now and start enjoying the results immediately. Sunfood is funfood!" — Jason Aberbach, founder of The Living Community Center, Tucson, Arizona

"David Wolfe, with **The Sunfood Diet Success System**, takes his rightful place with such notables as Cher Carden and raw-food 'guru' Aris Latham (**Sunfired Food Cookless Recipes**) in the forefront of live-food knowledge, healing, and wisdom, from spirit to emotions to the physical body. From the physiology chart comparing carnivores and vegetarian animals with humans, this book has it covered: life transformation, detoxification, even poetry. This book is a must read for anyone choosing to live 150 — or more — vital, strong, beautiful years on Earth." — Audrey Arbe, healer/psychic, columnist for **Inner Journeys**, producer/host of the award-winning cable television show *Aurora Borealis*

"The only thing I can say is: what are we going to do with all the other books we've been selling?! This book is amazing. It encompasses the entire field of raw foods. It answers every question." — Barbara Rogers, herbalist, Las Vegas, Nevada

"Thank you so much for your book. It is so powerful, so full of great Truths so little acknowledged, until now. I feel in my heart that anyone truly intent on becoming a better, more enlightened person could only benefit from the wisdom you so daringly offer within these pages. I know the Truth when I come face to face with it, and I don't hesitate for a moment to state that many profound Truths have come through you in the form of this book. Thank you and may you continue your diligent work of transformation — both of yourself and those who you touch, and the world at large." — Megan Oglevie, Sausalito, California

"Reading your book was like eating a fresh, ripe durian for the first time. At first you don't know what it is, but you know in some profound way it is really good! It starts to strike some familiarity with you but you can't place a finger on it. Maybe you had it when you were a little kid? No, you definitely would have remembered it if you had. Then suddenly, it hits you! You start realizing that in some mysterious way it is awakening past life memories! You had the knowledge and experience of the durian in a past life and now this powerful, aromatic, sweet, rich fruit has brought that knowledge and experience to your consciousness once again! You knew it all along, it was just locked up inside of you, and that first bite was the key that opened the door. David, this is your book, **The Sunfood Diet Success System!**" — Steve Adler, Sausalito, California

"This book advocates a simple, yet profound, plant-based diet that would heal many illnesses, support the growing organic food industry, shut down the abusive animal-farming cartels, and reverse much of the damage humans have done to this planet. It is a wonderful book and receives my highest recommendation." — John McCabe, author of **Surgery Electives: What to Know Before the Doctor Operates** and **Plastic Surgery Hopscotch**

David Wolfe is also the author of:

<u>Books:</u>
Eating For Beauty
Nature's First Law: The Raw-Food Diet

<u>Compact Discs:</u>
Vibrant Health, Youth, Abundance & The Best Day Ever

<u>Booklet:</u>
On Form And Actuality

David Wolfe is the publisher of:

The Sunfood Cuisine
(A companion recipe book to The Sunfood Diet Success System)

Dedication

This book is dedicated to my Aunt Dee-Dee.
You knew. You always believed. Thank you.

Acknowledgments

No one ever goes it alone. I thank every courageous spirit who has sought out this information and acted upon it. Thank you. You deserve the highest praise.

A special thank you goes out to Stephen Arlin and R.C. Dini whose incredible conviction has impassioned my life.

I would also like to thank the following people for their help, assistance, and friendship:

Fred Patenaude, author of **The Sunfood Cuisine** and editor of our magazine **Just Eat An Apple**, for his insights which helped formulate many areas of this book.

John McCabe, whose editing and ideas have made this book sparkle.

Angela Hartman and Susan Wildes, who have pushed me to bring this information to millions of people in a format all can understand, use, and apply.

Jolie Arlin, for her conviction and keen eye for detail.

Sequoia Neptune for her help in formulating the menu plans and several of the recipes and in indexing this book.

Table Of Contents

A Word From The Author

My name is David Wolfe. I am helping to create a whole new paradigm of health, wealth, happiness, success, prosperity, and possibility! In this book, we are going to find out just how good your life can be.

The material contained here is designed for all people, whether you are healthy, sick, searching, curious, looking for the next level, and/or seeking success physically and spiritually.

I cannot express how excited I am to present this information to all those interested in personal development and self-improvement. By availing yourself of this information you fulfill your destiny and simultaneously help fulfill my destiny of bringing **The Sunfood Diet Success System** to the world.

How I came to write this book is an interesting story. Both of my parents are medical doctors. My father had a general practice, then became an osteopath over his 35-year career. My mother is an anesthesiologist. As a child, I spent a lot of time at my parents' office. I used to play with my brothers beneath the chairs in the waiting room. I even used to travel with my dad on house calls.

I have seen the inside of the medical profession from a unique perspective. What I noticed was that people, over the long term, did not get better taking medicine. Instead, they got worse. When I was ten years old, I decided I was not going to take medicine anymore for any reason. And though I fought with my mother over this for many years, I did not submit. What I noticed was that when my two brothers and I would get sick, I would only be sick for one or two days, while their flus or colds would drag on for four or five days with the medicine. I learned then to just rest and drink only freshly-squeezed orange juice all day and soon I would feel better. That was a major revelation to me at that age and set me on the path to discover greater truths.

In my late teens I found that I was reacting to certain foods. I finally narrowed it down to dairy products. So, without really knowing anything about nutrition at that time, I cut out dairy products completely. And I immediately lost 10 pounds (4.5 kilograms) and felt amazingly better! I soon reached a point where I would not eat any food that contained any dairy products whatsoever — even if it was the tenth ingredient.

It was the discipline of completely letting go of all dairy products which set up a "blueprint" for more dietary progress. Therein I learned a valuable lesson: all disciplines affect each other. A powerful discipline can transfer over from one area of your life to any other area.

After letting go of all dairy products, I started to read every book and listen to every audio tape on the field of nutrition that we had in my house. I quickly found the book **Fit For Life** by Marilyn and Harvey Diamond which confirmed what I knew about the danger of pasteurized dairy products. I adopted the Fit For Life Diet and gradually moved over to a vegan diet by eliminating animal products from my life (the vegan lifestyle contains no animal foods or products which impact animal lives).

But I kept reading, I kept searching. All of my life I could not escape the feeling that I was missing something, overlooking something so obvious it had managed to escape me. Ever since the earliest days I could remember, I had a sense that I would one day discover some great secret.

Through reading I found out about The Raw-Food Diet. When I first discovered that one could live on 100% raw plant food, it was a revelation to me. It resonated with my core — it sent chills throughout my body. Within three months of eating raw foods, I knew I had found it. I felt as if the great secret of the ages had been revealed to me. For me, it was an Earth-trembling discovery. I knew this was the way to achieve my maximum potential. I knew instantaneously that it was my mission to bring this message to the world. I knew in that sparkling moment that I would revolutionize the personal development world with this information. I saw massive potential. Within three words — raw plant food — is the key to unlocking humanity's dormant powers.

I quickly found that this wonderful truth was not so evident to other people. And again I learned a great lesson. The greatest truths of the world, the ones which have shaken civilizations to their core, always appear insignificant to many other observers. But to the discoverer, the philosopher, that truth is priceless. To the one who has acted upon that truth and taken a new vantage, everything is clear and obvious. Through experience, a guess becomes knowledge, speculation becomes certainty. Part of the true world reveals itself and that in itself is a revelation.

I found out that just knowing to eat raw plant foods is not enough: breaking addictions plays a role, peer pressure steps in, the proper mind-set is important, detoxification is a factor, as are emotions, and balance. After many years of experimenting, reading, and communicating with thousands of others on this path of eating raw plant foods, I finally perfected what I call **The Sunfood Diet Success System** and wrote this book.

As you read through these pages, I think you may find yourself discovering the tremendous importance of this message for the future of the world; this information allows the Earth to heal and prosper. You may find new wonder and hope. You may perceive that your life can be transformed in a most profound way.

At this moment I am overcome with the emotion of gratitude for having reached the level of health I have been blessed to experience and for having the opportunity to present this health information to you. Thank you for choosing this book. I invite you as a guest into a new realm of possibility. I wish you the greatest prosperity.

Introduction

The Sunfood Diet is the promise that we can become something more — that there is a better way to live. You can be totally rejuvenated. You can walk the Earth barefoot again as you did as a child, feeling the blades of grass beneath your feet, touching the flower petals, chasing the butterflies, watching the ants, thinking clearly and calmly.

Within you is a power which will astonish you. Within you are the seeds of greatness, of beauty, of discipline, of excellence, of destiny. This is the last moment of the way you used to be. It is time to give yourself permission to reach the absolutely highest possible state of health.

What good are all the possessions in the world if you do not have your health? What good are material experiences if you do not have the intense vibrancy to enjoy them?

The Sunfood Diet is the product of a new will-to-health, a new will-to-life, arising from ashen foods like a phoenix all over the world. The Sunfood Diet identifies those foods that allow the body to work to its maximum potential. The Sunfood lifestyle teaches that robust health is the natural state; inspired energy is our natural birthright. It demonstrates how to purify your physical body and unlock the key to your maximum potential.

Sunfoods beautify the body, mind, and spirit. They carry with them the vitality of health and life — the vibrant Sun energy that nourishes all life on Earth. By taking in the energy of vibrant Sunfood you can overcome any health challenge. The Sun is a transformer. By eating Sunfoods you can improve your life in every way. When your health improves, every other aspect of your life improves simultaneously.

To strive for health, wealth, happiness, and success is as natural to your creative urges as it is natural for a tree to strive for its maximum fulfillment. In Nature, there are no limits to what you can have, be, or do. You deserve to reach the highest goal possible: vibrant happiness.

This book, **The Sunfood Diet Success System,** is first and foremost a philosophy. It is a study of secret fundamental things which are not part of everyday conversation. This message is about getting close to Nature and natural laws. It is the idea that people living close to Nature tend to be noble. Living close to Nature is the greatest wonder you can experience for your spiritual, emotional, mental, and physical health. The more natural you are, the healthier and happier you are (and there is no limit as to how healthy and happy you can become!).

Many books are filled with words about words, they are filled with researched research; the authors themselves have not experienced what they are writing about. What I teach is based on real-life experience. I have discovered powerful distinctions we can use immediately to dramatically improve our health today.

If you are tired of the crumbs and ashes of life, if a mediocre existence has become a burden upon you, then take this book to heart and read it deeply. For within these pages is a distillation of many wonderful principles of life transformation. These pages invite you to open your spirit to the full abundance life has to offer.

This is an abundant universe. Grasp your birthright. Success is a *massive abundance* of physical, mental, emotional, and spiritual health.

The divine power within you is the healing and creative power in your life. As long as you have a single spark of vitality within you, there is great hope. You are a physical, mental, emotional, and spiritual being capable of achieving incredible prosperity at all levels. You are priceless. Treat your body better than a Rolls Royce. No technology will ever surpass the magnificence of your own biological design.

The real lesson here is that you are in control of your destiny. The apple never falls far from the tree. If you do not like the health you are experiencing, you can change it! If you do not like the video being played across your mind, you can change it! If you do not enjoy the food you are eating, you can change it! You feel positive about yourself to the degree you feel you are in control of your life. You feel negative about yourself to the degree you feel you are not in control of your life. When you feel out of control, you experience stress, fear, and psychosomatic illness. Overcome negativity by understanding that you are always in control. No one outside of you controls how you feel; you are responsible. I congratulate you, because by reading this book, you have made the decision to take control; you have already begun to achieve vibrant health.

All books are not created equal. Of what account is a book that does not carry us away beyond all books? We learn for distinctions: little clues which improve the value of our lives. Each distinction becomes a fresh new opportunity. Tune into the information which contains the most distinctions. The best books contain a maximum amount of distinctions we can use immediately to produce incredible results now.

The most successful people in life have the best information. Through my organization Nature's First Law, I have been privy to some of the best personal-development information available. In our company library, we have some of the best, rarest, and most exclusive self-help information resources, gathered from around the world. Information drawn from these resources is contained herein. In fact, all the greatest transformative lessons I have ever encountered are planted here within these pages. The distinctions provided in this book have been proven by real-life testing. My own experience has made me a science project for these facts. My intense research has unlocked health secrets which can only be called "magical."

Nothing succeeds like success, and there is no better proof of something's worthiness than good results. The success, joy, and exuberance for life I enjoy each moment is proof-positive of the incredible power of the concepts in this book.

Stop listening to anyone, in any field, who is not getting the results that you desire. Stop. Read that sentence three times in a row. Would you go to a beggar for financial advice? Only listen to those who are getting the results you desire in any given area of life. I have achieved an extraordinary aliveness, and I will show you how you can achieve it too by the lessons provided within these pages.

The information within this book is meant for you to not only read, but to study and act upon. Expect the maximum possible value from each page. As you read, see, listen, and feel this message. Highlight your favorite passages. Take notes. Specifically: first read the book through entirely; second, read each chapter twice (before moving on to the next chapter) and highlight your favorite passages; third, immediately act upon the information by using the action steps provided at the end of each lesson; fourth, purchase and use a journal with which to record your progress.

The content of this book is revolutionary in scope. Any given person can begin to function at extraordinary levels once they have realized in which way lies their true line of progress. That line of progress is internal purification through the application of **The Sunfood Diet Success System**. Internal purification allows one to begin remembering how the mind works and how to use that knowledge to achieve superior health. A wise adage states, "All this struggling to learn, when all we have to do is remember." All the wisdom we require is already within us.

To direct this planet into a new era of massive prosperity, we are going to require a new level of physical health. A healthy body allows us to access the dormant areas of the brain. We access those areas as the pineal gland (the "spiritual" gland, located in the mid-brain), is purified through positive thoughts and food choices. When our brain (mind) is clear of toxicity, we can receive clear information, and then take action.

This is powerful information. The Sunfood Diet creates a whole new paradigm of success. Many, many people I have met have searched throughout the personal development, self-help genre of literature for a book on living foods and success. Many of the success philosophers of the newest age have missed this vital link. Only a few books hint of the connection, Anthony Robbins' **Unlimited Power** (Chapter X) is the foremost example which comes to mind. In his book, Robbins describes that a successful individual must be fueled by a healthy diet. *The connection between success and diet is absolutely crucial.*

The time has come to bring this diet information to the personal-development audience. I have tapped a magic power and I will show you how you can too. And so, I present to you the dietary approach to self-mastery and massive abundance:

THE SUNFOOD DIET SUCCESS SYSTEM
or
LIVING FOODS AND LIFE TRANSFORMATION
or
HOW TO UNLOCK YOUR MAGICAL POWERS

This book can show you how to achieve perfect health and perfect digestion as I have done. In the following 36 lessons are many seeds which you may nourish to discover a new destiny. This book is not only about diet, it is about a complete health transformation that begins with the proper frame of mind. I invite you to grasp the distinctions provided in these pages. Swallow this elixir of knowledge and experience the true beauty of living!

All confusion fades once the facts are known...

Lesson 1:
The Principle Of Life Transformation

"In order to have something, you must first be something."
— Goethe

"The outer situation is always a reflection
of the collective inner situation."
— Peace Pilgrim

You are not what you are, rather, what you are, is what you can be. The most interesting thing about life is that you can become more than you were before. You can become stronger, wiser, healthier than you ever dreamed possible. You can achieve your true potential. You can completely reform your physical structure, your intelligence, your emotional poise, your spiritual power. This book is about how to biologically transmutate the lead of life into the white gold of glory.

The Principle of Life Transformation is that life change comes from the inside out. All transformation begins with one person — you. As above, so below. Everything happening around you is only a reflection of what is going on inside you. If you want the world to change, *you* have to change.

We are all personally responsible for the state of the entire world because the world only mirrors our inner selves. Pollution, famine, and disease are reflective of the inner crisis gripping us individually, and therefore collectively. These "realities" are fragments of our collective consciousness projected outward upon our environment.

Your idea of the world (what you believe the world is) manifests everything in your life. When you change your idea of the world, the world itself changes. Essentially, your mission is not to set the world right, but simply to set yourself right. Then, and only then, will the world begin to be set right. I tell my seminar listeners:"The world does not change — we change."

Life transformation is an inner journey. To succeed in life you have to work harder. But not on your family, or on your friends, or on your job, or on whatever comes your way. You have to work harder on yourself first.

Your own happiness is your number one priority. Many have the idea that they have to undergo a process of stress and pain in order to provide for themselves and their families. They do so with the idea that at some future date they will all be happy. If this is you, please understand that you cannot make anyone else happy by being unhappy yourself. Only happy people make others happy. Instead of achieving to be happy, happily achieve.

When we strive to become better ourselves, everything around us becomes better too. The environment we live in will become better or worse depending on whether we become better or worse. The people we associate with will become better or worse depending on whether we become better or worse. You automatically achieve improved results, when you become an improved person.

It seems the whole works of humankind are backwards. Most are trying to convince, instruct, and purify everyone else — without first purifying themselves. To enlighten others we have to enlighten ourselves.

The best way to make others healthy is to become incredibly healthy yourself!

Health is not something we can get; rather, it is something we attract by the person we become. If we chase after health, it will elude us like a butterfly. However, if we calmly attract health by becoming the type of person who can be radiantly healthy, it will land upon us with a most radiant flutter.

Once we understand that life change comes from the inside out, and that it is in becoming something new that we achieve something new, then we decide to take full responsibility for our lives. The success philosopher Earl Nightingale expressed this understanding when he said: "All of us are self-made, but only the successful will admit it."

You will make incredible progress in your life when you accept 100% responsibility for everything that happens to you. You are where you are and who you are because of one person — yourself.

Take full responsibility for everything that happens in your life. As the saying goes: "When you point your finger at someone, you have three fingers pointing back at you." People accuse others of what they themselves are guilty of.

Winners take full responsibility for everything that happens to them — even when those things seem remote and are not directly attributable to their actions. Taking 100% responsibility for everything in your life transforms you into a new type of person because it forces you to research all "effects" back to their "causes." Understanding "causes" is the science of life transformation.

Our focus here in this book is vibrant, superior health. If you are suffering from ill health, there is only one person responsible — yourself. Blaming others will not empower you. Concepts such as the germ/virus theory are the end products of efforts to put the blame of ill health on someone or something outside of oneself — to remove responsibility from the individual. To achieve our goal of superior health, we must take 100% responsibility.

Action Steps:

1. Purchase and begin writing in a journal to record your progress through this book and beyond. Success philosopher Anthony Robbins says: "If your life is worth living, it is worth recording." Write down your wonderful thoughts. Begin now to describe your health transformation. Release worries, doubts, and fears by writing them down. What an amazing gift your journals can be to your children and their children — they can learn from you and feel a connection with you even when you are gone!

2. The first day you begin this book, take a "before" picture.

3. Instead of trying to remedy everything "out there," decide now to turn your focus inward to beautify your physical, mental, emotional, and spiritual potential. Write down the answer to the following questions in your journal: "What type of person do I have to become to experience radiant health?" "How do I become that type of person as quickly as possible while enjoying the process?"

4. Say to yourself daily:"I am fully responsible for my own great health. My daily habits create my great health." Write this affirmation on the first page of your journal and on your bathroom mirror.

*

"Correcting oneself is correcting the whole world.
The Sun is simply bright. It does not correct anyone.
Because it shines, the whole world is full of light.
Transforming yourself is a means of giving light to the whole world."
— Ramana Maharshi

Lesson 2:
The Foundational Law

There is a law which was decreed during the foundation of the world. It is the law upon which all things are based. It is immortal and true, even for the few. *The law is that things produce after their own kind.* It is the primal law of cause and effect: the Law of Production. "As ye sow, so shall ye reap" (Galatians 6:7). Those seeds planted must return to us their kind — in abundance. This law knows no exception. The Law of Production does not bend for anyone.

The profound truth is: one thing does lead to another.

Excellent food choices lead to more excellent food choices. Excellent habits create a fertile ground for more excellent habits. Excellent decisions lead to more excellent decisions.

If you sow that which is beneficial to all, you will receive that which is beneficial to you. If you sow compassion for all animals, you will receive the compassion of all animals. If you sow beautiful living, you will receive a beautiful life. We have the choice as to what vibrations we send out into the cosmos.

Once the seeds are planted they sprout and grow into realities. They produce after their own kind and, with concentration and emotion, spread prolifically.

In **The Dispersion Of Seeds**, Henry David Thoreau wrote: "Though I do not believe that a plant will spring up where no seed has been, I have great faith in a seed. Convince me that you have a seed there, and I am prepared to expect wonders."

Seeds are karmic substances; they have a potential, a destiny. "The seed is the word of God" (Luke 8:11). If you wish to reap a different destiny in any area of your life in the future, you need to plant new, different seeds today. Seeds grow into plants, and plants grow fruits, and the fruits spread more seeds.

The most fertile soil in the world is found in the human mind. No matter what one desires, it is not until the idea-seeds are planted in the garden-mind with nurturing emotion that they will come forth. To get a high quality of change, we must choose the highest quality seeds and provide them with an abundance of carefully selected nutrients. Those idea seeds given the greatest emotion will grow fastest and most abundant, perhaps even crowding out or overcoming weaker seeds. Strong emotion gives nourishment to thought seeds. Strong emotion sets seeds into vibration.

When you have an emotional thought, whether that thought is positive or negative, it will begin to materialize in your life. That is why it is so important to keep your mind focused with emotion on the things you desire and off the things you fear.

When the emotional desire for a thing is so intense that it illuminates every fiber of your being, then it shall be fulfilled.

As long as one nurtures the seeds of joy, achievement, and destiny, these things shall follow in abundance; however, if the poisonous prickly weeds of doubt and fear are allowed to take possession of the garden, they too shall follow. Poisonous prickly weeds grown in the garden-mind lead to negativity, hopelessness, inferiority complexes, and mental illness.

Growth, maturity, and reproduction is a pattern in Nature. Planting demonstrates how things produce after their kind — it is the Law of

Production in action. Use this knowledge now to begin cultivating within your garden-mind the seeds of exceptional health.

Action Steps:

1. Daily, as you arise, and also before you sleep, picture yourself in perfect health, happiness, and harmony. Picture yourself radiantly alive. Hold this picture with emotional desire in your conscious mind for 30 unbroken seconds. This will plant a seed. By consistent focus this seed will grow. The power and effervescence of superior health, happiness, and harmony will eventually come forth.

2. Begin to trace health challenges (effects), whether they be addictions, illnesses, etc., to their "causes." Record the answer to the following question in your journal:"What is the true cause of my foremost health challenge?"

The Law Of Production

The Law of our Fate
We choose our wealth.
Love brings love,
Health brings health.

Like produces like,
An effect resembles its cause.
Things produce after their kind,
It's one of the basic laws.

A smile brings a smile,
Peace brings peace;
And never will
This spiral cease.

As you sow,
So shall you reap.

Carefully choose
Which seeds you keep.

Abundant seeds
In the soil spread.
Fertile plants
Will grow when fed.

Things do follow
After their type.
You'll reap your crop
When the time is ripe.

For a future is found
In every seed.
It's "cause and effect"
...with godspeed.

The Law of Production,
The subtleness of mind;
Success breeds success:
Each creates its kind.

Lesson 3:
Thoughts Are Things

"All destiny begins with thinking."
— Percival

"The ancestor of every action is a thought."
— Ralph Waldo Emerson

"When any object or purpose is clearly held in thought,
its precipitation, in tangible and visible form is merely
a question of time. The vision always precedes
and itself determines the realization."
— Lillian Whiting

"We become what we think about."
— Earl Nightingale

You are not what you think you are, rather, what you think, you are.

Thoughts are things. Thoughts are seeds. Everything you do or think is a cause set in motion. Every thought sent forth is a never-ending vibration spiraling its way across the universe and returning to us what we have sent with interest.

Thoughts are energy. Energy pulsates, it sends ripples into the fabric of time and space, affecting all things.

Thoughts objectify themselves. Thoughts turn themselves into physical "objects." You magnetize into your life whatever you hold in your thought. The more often you think about something, the more quickly it will appear in your reality.

Thoughts are the foundation of everything you become. Everything you have in your life right now was once a thought in your mind. Thoughts shape your being and character. Everything which happens to you, which you attract into your life, is a product of your thinking. This means you are 100% responsible for your own life and death and nothing outside of you can bring illness upon you.

Thoughts are felt. Negative thoughts produce acid throughout the entire tissue system. Thoughts of envy, jealousy, fear, and resentment send waves of retentiveness and tension throughout the body. Those with a tendency to hoard typically suffer from constipation. Thoughts are things; they have a physical component.

Your subconscious mind cannot tell the difference between an emotional thought and an actual event. Your body reacts to an emotional visualization just as if the event actually happened! Do you remember times when you thought of something so intensely that your body tensed or relaxed as if you were actually there in the event again? Notice what changed...only your thoughts. Yet, you physically felt different by thinking stressful thoughts.

People who live with stressful thoughts are apt to become ill. Anxiety quickly weakens the whole body. Negative thoughts alone can create havoc throughout the entire nervous system. However, strong, pure, and happy thoughts build fortitude and beauty. The natural body is a sensitive, finely-tuned instrument which responds readily to the thoughts it is repeatedly presented. Habits of thought will produce their own effects (good or bad) upon the body.

We must aim to nourish the youthful spirit which can never die. Youth is not a time of life, but a quality, a trait of character, a state of mind.

Thoughts of fear, pain, and grief age the body. On the other hand, thoughts of joy, beauty, and triumph enliven the body. Positive thinking will do wonders and help keep us young.

What the mind thinks, the body expresses. You have the potential of having the body you want. The power of thought (through the aid of the subconscious mind) has control over every cell of the body. You can restructure and rejuvenate your body by rethinking yourself, by grasping on to a healthier vision of yourself. Send down a different body plan to your subconscious mind. With consistency, your body and experience will follow suit.

As a child, you come into the world unafraid and limitless, able to express yourself freely and naturally. Youthful freedom and joy are still with you in your mind. When you choose freedom and joy, you automatically have them!

Your mind is your first-mover. All actions, results, and forthcoming realities we experience in our lives begin with creations in our minds. All these "effects" are derivatives of thought causes. Your life's conditions are the effects of those thought causes.

The "heads I win, tails you lose" scenario is always of one's own making. The prisons people find themselves in are always first in their minds.

You are a creator of circumstance, never a victim of circumstance. There is no such thing as a coincidence. You are at the cause of all effects. We live in an orderly universe governed by definite laws. Everything happens for a reason. You have something positive to learn from each experience. To reach spiritual fulfillment, first you must understand this law.

"Where your thinking is, there too, is your experience" and "As a man thinketh in his heart, so is he" (Proverbs 23:7) are two wise sayings. Successful individuals become successful because they acquire the habit of thinking in terms of success. If you think successful thoughts, you will achieve success. If you think healthy thoughts, you will become healthy. Being healthy is a function of thinking healthy thoughts. Sound physical health begins with a "health consciousness" produced by a mind which thinks in terms of prosperity and dismisses all thoughts of illness and negativity. Empowering thoughts lead to wholesome patterns of behavior. Physical illnesses are essentially psychological in origin in the respect that, if the mind is thinking unhealthy thoughts, this leads to unhealthy actions which leads to an unhealthy diet and lifestyle.

It is your own habits of thinking which give you mastery in any field of achievement. Thought seeds produce after their own kind; it is a simple law. The way you think about things determines your level of success in any given area. One cannot think of failure, and then succeed. One cannot plant the jimson weed and get tomatoes.

Life-mastery requires mind-mastery. Mind-mastery begins with one discipline: Keep your mind fixed upon the things you desire and off the things you do not desire! Mind-mastery means using your will to control which thoughts and pictures you are allowing to dominate the computer screen of your conscious mind. It means focusing your conscious mind only on those thoughts and pictures which elevate you to divine heights.

Your ability to take control and selectively monitor the thoughts you allow to dominate your conscious mind determines how successful you will be in any endeavor. By undertaking the process of monitoring your thoughts and transmuting those thoughts into the empowering spectrum of life, you become enlightened.

The Cause Of Negative Thoughts

But how do we get control of our minds? How do we make sure that our dominant thoughts are positive?

Many people think limited, negative thoughts because they think they have to. They have thought negatively for so long that it has become comfortable for them. They know not the cause, nor the effect, of their thinking.

One cannot think negative thoughts and achieve positive results. Negative thoughts are destructive.

Remember: to achieve different results, we are going to have to think and do things differently. To eliminate negative thoughts, open your mind to a new understanding of what causes them. The primary causes of negative thoughts are the following:

Cause #1: Living with love withheld in the past or present. Many of us did not receive enough love from one or both parents when we were children and we carry these feelings of lack into adulthood. Some of us are living in situations right now where love is withheld and/or conditional. To reverse these situations, we can start by freely forgiving our parents, because they did the best they could, with what they had, where they were. Holding on to past injuries serves no purpose in creating a successful future. By applying **Lesson 1: The Principle Of Life Transformation**, we can begin receiving more love from those around us by becoming more loving ourselves and by expressing that love unconditionally.

Cause #2: Enduring destructive criticism in the past or present. Associating with those who criticize spoils the climate of our life. It is imperative to disassociate from people who have the tendency to make us feel inferior — this is absolutely critical to achieving excellent health. We are going to learn more about this in **Lesson 24: The Power Of Association**. The habit of replaying destructive criticism in the mind can be overcome by applying the Law Of Substitution (described below).

Cause #3: Ingesting too many phosphorus-rich foods. Food has a profound impact on the way we think, feel, and behave as you may discover through your own experiences in applying the diet plan described in this book. Flesh foods, as well as nuts and seeds (including rice and other grains), are high in phosphorous (and other acid-forming minerals) which has a contracting and acidifying effect on the body. These effects are reflected in our state of mind. We are going to learn more about the effects of flesh foods in **Lesson 8: Food And Karma** and how to balance the high-phosphorus foods, such as nuts and seeds, in **Lesson 14: Sapo-ty Brook's CaPNaK Chart**.

Cause #4: Ingesting excessive cooked and processed foods (food degraded by heat and flame). Cooked and processed foods have lost their energy and vitality, thus causing us to feel less energetic and alive. A physical state of low energy is associated with negative thoughts and emotions, whereas a physical state of high energy is associated with positive thoughts and emotions (see **Lesson 7: The Sunfood Diet**).

The Law Of Substitution

Once you know the causes of negative thoughts, you can purge them more effectively and use the Law of Substitution to totally eradicate them from your life. To remove a cloud of negativity from your mind, eliminate the causes mentioned, then just relax and substitute positive thoughts in their place. The Law of Substitution is essential to mind-mastery.

Consider the words of Brian Tracy in **Maximum Achievement**:
"The Law Of Substitution: This is one of the most important of all mental laws. It is an extension of the Law of Control. It states that your conscious mind can hold only one thought at a time, and that you can substitute one thought for another. This "crowding out" principle allows you to deliberately replace a negative thought with a positive thought. In so doing, you take control of your emotional life. This law is your key to happiness, to a positive mental attitude, and to personal liberation. It can change your relationships, your conversations, and the predominant content of your conscious mind. Many people have told me this law alone has changed their lives. Your conscious mind is never empty; it is always occupied with something. By using the Law of Substitution, you can replace any negative or fearful thought that may be troubling you. You can deliberately substitute a positive thought in its place."

One thought will always dominate your conscious mind. Sovereignty is never held in suspense.

Thoughts circling and spiraling on a self-destructive tangent always lead to failure. Negative thoughts always lead to negative emotions. You can delete these types of thought patterns immediately from your mind before they arise. Substitute these thoughts by rigorously holding to the beautiful visions of your goals or past successes. Vividly impress in your garden-mind all your desires, and remove all forms of limitation, fear, and doubt. Do not make one concession to any negative thought patterns. Negative thoughts dissipate your power.

The key to life-long happiness is to systematically purge negative emotions from your life — to eliminate anything which triggers negativity or stress in your psyche. A garden-mind encumbered by negative thoughts repels health and prosperity. Purging negative emotions is not optional, it is necessary to achieve a vibrant state of health. This means you have to get away from negative friends, associates, or relatives as soon as possible. You cannot let their negativity dissuade you from your greatness.

When you eliminate negative emotions you automatically become a truly healthy individual. Your major health goal should be to keep your mind consciously focused on health and to substitute all unhealthy thoughts with healthy ones. You can tell how powerfully you desire health by how willing you are to focus your mind on the health you want to manifest, and off of the illness, doubt, and weakness you do not want to manifest.

Beautify Your Thoughts

Beautify your thoughts. Thoughts are the headwaters of action, life, and manifestation. Make the headwaters pure and the stream of life will flow with reckless, pure abandon.

With the diet information contained in this book, you will be renewing your body, but first you must beautify your mind.

A healthy diet will help you achieve a healthy mind and life. But, even the best change in diet will little help an individual who is unwilling to alter their negative thoughts. In fact, one can never alter their diet beyond a certain degree until the thoughts change first.

Consider the wise words of James Allen in his classic book **As You Think**, "A change of diet will not help those who will not change their thoughts. When our thoughts are pure, we no longer desire impure food."

To beautify your mind, guard against negative thoughts. Thoughts of detriment, disappointment, depression rob your body of its vibrancy. Any thought of negativity, worry, or doubt diminishes your power; these thought types will alter the future against your favor. Build a fortress around you of positive thoughts and high-energy which repels even the most subtle infusions of negativity.

Use your garden-mind creatively to rethink yourself. You can change what and how you think about things in your mind and achieve incredible results. You can change what you imagine (the content of your thoughts) and how you imagine it (the size, color, volume, and tone of your thoughts).

You can accelerate the realization of your mental pictures by writing your thoughts and ideas down. Think on paper. Success philosopher Mark Victor Hansen says: "Don't just think it, ink it." This gives your thoughts more substance. It adds a reality to them making them more likely to manifest. Writing down your thoughts, ideas, worries, expenses, etc. allows you to let go of those concepts and releases more room and energy for other things.

You can also accelerate the realization of your mental pictures by eating lightly or fasting. This allows you to think and visualize with incredible clarity.

Master your thoughts. Keep in mind that a single thought can revolutionize your life. A single thought can make you prosperous beyond belief. Make yourself a powerful magnet by focusing your thoughts consistently on prosperity and happiness. Dwell only upon thoughts of health. Be cheerful by entertaining only cheerful thoughts. Your destiny is within your own hands. You choose the seeds, plant them, and harvest the crop. You are the gardener of your future, you are the forestal of orchards to come.

The greatest seed of all — your limitless potential — is with you at all times. Nourish this seed of your divine greatness through concentration of thought. There is no limit to who or what you can be.

One thing is certain in life, you have to think — thought is the very essence of the life experience. Since you are going to be thinking anyway, you may as well think incredibly positive thoughts! Great thoughts produce greatness. Perfect thoughts produce perfection.

Action Steps:

1. Get a clear picture on the computer screen of your mind of the achievement you wish to have, then continuously think about how to achieve it. What specific actions do you need to take? Record the answer in your journal.

2. For 21 straight days use the Law of Substitution to push out negative thoughts from your mind. Replace them with positive thoughts of your goals, aspirations, and the greatest successes of your past.

Thoughts Are Things

Thoughts are things and powerful things —
Incredible things they are.
A thought alone
Can send a stone
To a superabundant star.

A thought once thought
Exists and ought
Be revered as such by you.

What you are today
Is the result I say
Of what you perceive as true.

The thoughts that are in your head
Tell all, about who you are.
And if those thoughts don't uplift you,
You'll never get too far.

A thought once thought
Is felt and ought.
To soothe the joints and muscle.
The thoughts in your mind
Should be of a kind
To alleviate Life's stressed hustle.

A thought creates many changes
In your body's biochemistry.
The best action you can take
Is to choose those thoughts carefully.

Your body can't tell the difference
Between experience and state of mind.
The real secret is to control
The interpretation of what you find.

A thought once thought
Is real and ought
To be considered an action.
The thoughts you think
Should be the link
To your greatness and satisfaction.

A thought never heard
Is one-third a spoken word
And one-ninth of a word written down.

Think on paper,
For ideas are safer,
When before your eyes they are found.

Translate an idea into riches
Or other material things.
A thought creates the nest
From which the sparrow sings.

Animals think many thoughts,
That's why humans think they're dumb.
The difference is animals think
Just to have some fun.

Thoughts are things and powerful things
When attached to emotional desires.
Thoughts have carried the fairest of kings
And crumbled the greatest empires.

The thoughts that rule your mind
Say who you are to you.
Rule your thoughts and you shall find
You created you anew.

What you dwell upon grows,
What you think about shows!
Trust your instinct
Think the thought
Live the life
You've always sought.
Strike out boldly with your plans unfurled,
For a thought alone can move the world.

Lesson 4:
Beliefs

"If you believe that you can do a thing,
or if you believe you cannot,
in either case, you are right."
— Henry Ford

"Beliefs are prearranged, organized filters
to our perceptions of the world."
— Anthony Robbins

A belief is a habitual pattern of thinking about yourself and the world. A belief is a template of thoughts.

Your mind functions on the Law of Belief: whatever you believe with confidence becomes your own self-fulfilling prophecy. Believe it, and it will come to pass. "If thou canst believe, all things are possible to him that believeth" (Mark 9:23).

The power of belief is overwhelming: no matter how right or how true something is, if you believe you can't do it, guess what?...you can't.

Expectations

Your expectations in any area of life are dependent upon your beliefs. Whatever you believe to be true in terms of health, wealth, or spiritual growth will be reflected in your expectations about those areas. The world conforms to your expectations. You receive what you expect to receive.

You are where you are and what you are because of the beliefs you have about who you are. You are healthy or unhealthy, successful or unsuccessful, happy or sad because of the beliefs you have about yourself in those areas.

If you keep believing what you are believing, you will keep achieving what you are achieving. If you keep doing what you are doing, you will keep getting what you are getting.

We have, as part of our mind, a filter container called the Reticular Activation System (RAS). The RAS contains our belief system which sensitizes us to certain types of information from our environment that we are tuned in to see, hear, and feel.

Our experience of an event is not the actual event itself, but a representation of the event after it has been run through the RAS filter of our belief system. Because there are billions of pieces of information coming into our sphere every moment, our belief system determines what we are going to allow to enter our awareness — if it did not filter this out, we would be overwhelmed and surely driven insane by too much information!

We do not experience things as they really are! We experience things only through a filter and that filter determines what information will enter our awareness and what will be rejected. If we change the filter (our belief system), then we automatically experience the world in a completely different way.

From this understanding about the RAS, we may realize that little in the universe is absolutely known because what we think is real is actually only a reflection of our beliefs in that area. Two insightful sayings state: "You don't believe what you see, rather, you see what you already believe" and "Seeing is believing? No, believing is seeing." Complete

objectivity, in any field, may be impossible. We see that "objective science" is most often subjective (as we shall explore in **Lesson 9: Origins**)!

We do not know how the world really is, we only know what our beliefs
are about the world. Our perceptions create our reality. The reality of our
day-to-day lives consists of an endless flow of perceptual interpretations
which we, as individuals who live in a specific society, have learned to
hold in common with other individuals.

The world we think we see is only a view, a collective description of
the world, that we create through our belief systems. Accepting this fact
seems to be one of the most empowering things one can do.

The "reality" of our world is not as real, or as "out there," as we believe
it is. Reality is only a description. That which is held in our minds as the
real world is merely a description of the world; a description that has
been developing within us from our first moments. Overcome the illusion
— the world may be a far different place than we believe now.

Your beliefs determine what you consider real. To believe that the
world is only as you think it is now, is funny! How many times have you
had a belief in your life which turned out to be wrong? To be totally false?
How did those beliefs affect your life? Your potential? Remember, it is
our beliefs which shape and create our reality, so we must choose
resourceful and empowering beliefs for ourselves and others.

An individual's true beliefs are discovered by what they do, not by what
they say. What you *truly* believe is determined by the actions you take.
You always act and think in a manner which is consistent with your
beliefs. This is true even if your beliefs are totally irrational and ridicu-
lous. If you believe any "thing," then that "thing" is true for you.

Your beliefs affect your physical body. They shape how you look. The
cells are constantly changing and reformulating themselves based on the
thought template provided by your beliefs. The mind carves the body.
The physical body is nothing more nor less than the beliefs we have about

it. Not only do the beliefs themselves create the body we have, but the beliefs also induce the actions. The derivative actions have their effect too! The actions of diet, exercise, rest, play, and joy all have their influence.

The question is not: "What should I believe?" The question is: "What is useful for me to believe?" Beliefs are either effective or ineffective. They either help the achievement of our goals and spiritual desires or hinder them.

The mind is the greatest power in the world. The only thing limiting anyone is their self-limiting beliefs. Holding onto poisonous beliefs shuts out all of the abundance life has to offer.

Change your beliefs about what you deserve and you will attract a whole new reality around you. You can do this by creating a belief paradigm which allows you to live to your highest health potential — physically, emotionally, mentally, and spiritually in a manner which honors all life forms.

As young children we possess a perfect mind and a perfect memory. It is through limiting beliefs that this potential is dampened. When you overthrow limiting beliefs, you will be returned to a perfect mind and a perfect memory.

At any given time you may regain your extraordinary potential by identifying (in writing) all your disempowering beliefs and dissolving them in oceans of new knowledge and wonder. Simply refuse to limit yourself in any way. Ideally, we should proceed as if limits to our abilities did not exist.

When we have eliminated our own limiting beliefs, then we automatically help those around us eliminate their limiting beliefs. This is another aspect of The Principle of Life Transformation: a change of beliefs on the inside of your mind produces a change of beliefs in other minds.

One of the greatest gifts we can give to another is our own strong belief in their potential. By influencing their belief system, we help them achieve their true potential — which makes everybody better off. I attribute much of my success in life to the influence of my Aunt Dee-Dee, who consistently instilled confidence in my abilities. Perhaps the greatest gift one can bestow upon another is to instill confidence by saying: "I believe in you. You are something special. You can do it!"

Action Steps:

1. You have beliefs about how you look, what is a good weight for you, how much you should eat, what types of foods you should eat, and how much you should exercise. What are they? Write them down in your journal. Ask yourself:"How can I immediately and powerfully improve or replace these beliefs and enjoy the process? Write down the answers to this question for each belief, and act upon them immediately.

2. Identify 5 limiting beliefs in writing in your journal. Replace each limiting belief with a one-sentence empowering belief. For example, if your old belief was "I am too fat," change it to "I am daily making choices which make me look excellent."

3. Tell all the special people around you that you believe in them. Tell them how special they are to you. Sincerely help and support them. By the universal karmic law (the Law of Reciprocity), what you send out will come back multiplied. This is the way to receive the belief and support you deserve.

Lesson 5:
Goals

"Great dreamers' dreams are never fulfilled,
they are always transcended."
— Alfred Lord Whitehead

"Human beings, you and I, are goal-centered organisms.
We are teleological in that we are motivated by purposes,
by desired end states. We are engineered mentally
to move progressively and successively from one goal
to the next, and we are never really happy unless,
and until, we are moving toward the accomplishment
of something that is important to us."
— Brian Tracy, success philosopher

"Success is taking action towards your personal goals each day."
— Jim Rohn, success philosopher

"Feeling listless? Make a list!"
— Anonymous

Imagine a beautiful garden with brilliant Sun, crystalline water, friendly insects, and rich soil ripe for the planting. A garden, perfect in every respect, except, there are no desirable seeds present because you have not planted them. The only seeds sprouting are those weeds and shrubs planted by others, or by the wind and birds. Yet you continue to tend and cultivate those haphazard plants with your resources. This perfect garden, containing none of your own seeds, is what your mind is like when you have no definite goals. If you have no crop to nurture to an edible state, you drift along with the vagaries, whims, and goals of others.

If you are not working to achieve your own goals, you are always working to achieve another's goals. Everything you do, every day, is actually for the achievement of goals. What you may want to ask yourself is: Are they my goals? And: Are they worthwhile goals?

The mark of a winner is intense goal orientation. Napoleon Hill called this "definiteness of purpose." It is a direction you have selectively chosen for your life.

Few realize that a major cause of stress (the great destroyer of health) is having no clear goals, no future to await you, no plan to get somewhere in life. Setting goals allows us to chart the course of our life and control where we are going. The more control we feel we command over our future, the less stress we feel.

The very first step before you begin a journey is an undiminished decision as to where you are headed. First get clear about what you want and where you are going if you are determined to manifest the dormant powers within you. Decide. Dedicate yourself wholeheartedly to getting there. Chart your course; it is much easier to travel with a map.

If the success you seek is extraordinary, then you must begin immediately to set extraordinary goals. As long as you are going to dream, dream great dreams. As long as you are going for prosperity, go for it all! Spectacular success is always preceded by spectacular goal setting and mental preparation.

Release all limitations today! Set enormous goals! If your daily goal is just to make it home, eat unhealthy foods, watch TV, and go to sleep, you will achieve that. If your daily goal is to make it home, exercise, work on your favorite projects all night, and wake up in the morning with an abundance of energy, you will achieve that too.

Set goals which challenge your brain to think in new directions. Set too many goals. Set so many goals, it will take you a lifetime to achieve them!

And when you achieve a written goal, draw a star or check next to it. Keep track of your progress. Completing and checking off a complex, challenging goal gives one an amazing boost of satisfaction. Your own self-image will become more positive and confident as you check off each accomplished goal.

Work on yourself like a work of art through goal setting. Sculpt your character, physique, and future. Plan and determine the final masterpiece in advance. Set down your personal goals with tremendous clarity and intensity.

Set your goals, then plan how you are going to achieve them. Proper planning prevents poor performance.

Consider the following ratio:
Planning to action = 1:5 (one day of planning is worth five days of action).
Prevention to recovery = 1:5 (one day of prevention is worth five days of recovery).
The more you plan, the more effective your plans will become, and the more you can get done in less time. The more you prevent, the healthier you become, and the less time you need to ever spend on recovery.

Within his book, **Maximum Achievement**, Brian Tracy has outlined twelve steps to achieve goals:
1. Develop an intense desire to achieve your goals.
2. Develop a strong belief in your goals.
3. Write your goals down.
4. Determine how you will benefit from achieving your goals.
5. Analyze your starting point.
6. Set deadlines to achieve your goals.

7. Identify the obstacles that stand in your way.

8. Identify the additional knowledge or information you will require.

9. Identify the people whose cooperation you will require.

10. Make a plan to achieve your goals.

11. Visualize the achievement of your goals.

12. Persist until your goals are achieved.

The present does not spring from the past. The present springs from the future — your vision of the future! To predict the future, assess what is happening in your life now, develop a strategy to reach your goals, and create the future!

Humans have the divine ability to visualize, to see the future before it happens. We literally create the future through visualization. Positive, vivid mental pictures activate all of the laws of the universe and send things, people, and circumstances to us in harmony with those pictures.

You can go only as far as your vision permits. Expand your vision!

To expand your powers of visualization is to recreate the world. Through your imagination you can fly out amongst the stars, scale the majestic mountains of the world, enjoy the lush abundance of the tropics. Your imagination is the key to a brilliant life. Just as you can visualize amazing landscapes, visualize your goals clearly, consistently, and they will begin to manifest now.

When goals are visualized creatively, the rest of life is assured to be intensely interesting and endlessly exciting. This is because the sharper and more vivid a visualization, the quicker it will manifest.

Those who think about visionary goals, who use their garden-minds to erect fantastic visions of beautiful orchards, brilliant island vacations, perfect days, and radiant relationships, are living the most — they are getting the most enjoyment out of life.

A written goal describes clearly what we are seeking. Writing down a goal is making our desires known to the universe and starts the flow of abundance towards us. When we set our visionary goals down on paper, we give reality to them and solidify their entrance from the realm of pure potential into our lives.

Those who set goals are those who achieve them.

Anthony Robbins cites a famous goal study in his book **Unlimited Power**:

> "A study of the 1953 graduates of Yale University clearly demonstrates the power of goals. The graduates interviewed were asked if they had a clear, specific set of goals written down with a plan for achieving those goals. Only 3 percent had such written goals. Twenty years later, in 1973, the researchers went back and interviewed the surviving members of the 1953 graduating class. They discovered that the 3 percent with written specific goals were worth more in financial terms than the entire other 97 percent put together...The interviewers also discovered that the less measurable or more subjective measures, such as level of happiness and joy that the graduates felt, also seemed to be superior in the 3 percent with written goals."

When you take action and actually write down your goals and review them regularly, you dive into a strong current which will carry you to distant places. Unseen forces will come to your aid.

Writing a vision, idea, or goal down makes it a commitment. It tells the subconscious mind what you want to do. It compels the subconscious to figure out how to make your vision become reality. Remember: "Don't just think it, ink it." The more often you write down your goals, review them, and get into the habit of working on them, the quicker they materialize in reality.

You are capable, at any time in your life, of doing what you dream. *Everything you have in your life right now is only a duplication of what you subconsciously believe you deserve.* Many people are afraid to pursue their most important dreams, because they feel they do not deserve them, or that they will be unable to achieve them. That is not you; you can change your destiny. Once you have written your goals on paper, you automatically override thoughts of unworthiness and failure.

Think about your goals continuously. When your goals are clear, all the laws of the universe conspire in your favor to help you. Whenever you feel things are going badly, think about your goals! Uplift yourself by thinking about, visualizing, and feeling your goals!

To achieve your goals, you must become the type of person who can achieve those goals.

When I first started promoting a raw plant-food diet and lifestyle years ago, I was not the type of person who could bring this information to an enormous audience. But, in the process of my own transformation, goal setting, and goal achievements, I became a different type of person: a person brave enough, happy enough, and successful enough to take this information to the next level.

How you will achieve your unique goals is not always clear. In the same way, when you begin a garden you do not completely understand all of the implications involved. The garden's growth reveals the full manifestation of the goal. Like a tree which draws nourishment into its trunk, and transforms it with the assistance of Sun energy into whatever it needs (leaf, bark, sepal, petal, fruit, or seed) to fulfill its destiny, so too will you draw in knowledge and, with the assistance of focused energy, transform it into whatever you need to achieve your goals.

You can learn everything you need to know to accomplish your goals along the way to their achievement. The key is to keep taking action. Action attracts the knowledge you require and makes all things possible.

I tell listeners in my seminars:"Leap and the net appears." Use The Trial and Success Method: Learn from your past mistakes and adjust your behavior accordingly to achieve your goals — treat your past as a school, a vast resource to learn from to better yourself. Maxwell Maltz called this *Psycho-Cybernetics* in his well-known book of the same title. When the mind has a defined target, it can focus and direct and refocus and redirect until it reaches its intended goal.

Remember: The greater your goals, the greater the challenges which await you! Andrew Carnegie said: "Anything in life worth having is worth working for." When you set greater goals, you will face greater challenges. When you set the goal to reach an extraordinary level of health, people will oppose you! Peers may criticize you; family and friends will descend upon you; strangers will try to discourage you. You have to leverage your mind to handle these situations, maintain your focus, and enjoy the process!

At the bottom of it all, the final goal is that people just want to be happy. When all else is detoxified away, the pursuit of any goal is about achieving happiness.

To achieve the highest levels of health, maintain your happiness no matter what you are doing. Set happiness as your highest goal and organize your life around it. All beliefs, ideas, goals, and activities which diminish your happiness limit your potential. There is something in Nature which always attempts to guide you towards growing and achieving the greatest levels of happiness if you simply tune in, listen to, and act upon your intuition.

Always remember to keep your own happiness or harmony of mind as your number one value and all else will fall into place. The best way to make others happy is to be happy yourself! Your own happiness allows you to fully enjoy the abundance life has to offer. As long you choose your own peace of mind as your guiding principle, you will never make a bad decision on the way to achieving your dreams.

It is the possibility of having a dream come true which makes life most interesting! Get excited about your goals. Get excited about waking up in the morning! Become an irresistible force of Nature moving rapidly towards each set goal.

As your goals begin to materialize, you will enjoy life more, you will become more confident. You set into motion an upward spiral of ever-increasing achievement.

As you work diligently toward the achievement of your goals, you may discover the beautiful truth that, as you fill your spirit with positive thoughts, rewards, and exciting challenges, all weaknesses are automatically eliminated. Consider the story of business philosopher Cavett Roberts (whose success audio tapes I highly recommend). By middle age, Cavett's health was failing and he was given a death sentence by doctors. He quit his job as a lawyer, moved to Sunny Arizona, started selling real estate, and got so busy succeeding and achieving his goals that he forgot to die. He lived into his nineties, and outlived all his doctors!

No matter what your station in life at the present time, you can change your future in a moment with one powerful action. The actions you take, or do not take, each day shape your destiny. Each action or non-action is taking you towards a conclusion, a goal. Remember, you are always heading towards goals, the question is whose?

We are journeying entities, traveling in the garden of life, drawn to those destinations that are in harmony with our dominant thoughts. Goals are like orchards filled with ripe fruits, they pull us toward them. They breathe in new fragrant sensations into our being. They activate our imagination.

We are designed to set and achieve goals with the content of our life being the wonders we observe along the way.

The ultimate quest has no ending, and that fact gives it incredible value. The true value is not what we get, but what we become along the way. We journey to a goal, and then realize the journey is the goal.

Action Steps:

1. Set a health goal to continuously act upon the information contained within this book. Record this goal in your journal.

2. In your journal, write down 100 goals that you want to attain within the next year. Review them daily.

3. Take your top 5 yearly goals. For each goal write a sentence fulfilling each one of the 12 steps for goal achievement outlined by Brian Tracy earlier in this lesson.

4. Continuously write down additional yearly goals and long-term goals in your journal.

5. Check off each goal as you achieve it.

The Visionary

The beauty of the world,
Under sunshine, mist, snow
Settles upon dreams
Which nestle and grow,
In the slumbering visions
Of the secret and wild,
The supernal gods
In the feral child.

Vision — the strength,
It shapes and seeks:
The glide of the pen,
And a voice who speaks
To the mass of minds
Or a single face, with
Eloquent, astral, eternal grace.

Your vision is the promise,
You shall one day be.
Your ideal is the prophecy,
You shall one day see.

Nourished by seeds,
Of divine inspiration,
You become as great,
As the finest creation.

That which you love,
Shall come upon you.
That which you need,
Shall find its way too.

Vision — the master,
It guides and creates.
It plans for perfection,
And clearly states:
"The dreamers are the saviors
Of the world."

Those who cherish:
A beautiful vision,
A lofty ideal,
Have but one decision:

Inspire the dream,
To expand and rise.
Nourish that truth
Without compromise.

For those with visions
Of truth and right,
Even alone,
Have strength and might.

With a cluster of sparks,
The air of 'rudition,
That which is nourished,
Will come to fruition.

Vision — the power,
It molds and makes.
Hold it true so long
And evermore it shapes,
The reasons, minds, and the wills
Calling forth a thousand joys,
Disposing of a thousand ills.

Cherished in secret
Yet coming to pass,
Vision — the calm
In a pool of glass.

Tempest tossed souls,
Wherever you be,
Rest under the wing
Of the visionary.

In the Ocean of Life,
Isles of Bliss lay smiling.
The Sunny shore of your ideal
Awaits your arriving.

Keep your hand firmly poised
Upon the helm of thought.
Hold true to the vision
And you'll find what you have sought.

The Visionary's Epilogue

To humanity:
The seekers,
Never forget
Your dreamers.
Their ideals
Must never
Fade and die.
They live forever
And carry us high.
See in them
What you shall know.
Take from them
Some seeds to sow.
For musician, poet, painter, sage —
You are the architects
Of the golden age.

Lesson 6:
Faith

"Just as a green sprout never springs from seeds
that have been scorched by fire, so no virtues
will arise in people who have no faith."
— **Dasadharma Sutra**

Have you ever wondered why an electron spinning around an atom nucleus does not run out of energy? How does it operate in perpetual motion? The answer coming from the foremost progressive scientific minds is that the electron continually dips into the well of infinite energy and potential called the "ether." The ether is the cosmic force which provides life-force to all living things through the superconduction of mono-atomic elements inside living cells.

Through the great principle of faith we can tap the ether and draw forth any tangible item or intangible idea into the physical world. Faith is a superconductor which allows us to consciously tap into the cosmic, divine energy. Faith allows us to create things in the material world.

Faith is the ability to have trust in powers greater than yourself, to confidently stride into the unknown, and to believe in your own abilities — no matter what.

Faith is the fountain word; it is the principle of achievement. Faith promises all things; and it fulfills all things. To employ faith is to call upon the divine power and set it into action. "According to your faith be it unto you" (Matthew 9:29). Success philosopher Napoleon Hill described faith as the "élan vital" that gives inspiration. The power of faith becomes tangible as renewed cells and tissues, or in newly created things. Faith is the basic channel of Nature through which all things manifest.

Faith is essential to success. A lack of faith is essential to failure. Every belief we hold requires faith because we can never know anything for sure. Without faith, confusion, distraction, and inner uncertainty set in — leading only to failure.

"I would show unto the world that faith is things which are hoped for and not seen; wherefore, dispute not because ye see not, for ye receive no witness until after the trial of your faith" (Ether 12:6). Spiritual power overrides all. You can have, do, and be anything you want if only you dare to reach for it in faith. The divine power will make sure your faith is true by testing your faith. The stronger your faith and clarity, the quicker you will set yourself into the divine time flow where one is always in the perfect place at the perfect time.

If you are doing the work you were meant to do, then you can command that everything you require, whether known or unknown, will be there at the precise time you require it. What stops this process from occurring is doubt. What starts this process occurring is faith. Basically, all you need are two things: a goal and faith, and you will get where you are going.

The opposite of faith is fear and doubt. Doubt stops the full expression of your life potential.

Doubt

Forever clashing with the wise
Is the spirit that denies!

And to that Power never reposing,

Creative, healing
Doubt is opposing!

Doubt is a liar,
A burden endured.
From the gilden path,
Many are lured,
In treacherous compassion,
With flame-twisted word,
The mind becomes clouded, and —
Eden lies obscured.

The doubter can and shall never obtain anything. The abundance of the world is forever closed to the doubter. A doubter can never know truth, can never make a determined act. Doubt is pernicious as it destroys the climate of your life. If you be anything, be not a doubter. Only through faith are things granted. Faith is the one command which overrides doubt.

Embrace faith and you automatically master fear. Faith is the one power against which fear cannot stand.

Strong faith creates a positive attitude. Success seems to be connected with attitude. If your attitude is strong, powerful, attractive, and graceful, you can achieve any success you desire!

What the people need more than anything is faith: faith in themselves, faith in their fellows, faith in the power and goodness of Nature, faith in the healing powers of raw plant foods, faith in the divine powers.

All the greatest beings who have ever strolled through the Earth's gardens have been people of transcendent faith. Every one of them had a tranquil attitude and a calm belief in the helpful powers of invisible forces. These forces are always available to everyone!

Those who desire health must have faith, for those who have faith have everything.

Action Steps:

1. Plant the seeds of faith in the six individuals you associate with most often. Support them with faith, teach them to support themselves with faith. From faith flows all good things.

2. Open your journal and look at the top 5 yearly goals established in the **Action Steps** at the end of **Lesson 5: Goals**. As you read them, do the following:

   a. Write down all doubts which immediately come into your mind as you review each goal.

   b. Resolve, in writing, to dismiss away any doubts you may have associated with each goal.

   c. Write down exactly why you will faithfully persist until you achieve your top 5 yearly goals.

   d. Replace any thoughts of doubt or fear with faith. As long as you are doing it, never doubt it.

*

Now that you have reviewed the fundamental information I have shared in the lessons thus far, it is time to reveal to you the magic secret. In this next lesson, I am going to share with you an unprecedented health discovery. You are now ripe, through your own exposure and your own seeking, to make a dietary choice. You are now at that moment when you can make a leap of faith into a powerful stream of new information.

Lesson 7:
The Sunfood Diet

"And God said: Behold, I have given you every
herb bearing seed which is upon the face of the earth,
and every tree, in which is the fruit of a tree
yielding seed, to be your food."
— Genesis 1:29

"Kill neither men, nor beasts, nor yet the food which goes
into your mouth. For if you eat living food, the same will
quicken you, but if you kill your food, the dead food will
kill you also. For life comes only from life, and from death
comes always death. For everything which kills your foods,
kills your bodies also. And everything which kills your bodies
kills your souls also. And your bodies become what your
foods are, even as your spirits, likewise, become what
your thoughts are. Therefore, eat not anything which fire,
or frost, or water has destroyed. For burned, frozen, or rotted
foods will burn, freeze, and rot your body also."
— The Essene Gospel Of Peace, Book I
translated by Edmond Bordeaux Szekely

"When Mankind was created,
They knew not the eating of bread,
Knew not the dressing in garments;
Ate plants with their mouth like sheep;
Drank water from a ditch."
— Sumerian tale

"Hanuman was a monkey of the woods, he did not desire
fair women and he ate no cooked food."
— Hanuman is the monkey god of India featured in
the tale of the **Ramayana** from which this passage was quoted.

"Pious men eat what the gods leave over after the offering.
But those ungodly, cooking food for the greed of their stomachs,
sin as they eat it."
— **Bhagavad Gita**

"There is among the Indians a heresy
Of those who philosophize among
The Brahmins, who live
A self-sufficient life,
Abstaining from eating living creatures
And all cooked food."
— Hippolytus, Rome, 225 AD

"I am much more interested in a question on which
the 'salvation of humanity' depends far more than on
any theologians' curio: the question of nutrition."
— Friedrich Nietzsche, **Ecce Homo**

"It can be said that the greatest single cause of degeneration
in man is the use of fire in the preparation of foods."
— Arnold De Vries, **The Fountain Of Youth**

"Why all this cooking when there is really no cook like old Sol?
Cooked food is dead food — and remember, the whiter the bread
the sooner we are dead! Every attempt to improve on natural food
must prove a failure, and Nature will react at first acutely to any
interference with her beneficent laws of health. And if we continue
to disobey her laws by drugs or even surgery, the symptoms may
disappear for a while only to reappear in chronic or fatal
diseases...Man is the only creature that cooks his food, and he is
more subject to disease than any wild creature that dines on unfired
food. Tradition, gluttony, and increasing desire for strong stimulants

have caused man to prefer cooked food, which has seriously weakened his digestive organs. This is because cooked food can be swallowed so easily without chewing, whereas thorough mastication is essential to good health."
— Dugald Semple, **The Sunfood Way To Health**

"Your food determines in a large measure how long you shall live — how much you shall enjoy life, and how successful your life shall be."
— Dr. Kirschner, **Live Food Juices**

What we eat deeply and radically affects the way we think, feel, and behave. We are what we eat and we eat what we are. Food affects every aspect of our being. Food is the physical foundation of our body. If the foundation is unstable, all that is built upon it will be unstable. Everything you physically are was once the air you breathed, the water you drank, and the food you ate. The colloidal mineral structure of your body is built out of the foods you have eaten. If there is an alteration in the food, then it is reflected in the look and function of the body. Improve your food choices and you dramatically improve the foundation upon which your body is built.

Success is an accumulation of practicing fundamentals each and every day. Eating is a daily activity of vital importance which cannot be overlooked. A consistent habit of making excellent food choices is an absolute necessity for a successful life.

From average to exceptional is just a slight edge. The proper diet gives you a slight edge and a hundred times more. When you give your body incredible food, it will function incredibly.

To achieve your mission on Earth, you need excellent health and a supreme physical support system to get you there. Excellent dietary habits support your body and mind on the path to reaching amazing goals.

When your diet is pure, the planet freely bestows its wealth upon you. Diet is the mysterious key to life-long massive abundance. Diet is the key to the natural way of life. A wonderful life requires a natural diet rich in Sun-grown foods eaten in their pristine raw state.

If we think about it logically, when we arrived on the planet, we had no tools, clothing, or fire. How did we live? What did we eat? There must be some original diet, a diet we were biologically designed for, a diet which is the optimal diet for humankind.

Simplicity

"Success is nothing more than a refined study of the obvious."
— Jim Rohn, success philosopher

"Whatever must be proved is already doubtful."
— Professor Arnold Ehret

Simplicity is now, has always been, and will forever be, the key guideline of success.

The fact that there is more confusion, conflicting opinions, and false information concerning the field of diet now available than ever before is proof that there must be some simple truth beneath it all. There are always many opinions, but only one truth.

In science there is a principle called Ockham's Razor. This principle tells us that, amongst competing theories, the simplest is most likely to be true.

Natural Law is simplicity itself. A great axiom states:"Once you are complicated, you are ineffective." A great reason for my success and the success of others on The Sunfood Diet program is its incredible simplicity. Whatever simple reasoning cannot ascertain is nonsense and should be dispensed with! Nothing vital is complicated!

There is a poetry, a powerful truth, in simple facts. The simpler things are, the easier it is to live. Forager/gatherers were the original affluent society on Earth. The best things in life are free, for life depends on simplicity. The worst things in life are paid for with wasted life-force energy, for death depends on complexity.

People complicate things in direct proportion to their simplicity.

Anytime, if you feel you are being overwhelmed with information, simplify. Just get back to basics. All the greatest sports coaches the world has ever seen taught basics. Simple basics practiced over and over make enormous improvements in the long term. Here is the basics of nutrition: RAW PLANT FOOD.

Cooked food was not here when we first appeared on Earth.

Raw plant food is truly the most perfect food for human consumption.

The structure and function of humanity's teeth, jaw, digestive canal, sense organs, instincts of the young, psychological aversion towards killing, emotional feelings towards animals, as well as the cause and cure of disease and unhappiness, all demonstrate that humans are biologically raw-plant eaters (primarily consumers of sweet, non-sweet, and fatty fruits, and green-leafed vegetables). (See **Lesson 9: Origins** and **Appendix A**.)

Do you know the power of getting energy solely from plants? Every whole plant food is a symphony. The absorption and organization of Sunlight, the essence of life, takes place primarily in plants. The organs of the plant are therefore a kind of biological accumulation of Sun energy. Eating plant foods transfers the vital Sun energy directly to you, undiminished.

Raw plant foods are massively abundant. 99.99% of all food on Earth is raw plant food. In the grand scheme of things, cooked food is nonexistent, and animal food for omnivores and carnivores is minimal as the plant-eaters (mostly insects) are by far the dominant creatures on Earth.

Eating raw plant food provides you with an unlimited variety of food choices. There are so many raw plant foods on this planet that you could taste something new every single day for the rest of your life and still not even come remotely close to trying 1% of what is here on Earth! For instance, there are over 500 varieties of avocados. And there are at least 80 varieties of persimmons! There are even over 100 varieties of wild durian!

Raw plant foods fall into fourteen major categories:

1.   Fruits: Fruits are raw plant foods which contain the seed within themselves for the reproduction of their kind. Fruits may be sweet, non-sweet, or fat-dominant.

2.   Leaves: Leaves contain life-giving chlorophyll pigments, and are the best source of minerals. Most herbs are green leaves.

3.   Nuts: Nuts are the reproductive agents of certain trees. They are fat-dominant foods.

4.   Seeds: Seeds are the reproductive agents of plants. Depending on the type, they may be protein-dominant, or fat-dominant. Grains are seeds.

5.   Legumes: Legumes include all peas, beans, and peanuts, and are often sprouted before consumption. They are protein-dominant.

6.   Flowers: Flowers are the sexual organs of plants.

7.   Green sprouts: Green sprouts appear when sprouted seeds, or legumes, reach a certain point of growth and shoot forth green-leaves.

8.   Roots: Roots are the below-ground portion of plants.

9.   Shoots: Shoots are young plants spread by underground runners from their parent plants.

10.   Bark: The outer, protective layer of trees.

11.   Sap: The life-fluid of a tree.

12.   Stems: Stems are the fibrous, structural pieces of plants.

13.   Water vegetation: Sea vegetables are sea plant leaves containing bountiful minerals drawn in from the ocean, and up from the ocean floor. Spirulina and algaes of all types are included in this category.

14.   Mushrooms: Not a true plant food, this fungus grows in darkness, and is not directly nourished by the vibrant Sun energy.

What Is The Sunfood Diet?

The Sunfood Diet Success System is really The Raw-Food Diet Success System. I use the term "Sunfood" because it implies raw plant food grown under the vivifying influence of direct Sunlight in a wild, natural state. "Sunfood" has a refreshing, majestic quality to it. "Raw food" is ambiguous — "raw food" could mean anything raw.

The Sunfood Diet is a diet of abundance. **The Sunfood Diet Success System** demystifies The Raw-Food Diet, and presents a program which allows anyone to achieve the goal of succeeding with a raw plant-food diet.

Of all the raw plant foods on Earth, The Sunfood Diet requires that 80%+ of your food choices contain a balance of green-leafed vegetables, sweet fruits, and fatty plant foods. The other 20% can contain any of the fourteen kinds of raw plant foods mentioned above, or other foods that you feel are appropriate for you at this stage. This diet is not about denial, it is about success and achievement. The idea behind The Sunfood Diet is to eat at least 80% raw plant foods, and then move forward from there.

Benefits Of The Sunfood Diet

Every so often in history an idea comes along that revolutionizes everything which follows it. The discovery of The Raw-Food Diet is one of those ideas. The implications of raw nutrition on humankind are immense.

We do not just need information to achieve success, we need transformation. The Sunfood Diet rebuilds you at the most fundamental levels and transforms you in a most profound way. The Sunfood Diet is peerless. Once an individual enters its field, every other power opens up.

A diet of raw plant food puts you in touch with a new vital power. In the source of every vital power lies an endless abundance. A diet of raw plant food presents a whole new paradigm of health, wealth, success, and possibility. Since The Sunfood Diet is the natural way of life, it brings with it beauty, happiness, long-life, and prosperity!

We know that the more perfectly clean your body, the more perfectly it will radiate your super-natural powers. The first things to evaporate in a toxic environment are the super-natural abilities provided to us at birth. These powers are possessed by wild animals, and formerly by humanity. As soon as the body begins to be poisoned, the powers slip away. In any biological degeneration, the higher powers fade first. However, your natural superior abilities have not been totally destroyed by improper food, they are only dormant, and are capable of rebirth, regeneration, and resurrection.

One of the greatest values of The Sunfood Diet is that it opens you up to the idea that many of your other deep-seated beliefs may be totally false. The effects of adopting The Sunfood Diet disassembles your view of the world. Once you experience that eating cooked and artificially-grown food immediately detracts from the normal functioning of your body, you will begin to question many other aspects of your belief system. So, The Sunfood Diet acts like a battering ram crumbling away the stagnated belief systems of your mind. It allows you to grow in new directions you never would have predicted. You will be ready to try new things and to test new approaches to life's daily challenges.

As we learned in **Lesson 4: Beliefs**, we do not know what life really is; we only know how we represent life to ourselves. When you naturalize your diet, you automatically tune into a different energy band of life. You allow more information from your higher self to penetrate your conscious mind. And what you consider reality will change. Naturalizing your diet aligns and strips away mineral debris from the master gland in your brain (the pineal gland) allowing insights from infinite intelligence to flow more clearly into your thoughts.

Different foods fuel different perceptions of the world. Eating raw plant foods automatically tunes you in to a positive, prosperous energy band of life. In Nature, there are potions, mixtures, and solutions with which anyone may safely stimulate their minds to tune in to inspirational thoughts. Nature's stimulants cannot be improved upon. Nothing can compare to the aristocratic taste of a ripe cherimoya, nothing can touch the rush from fresh watermelons in the summer, nothing even resembles the energy derived from a meal of jackfruit.

Raw nutrition attunes you to the forces that surround us, permeate through our bodies, and that make up the essence of our existence. When you eat raw plant foods, your instincts become stronger. Your intuition becomes more reliable — clearer — and decision-making becomes effortless. I literally feel as if I have not made a bad decision in years; I go with my intuition every time; I have learned the only thing we have which is not an illusion is our intuition.

During the process of undertaking The Sunfood Diet, you will experience moments of instantaneous change. I recall one afternoon, several years ago, when my health partner, R.C. Dini, and I were juicing citrus fruits and feijoa (pineapple guava) at my home in San Diego. We were in the middle of drinking a pitcher, when we both simultaneously exclaimed, "I can see better!" And we could see better. My vision permanently improved that day.

During the process you will also experience subtle change. Over time the subtlety builds, and one day you will wake up profoundly transformed. *In general, food choices have a cumulative effect on the body.*

The digestion of cooked food takes more energy from the body than any other activity. You could run a marathon and still be walking and talking. However, an hour after a Thanksgiving dinner, guess what?...you are asleep! We know that all success is about transmuting energy. This message is about transmuting the energy used in digestion into achieving our goals.

On The Sunfood Diet you need less sleep. I used to sleep 8 hours a night. I was the type of person who had to sleep 8 hours. Since adopting The Sunfood Diet, my sleep needs decreased to 3 hours at a minimum to 6 hours at a maximum. On the average, judging from the information I have gathered, the people following this diet experience a decrease of 2 hours of sleep each night. In one year, that is an additional 30 days worth of extra time to accomplish goals and make a contribution to the planet.

The amazing thing about The Sunfood Diet is that it is something you can physically do. You do not have to think too hard about it, you can just do it.

After you have made the commitment to radically improve your diet, you subconsciously reinforce in your mind that your life has meaning and that striving for extraordinary health is worth the effort. You have made a commitment to really living life.

The strongest factor about The Sunfood Diet is that it compels you to live naturally and in harmony with the Earth.

If we pollute the planet after we eat with food packaging, then we truly are not living in harmony with the Earth. Eating raw fruits, vegetables, and other plant foods is the solution to world pollution. Landfills are filled with products directly or indirectly related to cooked and processed foods, such as: packaging, wrappers, bags, old stoves, microwaves, etc. One of the most startling revelations I experienced on this diet-path was that I stopped producing trash! My life has become more harmonious with the Earth.

By following this diet, you may one day find yourself in your garden or home planting seeds and growing plants. The home of the Sunfoodist is often surrounded with radiant plant life. Eating raw foods truly reconnects you to the fabric of life.

True progress in the field of nutrition has been made in this world. Solutions have been found. The confusion of nutrition is the most perplexing challenge humankind has yet faced. The Sunfood Diet solves the confusion of nutrition by simplifying our dietary essentials and presenting a balanced nutrition program consisting of raw plant foods, allowing any single person to achieve an extraordinary level of health.

Ayurveda, Traditional Oriental Medicine, & Macrobiotics

When people believed in the "Earth is flat" paradigm, every university taught its students that the Earth was flat. Every scientist and professor could "prove" to you that it was flat. Those scientists and professors were not lying to you — they just did not know. It took a few distinctions put forth by a few noble minds to dissolve away the basic assumptions of all those schools of thought. This is how knowledge moves forward — indeed, it is the only way that knowledge has ever moved forward.

The "Earth is flat" paradigm only allowed human understanding to proceed to a certain level, and no further. In the same way, diet systems such as ayurveda (from India), traditional Chinese medicine (and its macrobiotic offshoot) only allow human health to proceed to a certain level, and no further. The ancient systems have been dulled down over many thousands of years and no longer contain real vitality; the purpose of these systems was to help the average person reach good health. The purpose of The Sunfood Diet Success System is to help an average person become an extraordinary human being who experiences superior health, who encounters the highest forms of life, and who unlocks dormant powers. New distinctions have now surpassed the old system paradigms.

My goal has been to draw forth the best elements from ayurveda, traditional Chinese medicine, and macrobiotics and apply them to the Sunfood approach.

The insights on body-typing and nutritional balance coming from the ancient dietary systems and my own experiences with internal cleansing, tuning into food instincts, and eating a total raw-food diet have convinced me that the original creators of these systems were raw-food eaters. The original systems were certainly much more pure than they appear today.

Throughout its long history up to this day, the presence of raw-food diets has appeared in India. Many yogis currently living in the Himalayas eat only raw plant food, following in the spiritual traditions of their ancestors. During the Zhou Dynasty in China, it was recorded that: "The tribes in the east were called Yi. They had their hair unbound, and tattooed their bodies. Some of them ate their food without it being cooked by fire." This account continues on by describing tribes to the north, south, and west who did not eat cereals and who ate their food raw. From these accounts we know that raw-food diets were present in ancient China. This evidence again corroborates the concept that the original creators of the ancient systems were raw-foodists.

Cooked Food

After many years of careful study and investigation on the subject, I am convinced that the "the great change" which came over humankind occurred when humans took the power of fire into their own hands and began experimenting with eating cooked food.

Exactly when and where humans acquired fire is truly a mystery. Fire allowed early humans to begin to control their environment and spread out into more inhospitable places. Those with fire eventually overcame or passed it along to those without it. Whether it was the open flame or the tribal oven formed of red-hot stones paved into an oval hollow in the ground, fire became part of every tribe on Earth. But fire is a double-edged sword; unless one is careful with its power, it can turn on its master.

The world was given for us to turn into a paradise. To make this happen, cooked food needs to be understood for what it is, its consumption minimized, and its use eventually released from the human diet.

The assumption behind cooking is that the original form of Nature, as it exists, must be altered in order that it may be reformed to a new artificial form. The truth is that the original state is always superior. The bite-sized portions of an orange cannot be improved upon!

The raw-versus-cooked distinction is the most important insight in the field of nutrition.

Cooking alters organic molecules. When those molecules are ingested, they become part of the tissues. Thus cooking alters the tissues at a fundamental level.

When food is cooked it always becomes less than it was before, never more. Fire is a destroyer; it never creates anything. If you took a flame-thrower to this book, would it become more or less than it was before? Cooking only takes away. Eating cooked food is like spending millions of dollars on a brand new mansion, then burning it to the ground before you move in!

Understand: you are water — electrified water. Everything you swallow, must be broken down into a liquid to nourish you. The first thing to go with cooking is the water.

Cooked food is dense. It leaves a toxic ash, or residue, in the body after it has been processed as fuel. Over years and decades, this debris accumulates in the form of mucus and is deposited throughout the tissues. Eventually, the toxins reach a crisis level and clog and poison the system leading to heart attacks, strokes, and cancer. Disease arises out of the toxic residues left by cooked foods.

One of the primary ways your body experiences the world around you is by the food you eat. What does the body sense when one puts a charred piece of animal flesh inside it? The body feels death, pain, fire, destruction.

A cooked seed will not grow. Cooked food has no life-force energy. *Cooked food has no spiritual energy.*

People on a standard cooked-food diet go through life in a weakened condition with their vitality much below par, but they are not aware of this because they have never known anything different. They have no reason to believe their vitality and health are not what they should be. They cannot miss what they never had. People are falling day by day to weaker levels, while believing they are attaining a high standard of living.

Eating cooked and processed foods makes one groggy, affects moods, lowers one's level of awareness, and interferes with the body's optimal vitality. A poor diet results in toxic residues that have a long-range effect on longevity.

The nutritional properties of foods are degraded by the process of cooking. Heating converts foods into foreign substances which become harmful. Just like tobacco smoke, or brewed alcohol, these substances have no connection with the body's natural needs.

Cooked food is addictive (there really is no softer way to describe it).

An addiction is a desire for a substance that has no connection with the true desires of the body. Eating cooked food has all the marks of a physio-chemical addiction. This is a strong statement, but I think, as you experiment with eating more and more raw plant foods, you will find an interesting truth in it.

People are not truly attached to many of the cooked foods they eat. They eat them for flavor or fun. I have found with most people I have worked with that there are usually 5 or 6 cooked foods that they are actually addicted to and have trouble releasing. These usually include: bread, baked potatoes, coffee, potato chips, corn chips, tofu, candy (chocolate), cigarettes (not a true food), and/or fish. Typically these foods are attached to emotional anchors. When these foods are removed, emotional feelings come up to be detoxified out of the body. One may feel uncomfortable for the moment (as these feelings are released), but feel much better in the long-term. (More on this in **Lesson 10: Detoxification**.)

Cooked Food And The Environment

Cooking led to the animal and seed diet. The most frequent way people interact with animals is by eating them. The most frequent way people interact with seeds is by eating them.

The animal and cooked-seed diet led to grain farming which is stripping the fertile Earth of its minerals. Grain crops are collected, processed, cooked, fed to animals or eaten, and eliminated into the sewers and waterways of civilization. Erosion wears down unstable grain fields, washing minerals away. Farms are turned into deserts; jungles are turned into rice paddies. One way or the other, the soil minerals wash down and end up at the bottom of the ocean.

Eating raw fruits and vegetables radically improves the mineralization of the Earth as it encourages the planting of trees. Trees reach down 20 or 30 feet (6 to 9 meters) — sometime much farther (I have been told that wild grape vines reach down as far as 500 feet [150 meters])! Trees pull the minerals up into their stems, leaves, flowers, and fruits which fall to the topsoil increasing the mineralization of the soil for vegetables to

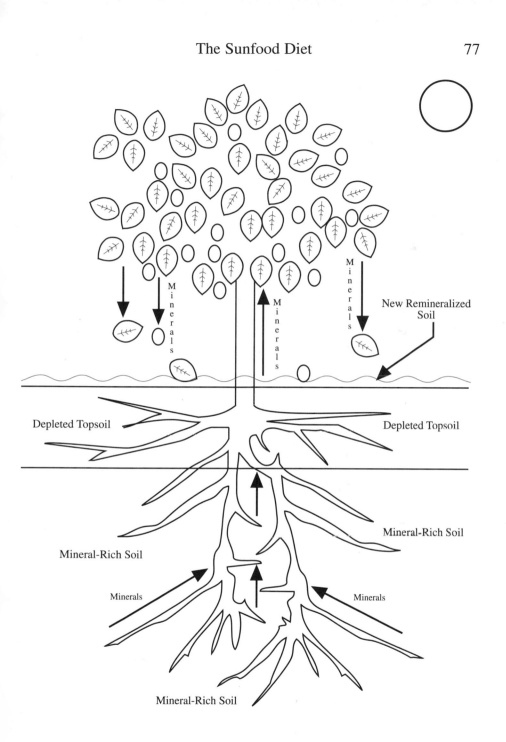

Tree Mineralization

grow. Deciduous trees, which drop their leaves each year, strongly min-
eralize the soil.

The cooking of food is by far the biggest waste of resources on planet
Earth. Viktoras Kulvinskas, in his classic book **Survival Into The 21st
Century**, reports that cooking destroys 85% of the value of food. When
I first realized this, I was staggered. But I did not understand the full
implication of this fact. You see, if 85% of the food value is destroyed in
cooking, then also destroyed are 85% of the time, labor, resources, and
energy which went into creating the foods. So this idea of eating raw
plant food impacts all agriculture, all business, all the economies of the
world, all politics.

Massive abundance is the true law of life. There is no shortage of food
on Earth! My date-farmer friend, Jamie Jones (a raw-plant eater for over
10 years), tells us, "The most vigorous date palms yield over 600 pounds
per tree per year. One date palm planted at birth could supply a person
with practically their entire lifetime supply of food." Probably everyone
would agree that eating only dates would not be ideal, but it does give us
an idea of how much food can come from just one tree! There is an infinite amount of food on this planet!

When I was a student at the University of San Diego, I had a job in cus-
tomer service at the campus bookstore. One day a nun came up to my
counter and we began talking. She described her recent trip to Haiti.
Apparently, each year she had been spending at least 3 months in Haiti
helping the impoverished children. She told me that Haiti had been deforested decades before. I asked her how that happened, expecting the
answer to be overgrazing, or too much wood demand for building homes
and shelters. Actually, neither was the case. She told me that Haiti had
been deforested because the wood was being used for cooking!

Most people who live in first world countries with gas stoves and electrical ovens have no idea that the other 90% of the planet is cooking with
wood. Cooking is a major reason for deforestation. In Africa, the tropical

forests of the mountain gorilla are being cut and cleared for cooking wood. Similar tragedies are happening on nearly every continent.

In third world countries, the cooking of food exposes people to the hazards of inhaling wood smoke or emissions from biomass fuels, such as cattle chips (dung). Emissions from wood and biomass fuels are major sources of air pollution in the home. Studies have shown that cooks inhale more smoke and pollutants than the inhabitants of the dirtiest cities.

Overcoming Disease

"Treat disease through diet, by preference, refraining from
the use of drugs; and if you find what is required in a
single herb, do not resort to a compound medicament."
— Baha'u'llah

"No matter from which angle we view health and disease,
we cannot escape from being entangled in the conclusion
that intractable disease is as old as cookery.
Disease and cookery originated simultaneously."
— Dr. Edward Howell, **Enzyme Nutrition**

Every living organism is vibrating at a certain metabolic level. If the internal energy of the organism drops below a certain level, then the immune system is compromised. Illness is an energy crisis in the body — the body no longer has enough energy to hold together its integrity. Purifying the body through a balanced raw-food diet raises the energy vibration, thus increasing the immune system.

Chronic disease has one true cause: toxemia. Toxemia is an accumulation of spiritual, emotional, mental, and physical waste, mucus, and various residues in the organism.

To combat disease by attempting to destroy germs is folly. Germs are found everywhere; they enter and exit the body, all the time, every day.

They co-exist symbiotically with the human body. Only when the human body is toxic, do germs become threatening. As the saying goes, "The microbe is nothing, the terrain is everything."

Chemical drugs and medicines do not heal, they only cause harm. All chemical drugs and medicines, with the exception of aspirin, have been (and still are) tested on innocent animals. Remember the foundational law? Things produce after their own kind. The torture and suffering of animals in useless attempts to find cures for diseases does no good, actually it can only do bad — it only produces more of its own kind: more torture and suffering...more disease.

True therapeutics involves releasing the power within each person to heal. It is not the disease which must be stopped, but the poisoning of the body by an unhealthy lifestyle. For a complete healing to take place, the body must experience: laughter, joy, excellent nourishment, and a new-found desire to learn and keep the mind active.

Relaxation is also a factor in overcoming disease. More people die on Monday morning than on any other day of the week or at any other time. Stress accelerates illness as it causes the eliminative organs and the muscular system to constrict and hold onto toxicity and metabolic waste. A proper diet will help immensely as certain foods (such as green-leafy vegetables) help to open up constricted muscles and certain other foods (such as juicy fruits) help to flush out the toxicity.

The emphasis here with diet is on removing the physical residue, on cleansing through proper diet. Once the physical body (the anchor) is put in tune — all the other bodies (mental, emotional, spiritual) line up and begin to cleanse as well. It is simple. It is real. It works.

A pure raw-plant diet assists the body's cleansing efforts in the most natural way by eliminating any toxicity from entering the system and by simultaneously moving toxicity through the lymph and blood and out of the body through the eliminative organs (the bowels, kidneys, skin, sinuses, and lungs). A purification of the diet enforces a self-healing and a radical whole-body rejuvenation.

As you apply the health and diet system in this book, you may find that the common cold, flus, fever, grogginess, etc., are all actually efforts by the body to eliminate physical waste; they are symptoms of a body in the process of healing itself. When you have mastered this health and diet system, you will have overcome the major illnesses. You will no longer experience colds, flus, fevers, etc. They will all be looked at as part of a past and unusual way of life.

Enzymes

"Enzymes are substances that make life possible.
They are needed for every chemical reaction that takes
place in the human body. No mineral, vitamin, or hormone
can do any work without enzymes. Our bodies, all our organs,
tissues, and cells are run by metabolic enzymes."
— Dr. Howell, **Enzyme Nutrition**

Enzymes are vital to all life processes. Enzymes are catalysts for all reactions in the body They embody the vital Sun energy in the body — they are transformers directed by hormones amongst a terrain of vitamins, minerals, carbohydrates, fats, and tissue proteins.

There are three classes of enzymes:
- metabolic
- digestive
- food

Metabolic enzymes operate in all the cells, tissues, and organs of the body and are an essential part of every activity.

Digestive enzymes are produced by, and appear in, the alimentary organs. They help digest carbohydrates, fats, and proteins. Amylases are enzymes that digest carbohydrates. Lipases are enzymes that digest fats. Proteases are enzymes that digest proteins.

Food enzymes come enclosed with all whole raw foods in their proper proportions. These enzymes are there to help digest the food (or to help ripen or decompose the food if it is not eaten). Food enzymes are destroyed at 118 degrees Fahrenheit (47.8 degrees Celsius). The dehydration of food below 104 degrees Fahrenheit (40.0 degrees Celsius) does keep most enzymes intact. Freezing and refrigeration hinders enzymatic activity. Freezing food destroys at least 30% of its enzymes and can destroy up to 66% of its enzymes. Fermented raw foods, including seed cheeses and raw sauerkraut, have a very high enzymatic activity and thus they have been used by natural health pioneers, such as Doctor Ann Wigmore, to accelerate healing and disease recovery.

Food enzyme shortages, sooner or later, result in physical degeneration and disease. When the digestive enzymes present in the body are insufficient, the body draws upon its reserves of metabolic enzymes from the major and minor organs and glands, weakening one's overall vitality. It takes ten metabolic enzymes to form one digestive enzyme.

Just because the dangerous effects of cooked and processed foods are not felt immediately does not mean they are not damaging. Humans have not adapted to cooked food in the way people assume. How can an animal, such as a field mouse, that has never eaten cooked food in its genetic history, be captured, fed cooked food, and still live? Did it instantaneously adapt to cooked food? Just because one can chew up something, swallow it, and live long enough to tell others about it, does not mean that person has adapted to it. White bread, for example, has only been around for the last 100 years. People eat white bread *en masse* and they are still alive. Does that mean humans have adapted to white bread? Cooked and processed foods have a cumulative effect on the body. The enzyme potential decreases over time. Once the enzyme potential is diminished beyond a certain threshold, the body wears out and the internal organs feel the damage.

After presenting a host of evidence demonstrating that all living creatures have a fixed enzyme potential which can be (and usually is) prematurely exhausted, Dr. Howell in **Enzyme Nutrition** writes: "Humans eating an enzymeless diet use up a tremendous amount of their enzyme potential in lavish secretions of the pancreas and other digestive organs. The result is a shortened lifespan (65 years or less as compared with 100 or more), illness, and lowered resistance to stresses of all types, psychological and environmental."

The generational introduction of substances foreign to the organism causes enzymatic adaptations to appear in the digestive fluids even though no physiological adaptation occurs. Different races of people throughout the world have developed enzymatic capabilities foreign to other groups in order to help digest their traditional cultural foods. These "enzyme mutations" are the body's way of accommodating itself to foreign food substances.

The enzyme mutation in a northern European person might give her/him an enzymatic capability to metabolize raw cow's milk, whereas a Mediterranean person may lack such an enzyme mutation, but possess an enzymatic ability to metabolize raw goat's milk. This capability would last until the person began to exhaust their enzyme potential. If the person drank the milk pasteurized, or if they over-intoxicated themselves with those substances (even if raw) then, over time, they would greatly weaken their enzyme potential, and no longer be able to tolerate such foods.

Even with enzyme mutations, the intake of animal foods is undesirable to the physiology of the human digestive apparatus. The shape of the teeth, jaw, width of the lips, shape of the cheeks, esophagus, stomach, duodenum, and colon, are not suited for animal foods (see **Lesson 9: Origins** and **Appendix A**).

Enzyme mutations come about as part of the Law of Vital Adjustment outlined by Professor Hilton Hotema in his book **Man's Higher Consciousness**. The body's Vital Adjustment to foreign substances taxes the system and is always accompanied by a Vital Reduction in the body's overall health and energy level. After a degeneration has occurred, the Law of Vital Adjustment can also work in reverse, as foreign substances are eliminated from the body, a Vital Increase occurs; the body is always capable, over time, of re-adjusting to its natural state because the underlying original biological design is still the same.

Genetic enzyme mutations in accordance with the Law of Vital Adjustment caused by generations of unnatural feeding have turned the human digestive fluids into an anomaly in Nature. The enzymatic activity in the human mouth and digestive system is far out of sync with anything in Nature.

Consider the writings of Dr. Howell, in his landmark work **Enzyme Nutrition**: "The digestive enzymes of civilized humans are infinitely stronger and more concentrated in enzyme activity than any of the metabolic enzymes — more concentrated than any other enzyme combination found in nature. Human saliva and pancreatic juice are loaded with enzyme activity. There is no evidence that wild animals, living on natural raw diets, have digestive enzyme juices even remotely approaching the strength of those found in civilized human beings."

Dr. Howell has demonstrated, through what he calls The Law of Adaptive Secretion of Digestive Enzymes (a manifestation of the Law of Vital Adjustment), that animals eating raw diets have no enzymes in their saliva, but they begin to when fed a heat-treated diet. Dogs taken away from their natural raw diet and put on a cooked-food diet had enzymes show up in the saliva in about a week. The opposite is true as well. When one returns to a natural raw diet, the frenzied enzymatic activity in the saliva eventually disappears.

Allergies to raw foods are connected with enzymes. Some people are allergic to oranges or strawberries, or some other plant foods. These foods contain enzymes which are like keys which unlock poisons the body has stored in locked "boxes." The allergy is actually a release of poison. If these foods are introduced slowly, and in small amounts, each "box" is opened and a little more poison is released. Once all the "boxes" are open, the allergy disappears.

Dr. Howell also uncovered a connection between enzyme deficiencies in the diet (cooked food) and a decrease in brain size and weight. This connection should be clearly understood by those interested in maximum brain performance — it is always best to maximize our potential.

Proper nutrition is the basis of mental power. The nutriment of the brain cells is derived from the blood corpuscles perpetually being pumped into them by the action of the heart. If the food stream is devoid of enzymes and impure, then the pump valves will be weak or out of gear, the stomach will become disordered, the liver will be corrupted, the lungs will become congested, and the brain will be starved, drugged, and poisoned, while all the thoughts that germinate therein will be improper and out of harmony with the Earth.

Thoughts of failure, world-weariness, morbidity, despair, and sorrow are all associated with states of low energy and enzyme depletion in the body caused by eating the wrong food. Low energy deeply affects the state of mind. If every mental disorder is accompanied by a physical disorder (psychosomatic illness), then it must also be true that every physical disorder (enzyme deficiency) is accompanied by a mental disorder (which can be healed by an enzyme-rich diet).

Recommendations For Rapid Results

Before continuing on with more specifics on raw foods and health, I want to provide you with specific foods, juices, and recipes to try now so that you may begin getting immediate results. Applying these suggestions demonstrates first-hand how raw plant foods work.

All these foods, juices, and recipes help detoxify our bodies while providing us with excellent nutrition. All ingredients should be raw and organic!

For Increased Energy
<u>Blend</u>:
5 oranges
5 tablespoons of flax seed oil

Peel the oranges, but maintain the nutritious white pith. Flax seed oil may be found in any natural food store. Blend the oranges and flax seed oil together. Do not bother removing the orange seeds as they are nourishing and contain anti-parasite qualities. Drink slowly. The fat in the flax oil allows the sugar in the oranges to release slowly over time. This provides excellent energy over several hours. This is a particularly beneficial blend to drink before a business meeting or as a starter in the morning.

For The Flu Or A Cold
Blend:
4 oranges
6 figs
1 medium-sized papaya

Peel the oranges, but maintain the white pith. Remove any stems from the figs (figs should be soft and ripe). Skin the papaya and remove all seeds. Be sure all fruits are at room temperature — putting cold refrigerated food into the body can weaken an already compromised immune system. Place all items in a blender. Add distilled water if necessary to thoroughly blend all ingredients. Drink this blend 3 times throughout the day, abstain from other foods. Oranges and papayas are alkaline fruits which provide excellent calcium and are rich in vitamin A (beta-carotene) and vitamin C (which, among other things, is an antioxidant). Flus and colds are typically caused by too much toxicity in the body, leading to a weakened immune system. These fruits help cleanse the gastro-intestinal tract of toxicity and simultaneously nourish the body. Figs are especially excellent mucus dissolvers and are ranked with an acid-binding value of 27.81 (one of the highest ratings of any food) in Ragnar Berg's Table in the book **Mucusless Diet Healing System**.

To Alleviate Stress or Anxiety
Juice:
5 leaves of kale
1/2 head of green cabbage
1/2 head of loose-leafed lettuce

Process all ingredients through a juicer. Drink 30 minutes before an event that has you nervous. If stress and anxiety is persistent, drink one juice in the morning, and one in the evening. Kale, green cabbage, and loose-leafed lettuces together provide a sodium-potassium balance which keeps us centered. Also, these three contain an abundance of alkaline minerals, especially calcium — which has a calming effect on the body. Lettuces have a soporific quality and can even induce sleep when taken in large quantities.

Or...

Breathing:

Oxygen is a food. Stress and anxiety are associated with shallow breathing. Relieve stress by taking 10 deep breaths in the ratio of 1:4:2 as described in **Lesson 22: Breathing (Pranayama)**, **Action Steps**.

For A Sore Throat
1/2 lemon
1 tablespoon of fresh ginger juice or raw ginger powder
6 ounces (0.2 liters) of distilled water
warmed up to 96 degrees Fahrenheit (36 C).

Mix ginger into the water. Squeeze lemon into the mix. Lemon is an excellent cleanser. Ginger works as an antibiotic and an expectorant, helping to relieve the sinus cavities and lungs of mucus. Drink this mix 4-5 times a day until symptoms disappear. The old home remedy also included 2-4 tablespoons of raw honey.

Or, if you are more active, try...
Juice:
3 apples
1 lemon
1 slice of ginger root

Peel the lemon, but maintain the white pith. Put all contents in the juicer. If desired, warm this drink to 96 degrees Fahrenheit (36 C). The apples are "soft" on the throat and provide you with sugar as fuel. Apples also contain pectin, which forms a gel in the intestines that helps remove toxins while simultaneously stimulating a bowel movement. A bowel

movement drains the lymph system, allowing lymphatic tissues throughout the body, including the tonsils in the throat, to alleviate any swelling.
Drink this juice 3-4 times a day until symptoms disappear.

For A Headache
Juice:
4 ribs of celery
4 ounces of fennel
1 apple
1 orange

Peel the orange, but keep the white pith intact. Process all ingredients
through a juicer. Drink immediately. Fennel is a wonderful, licorice-tast-
ing herb. The ancient Greeks and Romans used fennel to treat migraine
headaches. Fennel thins the blood. This allows obstructions — which
place pressure on the blood vessels (headaches) — to flow on and be
removed by the kidneys. Celery and apple are provided to maintain a
sodium-potassium balance in the blood. The orange is added for its alkalinity and calcium.

For Back Pain
Juice:
1 head of dark-leaf lettuce
1 head of broccoli
2 apples

Process all contents through a juicer. Drink once in the morning, once
in the evening. Back pain is associated with a high level of sodium (salt)
and phosphorus (acid) in the tissues. The high calcium content of the lettuce and broccoli immediately loosens constricted tissues. The high
potassium content of this drink provides a mineral balance against sodium. The apple is provided to sweeten.

Or...

Salad:
1 head of lettuce
1 large collard leaf
1/4 head of green cabbage
1 ounce (30 ml) of organic stone-crushed,
cold-pressed extra virgin olive oil
1 avocado
10 strawberries

Mix together and toss into a salad. Eat this salad twice each day: once for lunch, once for dinner. The high-calcium content of green-leafed vegetables loosens constricted tissues. Most back pain is associated with an acid condition of the body — calcium counteracts and neutralizes acidity. The strawberries are included because they contain organic salycilates, which are the basic ingredient of painkillers, such as aspirin.

For An Upset Stomach Or Ulcer
Juice:
1/2 head of green cabbage
2 ribs of celery
2 apples

Cabbage is rich in beta-carotene, vitamin C, sulfur, selenium, and especially the amino acid glutamine. Studies done by Dr. Garnet Cheney, who at one time headed the Cancer Division of Stanford Medical School, revealed the value of glutamine in healing ulcers. Dr. Cheney administered 1 quart (1 liter) of cabbage/celery/carrot juice a day to 65 ulcer sufferers. Within 3 weeks 63 of the patients were healed and 2 retained only minimal symptoms. I learned this one from Jay Kordich "The Juiceman" and have recommended it with success to many people over the years.

Or...

Salad:
1/2 head of green cabbage
1/2 head of purple cabbage
2 small avocados

Dice up the cabbage. Mix in the avocados. The sweet fat of the avocado is very soothing on the delicate mucous linings of the stomach and intestines.

Constipation

Constipation is caused by fecal matter that collects in the colon, dries out, and is difficult to move. Constipation indicates that a person has been eating too many cooked foods which are devoid of water and too few raw oils which lubricate the digestive tract. To prevent constipation in the future, eat chlorophyll-rich fibrous foods (green vegetables) with oil (flax seed, olive, etc.) as a dressing. This will softly broom and sweep the intestines alleviating this condition. Apples and pears may be added to this mix to help stimulate a bowel movement.

If suffering from constipation, try the following:
Lemon Water:
1 quart (liter) of distilled water
1 lemon

Constipation may be caused by dehydration. This may be brought on by stress, overexertion, or overexposure. Eating too much sugar can cause excessive urination and lead to dehydration and constipation. Drinking 3/4 to 1 quart (liter) of distilled water containing the juice of 1 whole lemon the first thing in the morning can stimulate a bowel movement and alleviate this condition.

Or...

Juice:
2 handfuls of parsley
4 ribs of celery
2 apples
1 pear

Process all contents through a juicer. If the constipation is more difficult, drink 12 ounces of this green-leafy vegetable juice first thing in the morning. Add more parsley to this mix if constipation persists.

For A Hangover
Juice:
1 head of romaine lettuce
1 stalk of broccoli
1 handful of spinach

Process all ingredients through a juicer. Drink immediately. Alcohol destroys the B vitamins. Romaine lettuce, broccoli and spinach contain excellent quantities of the B complex, including thiamine (B1), riboflavin (B2), niacin (B3), pantothenic acid (B5), pyridoxine (B6), folic acid (B9). I used to be quite a "social drinker" before I became a raw-foodist. As I began eating significant quantities of raw foods, I no longer would feel hangovers after a night of drinking with friends.

Or...
Fruit:
1 cantaloupe

Eat one whole cantaloupe. Cantaloupe is, overall, the richest fruit in B vitamins. Remember to buy organic foods and eat all the way to edge of the rind to get the maximum nutrition available in the fruit. Melons contain most of their vitamins and minerals near the edge of the rind.

Boost The Immune System
Juice:
2 cloves of garlic
1 slice of ginger
1 handful of parsley
4 pears
1 ounce (30 ml) of organic stone-crushed,
cold-pressed extra virgin olive oil

Process all ingredients through a juicer, except for olive oil, which can be stirred in with a spoon, or blended into the juice. Garlic and ginger are natural antibiotics that assist the immune system. Parsley is rich in iron to build strong red-blood corpuscles. Pear contains pectin which will stimulate a bowel movement, helping to drain the lymphatic system of toxins. Olive oil provides excellent monounsaturated fats the body needs to build strong white blood corpuscles. In my own diet, I include a habanero pepper in my immune system juice, you may want to try adding some hot pepper.

For Depression
Fruit:
Melons

To break a bout of depression, eat one or more melons in the morning for breakfast daily for 5-6 weeks. Eat them on an empty stomach and avoid other foods until 12 noon. Melons are rich in the B complex vitamins and these bolster the nerves. Spells of depression are often associated with moments of low blood sugar. Eat fruits throughout the day to keep the blood sugar up. Avoid complex carbohydrates (baked potatoes, french fries, breads, cakes, cookies, rice) and alcohol which can cause erratic blood sugar fluctuations.

Action Steps:

1. Begin today by treating yourself to luscious fruits and beautiful salads. Eating raw foods has a cumulative effect. The more raw foods you eat over time, the better you feel. The less cooked foods you eat, the better you feel. Do your best to increase your raw food intake and specifically decrease your cooked food intake each day.

2. Cut out 5 cooked foods from your diet today. List them in your journal. Notice the difference this decision makes in your life. Become more discerning in your food choices.

3. Seek out a source for organic (pesticide-free) foods. Support organic farmers by purchasing their higher-quality foods.

4. Invest in a juicer for you and your family.

5. Invest in one or more raw-food recipe books. Browse the Nature's First Law catalog and web-site at:

http://www.rawfood.com

Special Note: Raw plant foods (from herbs to fruits and everything in between) are the single most effective antidote to anxiety, depression, disease, fear, immobility, insomnia, pain, stress, and worry!

Lesson 8:
Food And Karma

The Teachings of Pythagoras:
"There was a man here......
He was first
To say that animal food should not be eaten,
And learned as he was, men did not always
Believe him when he preached, 'Forbear, O mortals,
To spoil your bodies with such impious food!'"
— Ovid, **Metamorphoses**

"Wer immer strebend sich bemuht,
Den konnen wir erlosen."
(Whoever strives with all his power,
We are allowed to save.)
— said the Angels in Goethe's **Faust**

Things don't just happen, things happen which are just. The universe is governed by a karmic law.

Karma is the total effect of an individual's actions and conduct during the successive phases of existence. The greater karmic forces include:
1. Individual karma
2. Past-life karma
3. Collective karma

All the things we have done or have not done in our lives add up to form our karma. Karma is energy. Your karma is what you actually are. What you are is all the thoughts and emotions you have released into eternity up until right now. Life is a mirror which magnifies. What you see out there is only a duplication of what you are inside. The vibrations you send forth are magnified by life and returned to you.

As we have discovered in **Lesson 3: Thoughts Are Things**, thought-fulness is a key attribute of super-success. The most thoughtful people draw all "effects" back to their "causes." They take full responsibility. They are aware of the karma associated with their thoughts and actions!

If we involve ourselves in the pursuit of discordant desires, then truly a karmic web is woven to capture us. We place our lives in jeopardy by our own discordant passions, pursuits, and blind ignorance of cause and effect.

A tremendous amount of destruction is caused by negative emotions and attitudes directly resulting from the karmic consequences of taking in negative karma (energy) through food.

Genesis 9:4 states: "But flesh with the life thereof, which is the blood thereof, shall ye not eat." Leviticus 3:17 describes: "It shall be a perpetual statute for your generations throughout all your dwellings that ye eat neither [animal] fat nor blood." Throughout history, many great religious leaders, spiritual teachers, yogis, and many of the world's religions have recommended a vegetarian diet, and they have done this for a good reason. The karmic consequences of eating animal foods dampens the spiritual powers while raising the emotions of fear and doubt in the mind.

If one exploits the animals and the Earth — the subtler truths of life will remain hidden — that is the fact, simple as that. The enslavement, torture, and death of animals for food, leather, wool, cosmetics, toiletries, down, medicine, etc. is leading humanity's fate to an ever-more perilous position. The mass destruction and exploitation of animal life is causing chaos in the spiritual world. Every animal exploited leaves a karmic ripple in the fabric of time which must eventually return back.

We should take only enough for our needs, otherwise the plants and the animals we have harmed would turn against us and cause us disease and misfortune. A thoughtful person is aware of this and strives to appease them, so that when the opportunity arises, the plants and trees, the worms and birds, and the rabbits and coyotes will send forth a positive karma to help that person along.

The book **Diet For A New America** by John Robbins describes in detail the correlation between eating animal foods and disease. Heart disease, the number one killer in the United States, is directly attributable to eating animal fat and protein. The incidence of cancer has been statistically correlated to the consumption of animal-derived foods. Colon cancer and other diseases of the digestive tract are directly caused by the overconsumption of animal foods and the underconsumption of raw plant foods. Environmental toxins accumulate in animals, especially in animal fats. All the toxins being poured into the atmosphere end up being collected in the tissues of animals. Eating those animals, whether they be insect, fish, or mammal, will give one a strong dose of toxins. In his book, John Robbins mentions that meat contains 14 times the pesticide level an equivalent amount of commercial plant food would contain; dairy products contain 5 1/2 times as much. The more animals people eat, the more likely they are to experience all sorts of health problems. That is a fact. The opposite is true as well. The more raw plant foods people eat, the more likely they are to experience all sorts of health benefits!

Some intellectual types have forwarded the argument that plants actually have a higher consciousness than animals and should therefore not be eaten. What this argument does not understand is that animals are simply transformed plants, thus eating animals brings along with it the karma of the plants they have eaten, plus their own karma. For karmic purposes, one does not have to kill plants, but instead simply eat their leaves and fruits. Sometimes a plant thrives better when its leaves are trimmed, and this actually associates a slightly positive karma to eating those leaves.

What I have discovered from my experience in the field of the raw-vegetarian lifestyle is that the whole question of carnivorism, omnivorism, vegetarianism, veganism, raw-foodism, and fruitarianism comes down to dietary fat. Good wholesome fat in our foods, not protein, is essential to good health and longevity (as we shall discover in **Lesson 11: The Secret Revealed**). Fatty foods are associated with strong karma. Humans are frugivores when they derive their fat from fruit (or other plant sources). Humans are omnivores when they derive their fat from animal sources. The truth is: we have been given a choice! We can rise or fall. I find that fascinating. The whole question is: From where are you going to get your fat? Which fat source has the least side-effects and is the most natural to eat? Of course, fatty fruits — the magic ingredient of The Sunfood Diet. For ethical, karmic, and health reasons, I recommend you get most of your dietary fat from fruits, such as avocados, Sun-ripened olives, and durians, or olive oil.

Fatty fruits have the most positive karma of all foods aside from mother's milk. All fruits with viable seeds have a positive karma. Green-leafy vegetables have a neutral energy associated with them. Hybridized or seedless fruits have a slightly negative karma, because their reproductive purpose has been eliminated.

Hybridized vegetables (carrots, beets, potatoes) have a negative karma associated with them (more details will be given on hybrid foods in **Lesson 16: Hybrid Food**). Not only are carrots, beets, and potatoes hybrids and not capable of growing wildly, but also they are roots which, if eaten, are typically killed (killing creates bad karma).

Consider the following chart. Use the chart to increase the karma of your daily meals. By following the chart to guide your food choices, you will be eating neutral karma foods daily to stay grounded. Between positive and negative karma foods is the area of the green-leafed vegetables. When one wishes to pass negative karma foods into a positive karma body, one must pass through the area of the green-leafed vegetables (eat negative karma foods with green-leafed vegetables). As long as the overall karma of each day's meals are positive you will carry forth a beautiful life.

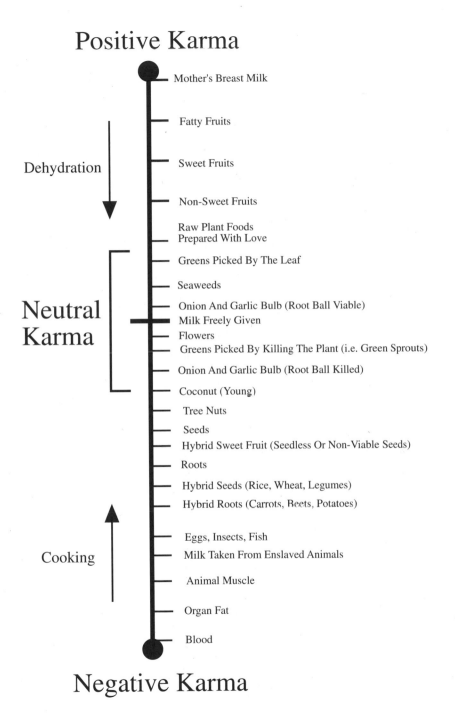

Positive Karma

Mother's Breast Milk

Fatty Fruits

Dehydration

Sweet Fruits

Non-Sweet Fruits

Raw Plant Foods
Prepared With Love

Greens Picked By The Leaf

Seaweeds

Neutral
Karma

Onion And Garlic Bulb (Root Ball Viable)

Milk Freely Given

Flowers

Greens Picked By Killing The Plant (i.e. Green Sprouts)

Onion And Garlic Bulb (Root Ball Killed)

Coconut (Young)

Tree Nuts

Seeds

Hybrid Sweet Fruit (Seedless Or Non-Viable Seeds)

Roots

Hybrid Seeds (Rice, Wheat, Legumes)

Hybrid Roots (Carrots, Beets, Potatoes)

Eggs, Insects, Fish

Milk Taken From Enslaved Animals

Cooking

Animal Muscle

Organ Fat

Blood

Negative Karma

The level of the food on the chart from positive, neutral, and negative corresponds to the energy (positive, neutral, or negative) of the karmic seed planted by eating that food. Raw foods have more karma than cooked foods. Cooking actually degrades energy and moves both positive and negative karmic foods to a more neutral level. Cooking degrades the energy in food and mitigates the karma. That is why people are better off, for karmic purposes, eating cooked flesh, than raw flesh and worse off eating dehydrated fruits than raw fruits. Cooking animal foods introduces a mitigating factor which disrupts and delays the karmic consequences, but eating animal flesh raw is not only dangerous, it has serious karmic consequences.

Many people have adopted vegetarian and vegan lifestyles, yet they still face health challenges because they have not grasped the distinction of "Sun-cooked" versus oven-cooked food. By cooking their food they degrade its energy. By switching to The Sunfood Diet (raw-foods and fruit) they will experience the highest levels of health, happiness, and harmony.

Fruit

"With all the time that humans have been around, I can't
believe the Earth is not covered with fruit trees yet!"
— Steve Adler, raw-food philosopher

Aside from mother's milk, fruit is the only food which possesses a powerful positive karma."Only fruits make you pure in thought, word, and deed." Fruits deserve special attention.

The fruits are the glowing visions of the plants and trees. All other things being equal, a diet rich in fruit is most conducive to the completeness of bodily development and perfectness of symmetry and beauty. Fruit will make you beautiful.

Even the Eskimos eat fruit! Berries — especially blueberries — grow abundantly in and around the tundra areas of the far north.

Eat fruit. Give fruit. Send positive affirmations out to everyone you find before you each day. Compliment them. It will help them out immensely and it will come back to you in many positive ways as well.

Fruit vibrates at a frequency to attract our attention. Fruit is the means trees have invented for traveling from one place to another. When you are attracted to, and eat, fruits, occasionally a seed will be carried within you to a fertile ground. Author and raw-food vegetarian activist, Jeremy Safron, insightfully describes that: "Fruits are the children of the trees."

Nature's Master Plan

Invest your Life
In every fruit,
Whose secret is unknown.
Your destiny
You shall see
In the fruit trees you have grown.

Eat the fruit and launch it far,
Out the window of a car!
Spread more Life,
As much as you can:
Fulfill Nature's master plan.

Our fate is aligned:
With the fruit of the vine,
With the fruit of the tree,
With fruit that grows
Next to the sea.

Love your food,
It all begins

With a fruit seed simply sown.
Nothing by chance;
It's a reflected dance of
Fruit seeds that you've thrown.

Fruit is your food —
Dispel each myth.
Align your fate, entwine it with:
Sumptuous fruit,
The deepest tan.
Fulfill Nature's master plan.

A fruit tree,
For those who see,
Is greater than any throne.
It's enchanting wealth
Can't be found
In any castle made of stone.

Fruit reveals the truth:
It frees the best in you.
Doing what you do best
Is best for Nature too!

Fun and family,
Life without need,
Spreading the vibrant, vital seed.
This is Life, at it's most.
Bring enchantment to every coast.

Propagate fruit
Far and wide.
Let Earth flower
On every side.

Take the seed

And hurl it far,
'Till it reach
The farthest star.

A call to you
As woman, man:
Fulfill Nature's master plan.

Karmic Sense

This world is meant to be, among other things, a sanctuary for all forms of wildlife. It is my duty as a Sunfoodist to protect, preserve, and defend all animals and plants, making no exceptions. I have personal convictions to uphold. All creatures are here with us as companions. Loving innocent life is a higher frequency of being. The Jain religion tells us, "Harmlessness is the supreme religion."

Every chicken killed, every calf stripped away from its mother, every fish plucked from its school, every monkey tortured in a cage is a burden of pain upon total humanity, and weighs heavy upon the karmic scales.

The factory-farming techniques of present-day civilization have created a frightening karmic debt and health danger for anyone still consuming flesh foods — especially if eaten raw. Factory-farmed animals are injected with, sprayed with, and fed, antibiotics, artificial hormones, and chemicals of all kinds; these toxins are still present in the flesh when the animals are slaughtered; they are passed directly into the body of the flesh consumer. Factory-farmed animals are kept in darkness and squeezed together in inhospitable cages. They are fed the most outrageous and unnatural foods imaginable. In the book, **Mad Cowboy**, former cattle rancher, Howard Lyman details that mad cow disease stems from the feeding concoctions of dead cows and other animals in the factory farms to the living cows. When those living cows are slaughtered and eaten, they pass the mad cow disease on to humans.

When one eats the flesh of tortured animals, or the milk of dairy cows, or eggs from factory chickens, one also ingests the fear, the pain, the exhaustion, and the sorrow of those innocent beings which manifests itself within the consumer as a negative attitude.

All the animals one has killed or eaten begin to form an ensnaring trap. Even done unconsciously, it does eventually catch up to us. Going 100% raw-vegan is the power to recall the karmic vibrations we have released into the world in ignorance and error (100% raw-vegan means letting go of all animal-derived foods and products from our lives). With deep desire we can correct our errors and throw off our past mistakes.

Just as you cannot make others happy while being unhappy, one cannot heal while inflicting hurt. Hurting animals to try and find a way to heal only inflicts pain, and never heals anything. This exposes the logical fraud of animal experimentation (vivisection).

All pharmaceutical medicines and drugs, with the exception of aspirin, are tested on innocent animals (read Hans Ruesch's book **Naked Empress** for information on this subject). Modern technological medicine represents a warfare against life. Pharmaceutical medicines and drugs are always harmful to you, the planet, and to innocent animals.

I will not cite animal experiments in this book because I am morally and ethically opposed to them. Animal experimentation (vivisection) is unnatural, unscientific, and always leads to destruction. I feel very strongly on this subject. Animals are beautiful creatures. I have an overwhelming obligation to save as many animals as possible from torture and death.

Once we know that we thrive on a 100% raw-vegan diet, then there no longer remains any reason to exploit animals! What incredible knowledge this is!

Eating raw plant food is a guiltless lifestyle. No pollution is created by using a gas or electric stove. Little, if any, packaging is thrown away. Little water is used to clean dishes and utensils. No animals are exploited to present delicious foods to you. Eating raw plant food is the only "win-win" dietary solution.

Living without the death of animals weighing on your spirit, increases your aliveness. Your aliveness is reflected in your physical body, which takes on a more perfect beauty and a new type of positive energy.

Every thought sent forth into action is a never ending vibration which wisks its way across the universe bringing us back a magnification of what we sent forth. By fulfilling our natural diet of raw plant foods, and by allowing only positive thoughts to govern our minds, only glorious vibrations will emanate from us and all earthly conditions will begin to sway positively in our direction. It is in this way that a new destiny is shaped for our lives.

The Sunfood Diet beautifies the body, mind, emotions, and spirit. Following this diet gives you glimpses of life in the state of instant karma: when an idea is thought, it is automatically transformed into actuality. After you adopt The Sunfood Diet, an amazing synchronicity will occur. Seemingly unrelated events will coincide for you to help you along in your growth and enjoyment of life! The more "raw" you are, the more you will experience synchronicity and serendipity. A 100% raw-vegan diet maintains you in that state of instant manifestation indefinitely. Remarkable coincidences become common place. Extraordinary circumstances begin occurring daily.

Remember: *Virtue is rewarded in this world.* Natural Law makes no false judgments. The karmic scales of all our deeds are constantly being weighed out. The universe is governed by laws — even if we do not know what they are. A true coincidence does not exist; everything happens for a reason.

Action Steps:

1. Set a goal to adopt a vegetarian diet. Decide to let go of animal-based foods. Start by going one day without flesh foods (i.e. no chicken or fish),

then go three days, then five days. Simultaneously eat more green-leafed vegetables, sweet fruits, and avocados. If you really need motivation, visit a slaughterhouse.

2. Next, set a goal to adopt a vegan lifestyle. The vegan lifestyle makes choices for foods, clothing, and other items which are not derived from animal sources.

3. Make a record in your journal of everything you eat in one week. Compare your food choices to the **Food And Karma** chart. Where is your overall balance? Are you developing a positive karma based on your food choices?

4. Read John Robbins' book **Diet For A New America**, Howard Lyman's book **Mad Cowboy**, and Jeremy Rifkin's book **Beyond Beef**. If you have teenage children, have them read the book **Old MacDonald's Factory Farm** by C. David Coats.

5. Spend some time enjoying cats, dogs, rabbits, and other animals. Discover the truth behind vivisection (animal experimentation). Watch the video **Lethal Medicine**.

6. Keep in mind that karmic energy may be balanced in other ways than from eating. Planting produces favorable karma. If one eats coconuts, tree nuts, and seeds, one should also plant coconuts, tree nuts, and seeds to balance the karma.

The Celestine Law

A celestial being,
A cosmic seeing.
New vision of Life
Now grasped;
False views of Life
Now dashed.
The glow of eye
Then seen,
The when, how, why
So keen.
The secret in this time
Revealed:
We chose which destiny
To wield.
For what you give out
Comes back!
Something has been
Keeping track.
Lest we should
Ever forget:
What you give is
What you get.
When you throw off
The karma inside,
By giving more
Than you can hide,
Your life-force
Will grow ever stronger,
And you may even live
A little longer!
Remember this secret,
So true,
And you will see Life anew.

Lesson 9:
Origins

Evolution: A Monkey's Perspective
(Author Unknown)

Three monkeys sat in a coconut tree
Discussing things as they are said to be.
Said one to the others: "Now listen, you two
There's a rumor around that can't be true,
That man descended from our noble race.
The very idea is a great disgrace.

No monkey has ever deserted his wife,
Starved her babies, and ruined her life.
And you've never known a mother monk,
To pass her babies on to another,
Till they scarcely knew who is their mother.

Here's another thing a monkey won't do:
Go out at night and get on a stew,
Or use a gun or club or knife,
To take some other monkey's life.
Yes, man descended, the ornery cuss,
But brother, he didn't descend from us."

"Those scientists who investigate the phenomena of life are as if lost in an inextricable jungle in the midst of a magic forest, whose countless trees unceasingly change their places and their shapes...Most of the questions put to themselves by those scientists who study human beings, remain without answer...Humans are made up of a procession of phantoms, in the midst of which there strides an unknowable reality." — Dr. Alexis Carrel, **Man The Unknown**

Introduction

Life is a mystery, so grand, so vast.
Origins are hidden, deep in the past.

Worn out, eroded,
Are they
Hopelessly unsuited?

Nothing is more fantastic,
Is anything more farfetched
Than slates of fossil stone
Which reality once etched?

Any philosophy of diet leads, typically, to a philosophy of human origins. It seems reasonable that the diet humanity originated on, should be the diet that best suits us. From research and experience we see that primitive diets do actually work because they are simpler, more natural, and the body has less confusion to contend with. Primitive peoples have more robust jaws and more beautiful teeth, which is reflective of their superior diet. But even primitive diets do have their limits. They contain cooked foods and animal foods which will only allow the body to reach a certain level of health and positive energy.

Some argue that humans have actually adapted through evolution to cooked foods and animal foods, but the thousands of gastro-intestinal and related diseases (which do not afflict natural creatures eating their natural diet) are positive proof that humanity's food choices have not been optimal.

This lesson challenges many of the false assumptions underlying the theory of evolution. It exposes the danger of "raw-food evolutionary diets" and describes that such diets do not lead to excellent health. With the theory of evolution proved faulty, *all* dietary systems based upon it must be reevaluated.

This lesson demonstrates that the form, function, and food choices of every plant and animal are not determined by evolution or adaptation over time. But that each organism has a form, function, and food supply ordained by design. When we humans follow our dietary design, the results are extraordinary.

This lesson also demonstrates concepts in lateral thinking and may be particularly interesting for those of a "success consciousness" who are always looking for unique intellectual angles and ways to think things differently. Understanding this lesson is not entirely necessary to succeed with The Sunfood Diet. Those who find the information here to be less than essential may move forward to **Lesson 10: Detoxification**.

Those who choose to study this lesson will find that many scientists and researchers have shattered the glass towers of evolution where hypotheses are based on hypotheses and fact and fiction are mingled in an ever-deeper confusion...the evidence of which I present.

Objectivity?

The challenge presented to all explorers of the microcosm and macrocosm is not to confuse the observed with the mind of the observer, not to construct a picture of external reality, which is only a mirror of the thinker. Can this challenge be overcome?

No one could accurately describe what happened on planet Earth yesterday, let alone what happened 100,000 years ago! History consists of what is *believed* about the past, not of what actually happened in the past.

The whole field of darwinism/evolution is based on the critical assumption that life is shaped by the outer environment. This generated the sociology of "the environment" as determining the character of living beings. And yet, in a pure sense, what is life? Life is the unfolding of the inner potential. Potential is fulfilled by action, just as a seed, with its inward certainty of bursting life and future fruit generation, is fulfilled by action through water, soil, and Sun. The environment does not determine the inner potential — it can only help or hinder its expression. The physical world of Nature is in reality the materialization of the inner spiritual potential of all living things. The inner world creates the outer world (**Lesson 1: The Principle Of Life Transformation**).

Science Or Philosophy?

"As the creation myth of scientific naturalism, darwinism
plays an indispensable ideological role in the war against
fundamentalism. For that reason, the scientific organizations
are devoted to protecting darwinism rather than testing it,
and the rules of scientific investigation have been
shaped to help them succeed."
— Phillip Johnson, **Darwin On Trial**

Today's fatalistic science includes science *and* philosophical deductions which are not science and are not supported empirically. The scientific observation of the world is simply empirical study. However, today's science implicitly contains philosophical deductions (loaded with ideas about the ultimate existential meaning of the universe, such as notions of how life began, what life is, etc.) not supported by empirical proof.

For example, we have the "common ancestor" idea, which sounds great to a materialistic mind, but is not supported by the fossil record. The common ancestor idea contains science (quantifiable similarities between species) *and* the philosophical deduction that they share a common ancestor — which has not empirically been shown.

Utilitarianism?

There is no evidence that the Earth's biological history or "evolution" (as it has been termed) is a mechanical process of increasing fitness and utility over time.

What of "survival of the fittest?" The philosopher Nietzsche pointed out, survival of the fittest happens, but is meaningless most of the time, because the vast majority of organisms do not fight, do not kill for food, and do not compete for territory in such a way that cause competitors to die out.

The utilitarian aspect of the darwinian theory is quite subjective. The utility of an "adaptation" is relative to the use sought to be made of it. A species without feathers has no need of feathers. A feather which gradually evolves would be a positive disadvantage over the "millions of years" necessary to perfect the feather. Furthermore, how did this process start? For an "adaptation" to be utile, it must be ready; while it is being prepared, it is inutile. But if it is inutile, it is not darwinian, for darwinism says evolution is utilitarian.

Why is it that the "lower" forms (e.g. the horseshoe crab), those which are simpler (less fit?) have not died out, and have not yielded to the principle of evolution? They remain in the same form they have had for vast expanses of the fossil record. Why do they not "evolve" into something "higher?"

The Fossil Record

The most conclusive refutation of evolution is furnished by paleontology. Simple probability indicates that fossil records can only be test samples. Each sample, then, should represent a different stage of evolution/adaptation, and there ought to be "transition types," not particularly of one species or another. Instead, what we find, in the actual fossil record, are genus forms (a genus is a collection of related organisms usually including several species) that have not developed themselves on the fitness principle, but appear suddenly and at once in their definite shape; that do not thereafter evolve towards better adaptation, but become rarer or finally disappear, while quite different forms arise again.

The mathematician Mandelbrot in his casebook **The Fractal Geometry of Nature** (about Chaos theory) describes two types of quantity variations recognizable in Nature:

1. The Joseph Effect. This means persistence: despite an underlying randomness, the longer a quantity grouping has experienced a condition, the likelier it is to experience more of that same condition. The Joseph Effect means that a certain genus of species, despite erratic conditions, may persist through countless eons, essentially unchanged.

2. The Noah Effect. This means discontinuity: when a quantity changes, it can change arbitrarily fast. Quantities can change instantaneously. They do not pass through all intervening points on their way from one point to another. The Noah Effect means that a quantum of species may instantaneously alter form and function.

Consider how Mandelbrot's observations are mirrored by Stephen Gould (quoted from **Darwin On Trial**), developer of the evolutionary "punctuated equilibrium" theory which attempts to explain away the embarrassing fact that the fossil record is devoid of transition types:

"The history of most fossil species includes two features particularly inconsistent with gradualism:

1. Stasis. Most species exhibit no directional change during their tenure on earth. They appear in the fossil record looking pretty much the same as when they disappear; morphological change is usually limited and directionless.

2. Sudden appearance. In any local area, a species does not arise gradually by the steady transformation of its ancestors; it appears all at once and 'fully formed.'"

All that we see about us impels us to the conviction that again and again profound and extremely sudden changes take place in the forms of living plants and animals. These changes are of a chaotic or cosmic origin and may be beyond human understanding.

Similarly, all active beings (including those reading this now) have striven towards their fulfillment by turning points or "epochs" in their lives — not by gradual evolution. Think about the events of your own life and decide which is a better description: a series of turning points or gradual evolution? The origins of the Earth, of life, of the free-moving animals, are such turning points or "epochs" of change.

Quantum physics is telling us things do not change slowly over time — they make quantum leaps. We jump from one level of experience to another.

Evolutionists never demonstrate what a smooth transition is — they never define it. A transition of macro-form should be demonstrated somewhere in a long sequence, say 50, 30, or at least 10 successive fossils in transition. Yet, with all the billions of fossils on Earth, no one has met this simple criteria for a fossil sequence.

We also do not find *any* genetic mistakes (one-shot mutations which failed) in the fossil record which is impossible if random mutation through natural selection (trial and error) is true.

By far the most abundant fossils in the world are the 14 types of ammonites — little shelled snail-like ocean species — which, as far as we can tell, have existed essentially since life began on Earth. Literally billions of these fossils have been found, but never have there been discovered any transition types, or smooth transitions, between any of these 14 types.

The first treatise which described that the basic forms of plants and animals did not evolve step-by-step, but were suddenly there, was given by Hugo de Vries in his work **Mutation Theory** in 1886. He described that we can clearly see (through scientific/utility analysis) how the "impressed living form" works itself out in the individual samples, but we cannot see how the "die was cut" for each whole genus. We cannot see how the genus appeared. Origins remain hidden from us.

We cannot ascertain how the Homo genus (Homo habilis, Homo erectus, Homo ergaster, Homo neanderthalis, archaic Homo sapien, Cro-Magnon, Homo sapien, Homo sapien sapien) appeared, yet it was suddenly there in the fossil record.

Evolutionists continue to argue the tired line that humans smoothly transitioned from one form to another and assume modern Homo sapiens arose merely 100,000 to 200,000 years ago (based on the present questionable dating system). In December 1997, **Discover** magazine reported the findings of a Spanish team working in Gran Dolina, Spain who uncovered an 800,000 year-old skull with remarkably modern features. The discoverer, Juan Luis Arsuaga Ferreras, stated, "It is so surprising we must rethink human evolution to fit that face." **Discover** magazine stated: "The Gran Dolina face is 800,000 years old and yet distinctively ours. It is almost that of a modern human."

The evidence is showing and will continue to show that all the Homo forms have existed together for thousands, or millions, of years without the gradual evolution through common ancestry concept.

The Homo life-form, like every other, originated in a sudden appearance or mutation (the Germans have the great word "Wandlung" meaning "instant transformation") of which the "when," "how," and "why" remains a secret. There exists somewhere in the recesses of time a sharp frontier on the hither side of which we see Homo as a completely formed type, endowed with a certain bodily structure, walk, and posture that has not materially altered up to the present day. All the ape-like remains (Australopithecus, etc.) and the hominid remains (Homo) found on Earth are still distinctly different, and bridging that gap to find a missing link remains elusive. No missing link can be found. This is because no missing link exists.

The fossil record is actually a liability which must be explained away by evolutionists. Pre-darwinian paleontologists were right on when they cited the lack of intermediaries as a conclusive reason for rejecting biological evolution initially. Stephen Gould has described "the extreme rarity of transitional forms in the fossil record" as "the trade secret of paleontology." Darwin wrote: "Nature may almost be said to have guarded against the frequent discovery of her transitional and linking forms."

Think about it logically, if there were gradual evolution, in the adaptation sense of the word, there could not be specific animal classes, but only a chaos of living singular forms left over from some "struggle for existence." Darwin posed this question to himself: "...why, if species have descended from other species by insensibly fine gradations, do we not everywhere see innumerable transitional forms? Why is not all nature in confusion instead of the species being, as we see them, well defined?"

The species we know today are all stable.

Common Ancestors?

"Darwinists assume that the relationship between, say,
bats and whales is similar to that between siblings and
cousins in human families. Possibly it is, but the
proposition is not self-evident...We observe directly
that apples fall when dropped, but we do not observe a common
ancestor for modern apes and humans. What we do observe is
that apes and humans are physically and biochemically more
like each other than they are like rabbits, snakes, or trees.
The ape-like common ancestor is a hypothesis in a theory,
which purports to explain how these greater and lesser
similarities came about. The theory is plausible, especially
to a philosophical materialist, but it may nonetheless be false.
The true explanation for natural relationships may be
something much more mysterious."
— Phillip E. Johnson, **Darwin On Trial**

Based on the fossil record, the general picture of plant and animal history is a burst of general body forms followed by stasis or extinction. We may hypothesize that relationships between these forms come from common ancestors, or from ancestors which were transformed by some means other than the accumulation of small mutations, or from some process altogether beyond the scope of human understanding at this point.

Neo-darwinism (the present-day evolution philosophy) has chosen the common ancestor idea as the key to understanding the relationship between the great classes of living beings. *This is a philosophical deduction based on materialist misconceptions and is not a fact.* If neo-darwinists truly wanted to be scientific, they would have to define the common ancestry idea as an empirical fact rather than as a "logical" deduction from material classifications of species.

Primates And Diet

Omnivorous feeding patterns among primates have been used to justify omnivorous eating by humans through evolutionary theories (if chimps eat animal foods and humans evolved from chimps, then humans should eat animal foods). These comparisons are specious, not only because the common ancestry idea is faulty, but because of the objectivity problem.

In his phenomenal book, **L'Homme, Le Singe, Et Le Paradis** (Humans, Primates, and Paradise), Frenchman Albert Mosseri cites professor Henry Bailey Stevens' insightful observations:

(Translation): "In his study, **Pyramid of Life**, professor Henry Bailey Stevens writes: 'Short term effects appear in tropical monkeys, where humans deranged their natural habitat. Civilization, with its growing demand for monkeys for lab experiments, completely changed their behavior. We must keep that in mind during interpretations. For example, we never saw in the past a monkey kill for food. Now in 1960 Jane Goodall Lawick went on an expedition to live a year with the chimpanzees in Tanzania. The chimpanzees got used to her presence and lost all apprehension. During this period, they had also the occasion to observe her own behavior and diet. They are gifted imitators, so they were able to admire human ingenuity When she announced that some young chimpanzees in the group killed 4 monkeys, one antelope, and a pig, we saluted this as a scientific contribution. Alas, it was only a deviation due to what our civilization reflected on the chimpanzees.'"

The point here is instructive. Many chimpanzee groups — especially the bonobo chimps (the most genetically similar to humans) — do not engage in hunting behavior. It is extremely likely that the chimpanzees of Gombe (Jane Goodall's research group) and other chimp groups learned their much-publicized killing and meat-eating behavior from humans; probably originally deriving such practices from local human tribes whom they lived amongst for thousands of years.

Among the more remote anthropoid apes, such as orangutans, we find no hunting behavior. Studies of orangutans have revealed they might rarely eat insects or bird's eggs, but do so initially in their youth out of curiosity and, as adults, occasionally due to hunger.

Amongst omnivorous eating patterns of some primates we find the folivorous gorilla. No one who looks into a gorilla's eyes — intelligent, gentle, vulnerable — can remain unchanged. Gorillas are a shining example of the raw-vegan diet amongst an anthropoid ape in Nature.

Dr. George Schaller, in his incredible book **Year Of The Gorilla** describes: "I never saw gorillas eat animal matter in the wild — no birds, eggs, insects, mice, or other creatures — even though they had the opportunity to do so on occasion. Once a group passed over a dead duiker without handling the fresh remains, and another time a group nested beneath an olive pigeon nest without disturbing a single egg." Gorillas have been observed to remove insects from vegetation before eating it.

Diet And Evolution?

At its inception, each new genus form is associated with a definite energy and a specific physiological design. Its functioning environment, physical form, social life, physical life (i.e. how to spin web), and food/fuel choice are pre-determined within a narrow variable range. These are not subject to change and do not (actually cannot) adapt beyond a certain threshold.

The Homo genus has a specific biological design for food/fuel, as do all other genus forms.

Those who espouse evolutionary diets have as their base tenet the assumption that we have adapted to a specific diet through millennia of certain feeding behaviors. These behaviors vary widely and can never be precisely known. They can only be guessed at, as both frugivorous plant eating and omnivorous feeding teeth-striation patterns have been discovered amongst various fossils in the Homo genus.

To a degree humans have adapted. Enzymatic adjustments or mutations have occurred amongst the different human races to help accommodate foreign foods. For example, Caucasians have the ability to enzymatically breakdown alcohol, whereas Native Americans do not have the enzymes to do so easily (Dr. Bert Vallee and other researchers at Harvard Medical School have isolated 15 different types of alcohol dehydrogenase (ADH) liver enzymes. They discovered that the number and variety of these enzymes vary between individuals and ethnic groups. The number and variety of these "isoenzymes" appear to be genetically controlled).

In spite of enzymatic mutations, amongst all the races, no "macroevolutionary" change has occurred to the human digestive organs (the teeth have not sharpened, the bowels have not de-sulcified and shortened, the liver has not enlarged), even in spite of humanity's recent history of chaotic dietary patterns.

Different races and blood types display patterns of enzyme mutations allowing certain groups to metabolize certain foods, while other groups lack those enzymes. This understanding underlies the blood-type theory. This theory describes that our blood type (of which there are four different varieties: O, A, B, or AB) exerts a powerful influence on the foods which digest and assimilate well for us. The theory states that Blood type O is for omnivore (an eater of both plant and animal foods).

I am a blood type O and have had no problem eating a 100% raw diet since January 1995, and plant foods only since January 1993. Brian Clement, director of the Hippocrates Health Institute, is a blood type O and has been a vegetarian for over 35 years. Dr. Gabriel Cousens is a blood type O and has been a raw-food vegetarian for over 15 years. There are many other examples I could site.

In my own experience counseling people on diet, I have found the suggestions of what foods are agreeable and disagreeable based on one's blood type to be often applicable to cooked foods and rarely applicable to raw foods and raw-food eaters. I have also found that people of blood type A tend to burn sugars (carbohydrates) more slowly and can generally handle more sugars in their diet. People of blood type O tend to burn sugar more rapidly and do better eating less carbohdrates and more fats for energy.

Obviously different blood groups, races, and ethnic groups share different affinities for natural foods (e.g. northern Europeans tend to like green apples, southern Europeans tend to like red apples). Each group has different enzymatic capabilities to digest their traditional cooked staples. So there is a partial truth in the blood-type theory; however, the blood-type theory makes no distinction between raw or cooked foods, nor does it address blood type O's who thrive on a vegetarian, vegan, or raw-food diet — indicating a flaw in its reasoning.

If we look closely, we see that eating animal foods (protein flesh, milk), or ingesting alcohol, requires enzyme mutations present in some groups, and absent in others. This means that these foods were added later in our history on the planet and were not originally present. All the enzymes originally present are still with all of us now and are designed to breakdown raw plant foods, especially green leaves and fruits (sweet, non-sweet, and fatty).

As mentioned in **Lesson 7: The Sunfood Diet**, **Lesson 8: Food And Karma**, and **Appendix A**, the structure and function of humanity's dull canines and grinding teeth, the pouchy shape of the lips and cheeks, the elongated digestive canal, the sensitive nature of the sensory organs, the method of nourishment for the young, the pattern of children's develop-ment, mental set, emotional feelings, as well as the cause and cure of dis-ease and unhappiness, all demonstrate that humans are biologically plant eaters (eaters of sweet, non-sweet, and fatty fruits along with green-leafed vegetables). Humans descend from the natural state into omnivorism when foods, especially fats, are drawn from animal sources (more on this in **Lesson 11: The Secret Revealed**).

Omnivore theorists believe that because an animal can chew something up, swallow it, and live long enough to tell others about it, then that ani-mal is an omnivore. For example, the herbivorous cow has been fed the flesh of other dead cows, mixed in with its feed, for at least a century by the cattle industry. Cows still continue to survive on such food. Yet, an omnivorist would argue that the cow is no longer an herbivore, but is now an omnivore, because it can eat something aside from common grass. Almost any animal, can eat just about any type of so-called "food," and still live, but that does not mean it has "evolutionarily adapted to," or is designed for, that food!

Every natural species can tolerate a vast amount of improper food (fuel). That is why dogs, mice, rats, cats, birds, etc. can tolerate large vol-umes of denatured, dead, and improper food even though they have never seen these types of foods in their genetic history. The cells and tissues composing the anatomy of these organisms always display an amazing degree of resilience, elasticity, and buoyancy. However, every living organism can "adapt" itself up to a certain point only, and beyond that point follows illness and degenerative disease. And every "adaptation" along the way occurs at the expense of a repression of the body's func-tions of elimination — each "adaptation" has its price. Professor Hilton Hotema termed this the Law of Vital Adjustment, and later specified it as really the Law of Vital Reduction. This is how the body builds up a tol-erance to food and air pollution: the body's eliminative functions must first be weakened before it will submit to inimical foods and environ-ments.

The most amazing thing about human life is that we can discover our form, function, and food choice design and choose to follow it, therefore actualizing the highest potential of our species. That is the purpose of this book. We will discover the specifics of our natural food choice design in **Lesson 11: The Secret Revealed**.

Natural Selection And The Species Boundary

Returning back to the discussion of evolution, we find that natural selection (the primary agent of species creation under the evolutionary theory) is a tautology — it can be made to explain anything. For example, evolutionists claim plant-mimicry among insects is beneficial and will be selected for, but they also claim that warning-warrior colorations, such as insect stripes, are beneficial and will be selected for. Yet if both these hypotheses are true, any kind of coloration on the insect will have some beneficial value and will be selected for. Natural selection cannot make unique predictions, but is used retrospectively to explain everything.

Natural selection, as observed in operation, permits variations only within species boundaries. It operates also to preserve those boundaries. The theory that natural selection has the creative power needed to fuel the changes necessary to turn one species into another is unsupported by the empirical scientific evidence.

The claim of "evolution in action" is simply the observation of local fluctuations of genotypes within a single species. To be more specific, we know certain circumstances favor drug-resistant bacteria as opposed to normal bacteria, or big-beaked birds as opposed to little-beaked birds, or black-peppered moths as opposed to white-peppered moths. In such circumstances, the population of normal bacteria, small-beaked birds, and white-peppered gypsy moths may become reduced as long as circumstances adverse to them prevail, but they do not disappear. As circumstances change, their portion of the genome may again come to predominate, and the population can fluctuate back.

How far can a new species vary? Consider this fact: no one has yet bred a new species artificially. Species have inherent biological limits. The hybridization of the beet vegetable is instructive. Wild beets have a sugar content of less than 4%. Hybrids were developed from wild strains which increased the sugar yield to 17%! However, biologists have never been able to get beets of a higher than 17% yield. By breeding high-yield varieties together they often get throw-backs to the wild stocks. 17% is a barrier.

Nature has to economize in one area in order to expand in another area. This is a basic law of compensation which limits variability. This opposes evolutionary theory which suggests each organism has an infinite genetic plasticity which, coupled with mutation and natural selection, can stretch a bacteria into a human given enough time.

The Random Mutation Theory

Let's think logically: natural selection implies the selection of certain traits from a larger pool of traits within a group. Thus, over time, it is a mechanism which reduces biological diversity. Obviously, the diverse natural world itself represents the opposite. The random mutation theory has to provide the favorable characteristics to create diversity. Micromutations, we are told, stem from random mistakes in copying the commands of the DNA's genetic code. To say that such chance errors could construct even a single complex organ, such as a stomach or an intestinal tract, is like saying a dictionary could result from a print shop explosion.

Just how the unique bone structure of birds could have evolved gradually through natural selection and mutation from the standard vertebrate design is fantastically difficult to imagine and even more difficult to prove. All micromutations have to appear simultaneously and work together at every step along the way. For instance, the spine and bone structure are absolutely vital to every moment of the organism's existence — even the slightest mistake or variance leads to death.

One eminent scientist of the mid-twentieth century, who concluded the theory of evolution had fallen apart, was the geneticist Professor Richard Goldschmidt of the University of California at Berkeley. In his book, **Darwin On Trial**, Phillip Johnson describes Goldschmidt's now-famous challenge to the neo-darwinists, listing a series of complex structures, from mammalian hair to hemoglobin, which he concluded could not have been produced by the accumulation and selection of small mutations. Goldschmidt described how the idea that an accumulation of micromutations could lead to new organs and species is a mathematical impossibility.

Beyond Natural Selection And Random Mutation

"A very large yet undefined extension may safely be
given to the direct and indirect results of natural selection;
but I now admit...that in the earlier editions of my **Origin of Species** I probably attributed too much to the action of natural selection or the survival of the fittest...I had not formerly sufficiently considered the existence of many structures which appear to be, as far as we can judge, neither beneficial nor injurious, and this I believe to be one of the greatest oversights as yet detected in my work."
— Charles Darwin, **The Descent Of Man**

We know that close contact with other living beings unites patterns of thought, emotion, biological appetites, and impulses. And that people *do* resemble their pets and vice versa. Biological theories have not been able to explain the "Power of Association" scientifically.

Natural selection is the most famous mechanism that can cause biological adjustments in organisms, but it may not be the most important element. Other factors that cause changes in species include: directed mutation and/or geographic morphism.

Experiments have shown bacteria can mutate in beneficial ways, due to directed mutation, without natural selection. Consider the results of the following experiments conducted on E. Coli bacteria. Researchers Dr.

John Cairns and Dr. Barry Hall independent of each other confirmed that when bacteria are deprived of certain nutrients, such as the amino acids tryptophan and cysteine, they are able to, under hostile conditions, give rise to offspring which can internally synthesize these nutrients. This is a directed mutation. (See Cairns, J., "The origin of mutants," **Nature**, 335:142-145 and Hall, B., "Spontaneous point mutations that occur more often when advantageous than when neutral," **Genetics**, 126:5-16, September 1990). If simple bacteria can synthesize their own nutrients, imagine what humans can do!

Environmental factors directly affect the structure of living organisms — this phenomena is termed "geographic morphism." Within each landscape, the forms of plants and animals have local characteristics which can be, and often are, picked up by transplants of plant and animal strains and stocks from other landscapes. For example, in the 19th century it was discovered that for any given inhabited area of the world there was an average cephalic index (the ratio of the greatest breadth of the head to its length from front to back) of the human population. More important, it was learned, through measurements on immigrants to America from all over Europe, and on their American-born offspring, that this cephalic index corresponds to the geographical location, and immediately makes itself manifest in the new generation. Thus, long-headed Sephardic Jewish people and short-headed Ashkenazi Jewish people, after arriving in America, produced offspring with a specifically American cephalic index.

From intuitive observation, it is apparent that the landscape exerts an influence on the plant and animal life within its bounds. The mechanism of this influence is beyond our scientific understanding at this time. The source of it, however, we know: it is the cosmic unity of the totality of things, a unity which shows itself in the rhythmic and cyclic movement of Nature.

Embryology

If evolution were correct, then we should find that the embryonic development of animals would replay a synopsis of the whole evolutionary picture. Organisms should start out in life as relatively similar, and then form their differing features later.

In reality, the embryonic patterns represent a mysterious puzzle for the evolutionary theory. Although it is true that different vertebrate types pass through an embryonic stage at which they resemble one another, they develop to this stage very differently. Each vertebrate egg, upon fertilization, undergoes cell divisions and movements characteristic of its class: fish follow one pattern, amphibians another, reptiles another, birds another, and mammals yet another.

Embryologists have known for many decades now that vertebrate embryos develop along different lines which converge in appearance midway through the process, then diverge again until they finally develop — in totally different ways — similar organs, limbs, and bones.

Darwin thought embryology was a guide to evolutionary genealogy. If this were so, then embryology is telling us vertebrates have multiple origins and did not inherit similar characteristics from a common ancestor.

Are Species Real?

Up until now, I have used the word "species" in its traditional sense (the way neo-darwinists have defined it for decades). The traditional definition of "species" connotes organisms which can breed together. There are major problems with the definition of the word "species." Pleomorphic organisms and all animals and plants which reproduce asexually fall out of the species categorization. This presents an enormous population of living things on Earth and an enormous problem for neo-darwinists. How do we classify such organisms? Another problem with this definition is that extinct populations of fossils do not breed, so we do not know whether they could breed together and do in fact represent one or more species. This also can never be tested. And what of living populations that are genetically identical but cannot breed together, such as varieties of the fruit fly? And what of the offspring of a horse and a donkey (a mule) which is fertile, even though most are not? A bull can be crossed with a bison to produce fertile offspring, and this also violates the definition.

Even defining a species by chromosomal similarities may prove impossible. Italian researchers have discovered a strain of mice with only 16 chromosomes instead of 20. But Silvia Garagna, a zoologist from the University of Pavia involved in the research, has stated: "We have not found a new species. We have just found a new chromosomal race within the mouse species." (See **The San Diego Union Tribune**, "Of Mice And Scientists...", Section E-1, December 17, 1996.)

When the definition of "species" is thrown up to the wind, then statements such as "all the species of Galapagos finch have evolved from common ancestors" loses any value.

Claims of new species forming within the present day continue to be asserted by neo-darwinists. In all of the examples they offer, however, what we actually find are two types of situations.

The first type involves blurring the definition of what they have defined a species as and replacing it with a definition so poorly defined that any sub-species variation can be claimed as "speciation." The Galapagos finches are an excellent example of sub-species variations claimed to be different species. Jonathan Weiner, in his Pulitzer-prize winning book **The Beak Of The Finch**, describes researchers Peter and Rosemary Grant's observations that different finch "species" do breed together and produce fertile offspring.

The second type involves chance mutations where the chromosomes suddenly double (as in plants), or change in some other way, but these mutations have never been shown to reproduce themselves into a new species.

The fact that a "species" cannot be precisely defined disassembles the entire darwinian classification system which relies on categorization.

The Fallacy Of Radio-Isotope Dating

The vertebrate sequence
A reflection in rock
Obscured by the ages,
A frozen time clock.

But how many years,
Into the din,
Dates each fossil
We're examining?

More than anything else, evolutionists do not like having their dating system challenged. The present dating systems for organic material and rocks are so ingrained into the present scientific consciousness in the fields of biology, anthropology, paleontology, etc., that to question their veracity is bound to raise emotions. As strange as it may sound, radioactive dating — the most crucial leg of the neo-darwinian support structure — is perhaps the least scientific and the most flawed of all evolutionary postulates.

Richard Milton, in his phenomenal book, **Shattering The Myths Of Darwinism**, outlines the history of present-day dating systems and their flaws, some of which I have outlined in the section below, along with my own research:

In the 1940s, American chemist Willard Libby developed the radiocarbon method of dating organic materials. His system was based on carbon 14, a radioactive isotope of carbon 12. Carbon 14 begins to decay as soon as it is created at a half-life rate of 5,700 years. When a plant or animal dies, it stops taking in carbon 14 from the land and atmosphere, so the amount of carbon 14 in its body begins to decay, while the ordinary carbon 12 remains the same. All other still-living organisms, argued Libby, still retain the same proportion of carbon 14 to carbon 12. This proportion does not change as long as the organism is still alive, thus it can be determined, based on the proportion of carbon 14 to carbon 12, how long ago the organism died.

Willard Libby made the crucial assumption that the total amount of carbon 14 in the atmosphere has remained constant over time.

Studies by researchers Richard Lingenfelter, Hans Suess, V. Switzer, and Melvin Cook (done independently) have determined the proportion of carbon 14 to carbon 12 in the atmosphere is increasing (see Lingenfelter, R., "Production of C-14 by cosmic ray neutrons" **Review of Geophysics**, Feb. 1963, 1:51; Suess, H., "Secular variations in the Cosmic-ray produced carbon 14 in the atmosphere and their interpretations" **Journal of Geophysical Research**, Dec. 1965, 70: 5947; Switzer, V., "Radioactive dating and low level counting" **Science**, Aug. 1967, 157:726; Cook, M., "Do radiological clocks need repair?" **Creation Research Society Quarterly**, Oct. 1968, 5:70). Melvin Cook found, at present, carbon 14 is increasing 38% faster than it is decaying. The Earth's atmosphere is accumulating carbon 14.

If carbon 14 levels are increasing, the amount of carbon 14 the animal had before it died will be higher than assumed. This assumption will cause test samples to appear younger than they actually are, causing inaccuracies. Also, the carbon-dating system is not usable after 57,000 years because after 10 half-lives, very little carbon 14 is left in the sample to examine.

Researcher Melvin Cook has also demonstrated that uranium-lead and potassium-argon methods for dating inorganic rocks are also severely flawed. Cook's findings have been supported by other reputable scientists in the peer-reviewed literature. Funkhouser and Naughton demonstrated the flaws in uranium-lead methods by dating volcanic material known to have been formed in a Hawaiian volcanic eruption in 1801. The dating system showed these new materials to be 3 billion years old (see Funkhouser, J., Naughton, J. **Journal of Geophysical Research**, July 1968, 73: 4606). In another related study, Professor McDougall of Australian National University found, through potassium-argon dating, ages of up to 465,000 years for rocks known to be less than 1,000 years old (see **Nature**, 20 March 1980, p. 230-232, 12 November 1981, p. 123-124).

Most people do not realize that the 4 billion year age estimate of the Earth derives exclusively from methods of assessing radioactive uranium decay (and the decay of similar elements). No other dating system presents an age of the Earth even in the ballpark of 4 billion years.

The uranium dating system works by tracking lead isotopes which are formed from the decay of radioactive uranium 238. Uranium 238 decays into lead 206, which is distinct from common lead 204. The half-life of uranium 238 is 4.5 billion years; thus, a sample of uranium 238 should become half lead 206 in 4.5 billion years. From this relation, rocks are dated. The amount of uranium 238 and lead 206 in the sample are compared. The problem with this dating system is that lead 206 can be formed by other processes! While uranium 238 is decaying, it is also releasing neutrons which bombard surrounding particles, including common lead 204. By absorbing neutrons, common lead 204 can be converted into lead 206.

Uranium 238 and other isotopes are not metals in their natural form, but appear as water-soluble uranium oxide which can wash from one place to another, thereby enriching some sites and depleting others, throwing off the dating accuracy yet again.

The problem with radioactive dating is there is no independent means (outside of the radioactivity paradigm) of verifying the ages of samples. Most rock samples, when dated, present a range of dates which appear as a bell curve. Along the curve some ages are too old and some are too young and ages are chosen subjectively often because they "feel right" within the context. Consider the McDougall study (cited in **Nature**, also see and compare **Nature**, 18 April 1970, 20 September 1974, 4 December 1975, 28 October 1976), where the "scatter" of dates conducted by different groups of researchers ranged from 0.52 million to 17.5 million years ago for a sample of KBS Tuff rock material used to date the age of the Lake Turkana Man fossils. The dates for rock samples taken from the KBS Tuff were all over the place. The date of 2.6 million years arrived at for the KBS Tuff sample was eventually chosen, to end the whole debate, because it was apparently "reasonable" to the scientists involved.

The assumptions behind radioactive dating cannot be applied to a system that is not understood within the unrestricted world of physics in Nature. When we pull out the dating system and really understand that the entire methodology for dating the Earth, the fossils, and even the universe itself is flawed, then we may, perhaps for the first time, appreciate the incredible mystery of Life. The Earth could have been here for trillions of years, millions of years, or a few thousand years — the truth is...nobody knows.

Raw "Evolutionary" Diets Don't Work In Practice

If humans are truly omnivorous, then, in the natural state (naked, with no tools or traps, and no fire), humans should be capable of, and enjoy, capturing and eating wild game and fish, worms and insects, eggs and honey. Such raw animal-food diets are promoted out there in the world. At the head office of Nature's First Law, those diets are called DUM (Dead Uncooked Meat). "Instinktive eating" is one such philosophy as promoted by a staunch evolutionist Frenchman named Guy Claude-Burger.

Eating raw animal flesh is better than cooked animal flesh *for a time* and people will feel better until the body begins to accumulate the unmitigated death energy (karma) of the animals, and then the trouble starts. I cringe when I receive e-mails from young people who are new to raw foods and have been convinced to eat raw animal flesh for strength and health. They have no idea of what they are getting into. I have seen people on raw animal-food diets over the long term and have seen lives destroyed by the negative energy of such foods. I have personally seen that eating raw-animal foods, especially as more than 5% of the diet, leads to major problems including: extreme anger, body odor, immobility, infertility, repeated illnesses, and rampant parasite infections.

Raw animal-food consumption seems to be associated with a poverty consciousness — a subconscious belief that lack and hardship is a law of life. Repeatedly thinking about demineralized food and deficiency is another facet of a poverty mentality. Thoughts of lack create lack. Thoughts of abundance create abundance! Feelings of fear along with thoughts of lack, deficiency, and doubt lead one to create a reality where those thoughts thrive — a raw animal-food diet.

A few people opt for raw-animal food because of food addiction and an unwillingness to detoxify. They want The Raw-Food Diet without detoxification, but do not understand that something for nothing disobeys the karmic law. They replace cooked-food stimulation with another kind — raw, dead-animal food. Eating raw flesh as food always leads to food obsession. I have seen this repeatedly. Typically, on the raw-animal diet, people become so unbalanced, confused, and filled with negative energy, they go back to cooked food (usually they have been eating it all along) to degrade the karmic energy of eating animal foods.

Those who stick with raw-animal foods long enough eventually break down. The case of Guy Claude-Burger's wife, Nicole, is instructive. From the Internet I downloaded the following:

"...there was a letter from Montrame which explained (their version) of the reasons and the course of events of Mrs. Burger's death. The letter explained that both Burgers acquired the habit of eating lots of meat during an experimental phase, after they and their friends discovered the beneficial effects of raw meats, particularly for people who suffered from cancers. After some time Mr. Burger developed one small cancer-like melanoma on his legs, which was removed by surgery. He stopped eating meat for some time, then. After some time, Mrs. Burger, who already was in menopause, did get her period again. The reason was cancer. But Mrs. Burger was addicted and couldn't break the habit of eating meat, she didn't believe in her husband's new theory that meat can also cause cancer. She ate it every day and after Orkos stopped delivering it to her, she ordered through other people.

One has to know, that she had lots of bad stress during that time. She worked a lot, regularly sleeping only 3 hours per day and her husband was in jail at that time, because of charges of working as a doctor without admission. (These were dropped much later). So Mrs. Burger became sicker and sicker and lost a lot of weight. And then she resorted to conventional medicine. She was treated with chemotherapy and artificial food for gaining weight, containing milk products. Probably caused by that she got pneumonia, from which she recovered when she started Instinkto again, but it was too late, she died some days later. This kind of addiction can happen with all kinds of natural foods, but especially easy with meat and other proteins..."

Eating a meat-based diet, especially a raw-meat diet, leads also to parasitic infections and a "parasite consciousness." I was once talking to a long-term raw-foodist on the phone and he had a most insightful observation. He said to me, "David...parasites rule the Earth. They have infected the entire population and are bending it towards ever more chaotic dietary patterns so that their consciousness may dominate the world."

The mythology of the "wonderfully healthy meat-eating Eskimo" has been shattered in the past twenty years. The Eskimos have the highest suicide rate of any ethnic group on Earth. Typically, they suffer from such severe teeth problems that the pain eventually drives them to suicide.

Raw fish is not a safe choice. I have repeatedly seen how raw-fish diets lead to parasite-worm infections and/or mercury poisoning. This is because animals accumulate and concentrate toxicity from the environment and few places on Earth are entirely devoid of pollution. It is especially true with fish, as they live in and constantly filter impure water leaving toxins in their tissues. Because toxicity is channeled to the liver of animals, fish liver oil is likely to contain large doses of poisons. We must keep in mind that, either we filter out what we are allowing into our bodies, or we ourselves will become a filter.

Recently, a long-time raw animal-food eater from Hawaii, who was eating up to 5 pounds (2.2 kilograms) of fish a week, discovered he had a mercury level of 16, where 1.5 is considered a dangerously high level. If you or someone you know has eaten large quantities of fish, raw or cooked, please consider testing for mercury.

The truth is that flesh-eating is a bad habit. We appeared on this planet as a raw eater with a specific food design. We are not designed to eat raw animal foods and that is why these diets lead to trouble.

Does biting into a raw fish with its slime, scales, and watching eye sound appetizing? Of course not. Does eating bugs out of a garden sound enticing? No way. No one has the propensity to go outside of their home at 3:00 am and chase a rabbit down, kill it, and chew it up with their teeth. *Raw animal foods cannot be eaten naturally and that is truly the final settlement on the issue.*

Conclusion

As I have demonstrated, radio-isotope dating is inaccurate, "smooth" transitions are riddled with irreconcilable gaps, natural selection cannot form a new species, the fossil record contradicts the darwinian theory, there are no missing links, etc. These truths indicate that the theory of evolution is flawed and predicated on wrong assumptions.

Along with evolution collapses the major philosophical basis for humanity's omnivorous and cooked-food diet. Are we supposed to understand the theory of evolution to know how to eat? Such a proposition is absurd on its face. Eating naturally is an intuitive knowledge, a natural propensity. Raw plant food stands as the obvious form of food for humans.

We arrived on this planet with a design to eat raw plant food and that is still our design now. This fact is proven by the extraordinary results, one will achieve following The Sunfood Diet program.

Action Steps:

1. For more information on the theory of evolution and diet, please read my booklet: **On Form And Actuality: A Refutation Of The Theory Of Evolution And Adaptation.**

Evolution: A Monkey's Perspective Revisited

One day the monkeys played
Amongst the trees,
When their fellow appeared
From a canopy of leaves.

"There is a rumor about,
Have you heard?
It's being touted
As the new holy word:

That humans are descended
From our noble tribe.
The arrogance of this
I can hardly describe.

Our joy and laughing,
Our natural bliss,
Is something the humans
Seem to totally miss.

Our zest for life,
Our radiant glow
Is this something
They can ever know?

They claim they've found
The secret design,
But the simple word: "species"
They cannot define.

Where are the transitions
The claims between form?
Nature is ever-changing
Yet stasis is the norm.

Guesses upon guesses
And the ages of rocks,
A blind watchmaker run
By atomic time clocks.

The theory is so boring
And mechanically untrue,
Science can't pollute the Earth
And understand it too!"

The monkey paused,
To stretch and yawn
Took a deep breath,
And continued on:

"Trust in faith and
Common sense
Have no place
In their science.

They don't understand
The reality they picture
Is but a reflection —
Of the thinker.

Divine and regal,
Is the grand-ancient world
The creation riddle
Cannot be unfurled.

Out there is a different place,
Older, greater, deeper by far
Than the twinkling of
The farthest star.

The harm to the Earth
Might be absolved,
But her mysteries
Will never be solved."

They chewed on fruits
In the soft, warm breeze.
As a waft of smoke
Caused a monkey to sneeze.

"Here they encroach
On our Paradise Found
They'll slash and burn this
Place — to the ground.

They don't think
Beyond the fringe
Of the tiny world
They're living in.

They cut then build
Another sharp fence,
When all they need is
Water, leaves... silence.

Materialist obsessions,
The Survival of the fit
Has turned the Earth
Into a fire pit.

And it becomes clear,
The deeper one delves...
That they've brought this
Misery, upon themselves.

Their race is declining
Into brutal passions,
Of which this theory
Is the latest of fashions.

The Earth is weary.
Of misdirection
This theory dies first
By natural selection."

Into the distance
The raindrops poured
Pattering the leaves
Between each word.

"Fancy theories,
Can never express,
The ancient dreams
Of this old forest.

Those splendid secrets
The poetry of facts.
Shouldn't lead them to worry
But simply relax."

The wise monkey grinned
As he declined some food
And all ears turned
To hear him conclude:

"Humans are something,
A different breed,
And compared to them
We have all we need.

You'll never see a monkey
Be hostile or rude,
You'll never catch a monkey
Cooking her food.

So to answer the charge
Of this latest fuss,
Tell them humans have descended alright
But they haven't descended from us."

Lesson 10:
Detoxification

"Know thou that the human soul is exalted above, and is
independent of all infirmities of body or mind. That a sick
person showeth signs of weakness is due to the hindrances
that interpose themselves between the soul and the body, for
the soul remaineth unaffected by any bodily ailments.
Consider the light of the lamp. Though an external object
may interfere with its radiance, the light itself continueth
to shine with undiminished power. In like manner, every
malady afflicting the human body is an impediment that
preventeth the soul from manifesting its inherent might and
power. When it leaveth the body, however, it will evince
such ascendancy, and reveal such influence as no force
on earth can equal. Every pure, every refined and
sanctified soul will be endowed with tremendous
power, and shall rejoice with exceeding gladness."
— Baha'u'llah, **Gleanings From The Writings Of Baha'u'llah**

"The constitution of man's body has not changed to meet
the new conditions of his artificial environment that has
replaced his natural one. The result is that of perpetual
discord between man and his environment. The effect of
this discord is a general deterioration of man's body,
the symptoms of which are termed disease."
— Professor Hilton Hotema, **Man's Higher Consciousness**

"Long-continued violation of the Laws of Being is the cause
of disease; long-continued perseverance in obedience is
the only means by which health can be recovered."
— Dr. Herbert Shelton, **Hygienic Review**

The Physiology Of Detoxification

In a world given to superstition, we must always get back to basic simple concepts.

Over a lifetime of eating cooked foods, the body gets "silted up." This silt consists of the residues of an improper breakdown of cooked food, the elements of which are spread throughout the body. These obstructions act as blockages in the electrical circuitry of the body.

Dr. C. Samuel West, chemist and lymphologist, in his amazing book **The Golden Seven Plus One** describes that the primary obstruction in the body of the typical person is protein trapped in the intercellular fluid between the cells. He discovered that: "If the blood proteins cannot be removed from the spaces around the cells by the lymphatic system, they can cause our death within just a few hours."

The whole process of detoxification consists of removing these obstructions from the lymph fluid (intercellular fluid) and washing them out of the body. As your body is lightened of obstructions, your health will rise accordingly.

Within a few hours of eating food, the quality of the blood is changed. Dr. Michael Klaper, in his video, **A Diet For All Reasons**, shows an example of thick, heavy blood drawn from a person on the standard cooked meat and pasteurized milk diet. Surgeons know that the blood is almost immediately thickened by eating heavy foods, making it dangerous to operate, that is one of the main reasons why they will only operate after the patient has fasted on water for at least 8 hours. Eating raw plant food thins the blood, as does fasting.

The average person has approximately 1.2 gallons (4.5 liters) of blood. But each person has four times as much lymph fluid as blood. Your lymph fluid bathes every cell. Because the blood feeds and draws waste from the lymph fluid directly, the process of detoxification begins as soon as the blood is thinner than the lymph fluid, allowing trapped toxicity in the lymph to diffuse back into the blood to be detoxified. The principle of diffusion states that things move from areas of greater concentration to areas of lesser concentration.

Clean and light foods allow the blood to become clean and light, which in turn allows the lymph to become clean and light. Over a period of years (at least three) on The Sunfood Diet, as the body is purified, it will change from a solid, rigid, weakened condition to a comparatively elastic, fluid, and energetic state. Yoga, exercise, and massage speed up this process by stimulating the circulation of blood and lymphatic fluid.

As the lymph unburdens itself of undigested proteins, toxins, chemicals, and other undesirables, the substances flow into the blood. Instantly a poison may be all over the circulatory system before it is filtered out as waste. This is why some may have sudden cold or hot flashes, fevers, diarrhea, rashes, desires for poor foods, tastes of old medicines, mucus discharges, and other symptoms, while detoxifying. These physical eliminations also carry with them emotional releases, such as anxiety, depression, and other imbalances. These are good signs, you want those poisonous substances and emotions out of your body. Don't worry about them, embrace them as part of the process. Other detoxification symptoms may include: bad breath, coughs, cold symptoms, drowsiness, headaches, momentary aches, nausea, unclear thinking, and/or weight loss.

While detoxifying, the body makes use of all its eliminative organs: the bowels, mouth, sinuses, skin, and kidneys, thus releases will occur in those areas. The urine, in general, is an excellent reflection of the blood; urine is purified blood. Turbidity in the urine is indicative of toxicity being released from the blood. Clear urine is a sign that the blood is clean at that moment.

Remember, as soon as anything cooked enters your mouth, detoxification stops immediately. Symptoms of detoxification will clear up almost instantly upon eating cooked food, as the blood is thickened and the lymph's waste elimination halted. If you feel you are detoxifying too rapidly, you may want to introduce heavier foods to slow the detox process down. Eating lightly cooked foods or steamed vegetables will slow detoxification. Eating more young coconut, avocados, nuts, and seeds with green-leafed vegetables will thicken the blood to a degree that slows detoxification; this will allow you to remain on the raw diet, but also to comfortably detoxify.

During detoxification, blood pressure may increase as thick, soupy materials pass out of the lymph into the blood. This will pass over time on a natural diet as the lymph and blood unburden themselves and normalize. An elevated blood pressure is caused by obstructions in the blood vessels (cooked fat, cooked protein, chemicals), an increased thickness of the blood, and/or a constriction of the arteries due to stress, all of which cause the heart to work harder to push blood through the vessels. Nutritionally, the blood pressure can be quickly decreased by adding garlic bulbs and onions into the diet. These foods help thin the blood so as to lower blood pressure.

Healing Through Detoxification

The major diseases and illnesses are diet related. Detoxification through a raw plant-food diet is the physical path back to perfect health. If diet is ignored, the maximum benefit of other therapies will not be achieved.

There is no magic pill, but there is a magic process. For you, detoxification can be the greatest event of your life. As you become more aware of your body's true condition, you will intuitively be presented with intelligent plans, renewed strength, and energy with which to retrace the steps back to physical perfection. You will be healed naturally through detoxification.

Hering's Law describes that all diseases retrace their history during the healing process. Specifically, the following pattern occurs:
1. Healing begins deep within and works its way out.
2. Healing occurs from the head down.
3. Symptoms occur in the reverse order from the way they developed.

The process of detoxification is non-linear. It travels in circles and waves and heals you in cycles according to Hering's Law. Depending on your previous diet, you may feel worse before you feel better, as toxicity is washed out of the body. If one is coming from the Standard American Diet (SAD), a powerful detoxification may occur. If one is more purified on a vegetarian or vegan diet and eating organic food, the detoxification may be more mild.

Just as it takes years for your tissues to become encumbered by improper materials, so too does it take years to dissolve and eliminate these improper materials. In general, I have found that it takes one month on a 100% Sunfood Diet to reverse one year on a cooked, toxic diet. So, for example, if one is 45 years young, then it will take 45 months to detoxify the body on a 100% Sunfood Diet.

Every living organism strives always to remove obstructions and achieve perfect health. When you start removing obstructions from your body, radiant health appears. Obstructions are the residues left over from a lifetime of improper foods and negative thoughts. Illnesses are caused by obstructions. Symptoms are caused by the body's attempt to detoxify obstructions. Death is caused by a suppression of detoxification.

Detoxification is a skill. This is an "unwinding" process — seek the best way to unwind yourself out of the old habits. Nurture yourself through this process.

When I began to study the psychology and science of physical detoxification, I used myself and my situation as the test of what was true. You must do the same. Listen to your inner voice.

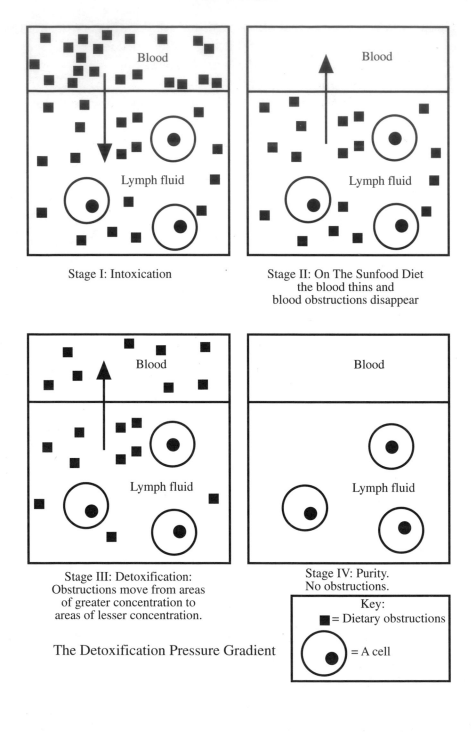

Stage I: Intoxication

Stage II: On The Sunfood Diet
the blood thins and
blood obstructions disappear

Stage III: Detoxification:
Obstructions move from areas
of greater concentration to
areas of lesser concentration.

Stage IV: Purity.
No obstructions.

The Detoxification Pressure Gradient

Key:
■ = Dietary obstructions
⬤ = A cell

Diffusion Pressure

Success philosopher and author, Og Mandino, used to say that, "you are not a human being, you are a human becoming." You are constantly becoming something different. Remember, the human body is constantly recreating itself out of the air, water, food, and thoughts you ingest. Studies show 98% of the atoms in the body are completely replaced in two years. In seven years, 100% of the body is replaced. In just a few years you can completely reconstruct your entire body from totally brand new high-quality materials! It is never too late for anyone. You can regenerate!

The body is a self-sustaining, wonderfully regenerating organism which wears out due to high levels of toxicity. This toxicity comes through diet, negative thinking, and disempowering belief systems. Detoxification ("letting go") at all levels heals all things.

The Mucous Lining

Your entire digestive tract and breathing apparatus is lined with a very sensitive, naturally transparent membrane. This mucous lining becomes irritated on a diet of cooked foods. An irritation of the delicate lining causes sensitivities or allergies.

The mucous membrane is always trying to diffuse impacted mucus and cooked-food residue up from the colon, intestines, and stomach to the less impacted areas of the digestive tract, such as the throat, mouth (tongue), and sinuses, through the simple process of diffusion (the movement of particles from an area of greater concentration to an area of lesser concentration). This is why Professor Ehret called the tongue the "magic mirror" because as soon as the body has a chance to diffuse toxins out of the lower digestive organs (through fasting or sleeping) it will do so and mucus will migrate up through the stomach lining, esophagus lining, and into the mouth. The tongue will become coated, the breath will turn foul. The coating on the tongue, then, becomes a key indicator as to how much constipated mucus has accumulated in the digestive organs.

Constipated mucoid plaque in the colon is the product of decades of eating improper foods. To achieve excellent health, mucoid plaque has to be flushed out of the colon through raw foods, colonics, and fasting. Even if bowel movements are regular everyday, mucoid plaque can still be present, clinging to the colon walls, and should be addressed.

Mucoid plaque also builds up from incomplete bowel movements caused by not fully squatting while eliminating. Sitting on the standard toilet pinches the colon, hindering complete elimination. Consider squatting on the toilet, or purchasing a small foot-stool which raises the knees into more of a squatting position when sitting on the toilet.

Parasites

By far the greatest variety of parasites afflicting the present population of the Western world comes from animal foods. Almost every variety of commercial meat available is loaded with parasitic worms. Also, parasites are present in tainted water sources. Parasites thrive in an unhealthy body. They feed on excessive toxicity (constipation) in the colon, particularly cooked starch and decaying cooked animal foods. In that way they are somewhat beneficial; they help detoxify the colon by breaking down substances the body cannot deal with into waste the body can eliminate. However, when the body becomes so weakened from a toxic lifestyle that the parasites breach the digestive tract and enter the internal organs of the body, major problems arise. Liver flukes, pancreatic flukes, eggs in the brain tissue, eggs in the liver (occasionally mistaken as liver cancer), etc., all have their role in the manifestation of the major diseases.

The way to eliminate parasites is to stop taking in animal products of all kinds. Only pure or distilled water should be introduced into the body. Adopting The Sunfood Diet along with special care to send "hot" foods through the digestive tract regularly such as: garlic, onions, hot peppers, ginger, etc. will eliminate parasites. These foods may be mixed in juices (see **Appendix C: Sunfood Recipes** under **Molotov Cocktail**), or eaten whole with raw plant fats, such as walnuts. Black walnut hulls have been used as a treatment for ringworms for thousands of years. Colon hydrotherapy will also help flush parasites out of the system. I have worked with people who have passed worms in excess of 1 foot (0.3

meters) in length, and upon passing them, they experienced a subsidence of disease symptoms.

When freshly picked, raw plant foods have excellent microbes and bacteria for our digestive tract. They do not typically have harmful parasites on them, unless picked near contaminated water sources, or grown in soil saturated with toxic fecal matter.

Colon Hydrotherapy

Colon hydrotherapy speeds up detoxification. It allows a great amount of toxicity to be flushed out quickly, so we can continue with our daily lives without enduring extreme detoxification symptoms. I recommend beginning The Sunfood Diet and/or any healing regime with a series of colonics. Colon hydrotherapy is simple, painless, and discreet.

Trips to the colon hydrotherapist may replace trips to the doctor. The habit of regularly visiting a colon hydrotherapist will extend your life and increase your health. The raw-foodist Dr. Norman Walker had two series of 6 colon cleanses done every year of the second half of his life...he lived to be at least 109 (some say older). I've found that one colonic every 4-6 months has been effective for me. At the initial stages, I would recommend a series of 4 to 6 sessions even if you feel like you do not need it.

The primary goal of colon hydrotherapy is to remove encrusted mucus (which feeds parasites and poisons the system) from the colon wall. The secondary goal is to allow the liver to flush and release. The first time I ever had a colonic done, at the very end of the session, my liver released a yellow fluid (a standard colon hydrotherapy machine displays a clear tube which allows one to see exactly what is being eliminated from the colon). I felt a jump in vitality immediately. I later intuitively concluded that what was released was beer residue of some type, because I could never drink a beer again after that moment.

Colon hydrotherapy is a way to keep our colon mechanically operating properly, it is not a crutch to help us eliminate. Good elimination comes from eating a healthy raw-food diet rich in green leaves and fruit.

The growth of healthy bacterial flora can be assisted in the colon by eating raw foods, especially unwashed garden plants, wild plants, and/or fermented foods. A probiotic (a culture of beneficial bacteria) in powder or liquid form and a supplement of soil-based organisms will work more effectively to restore harmonious digestive conditions and reverse problems with an overgrowth of harmful bacteria. The best combination of probiotics and soil organisms in a matrix of raw-alkaline nutritionally-packed superfoods can be found in a product designed to my specifications by HealthForce founder, Jamey Dina, N.D., called **Nature's First Food** (please see the **Resources** section at the end of this book or call 888-RAW-FOOD for more information about this product).

Aside from colon hydrotherapy, you may also speed up the detoxification process by doing enemas coupled with fasting on lemon-water or green-leafy vegetable juice.

You alkalinize your blood by taking in green-leafy vegetable juices, which increase the blood's electricity. Electricity increases the solubility of the blood. The more solubility in the blood, the more undigested and misappropriated minerals it can suspend, remove, and metabolize or eliminate. Chlorophyll and the alkaline compounds in green-leafy vegetables can combine with heavy metals and foreign chemicals in the body to form salts which will allow the body to wash them out. I have coached and worked with many people who have overcome mercury and chemical poisoning by eating raw plants foods, especially green-vegetable juice.

Liver

Even if the diet is toxic and deficient, if the liver is still functioning at a high rate, the body will compensate for deficiencies through biological transmutation. Louis Kervran, in his fascinating book, **Biological Transmutations**, demonstrates that living organisms have a limited ability to transmutate one element into another alchemically. That is, they can convert organic silica into calcium, or magnesium into calcium, or sodium into potassium, or manganese into iron, etc. Biological transmutations most often occur in the green leaves and roots of plants. In the human body, such transmutations occur in the liver and intestinal flora. It is extremely important to keep the liver functioning at an optimal level. If the liver function drops below a specific level, biological transmutation stops, and one's health is compromised.

One of the main goals of detoxification is to get the liver clean. The liver can completely rejuvenate itself even if only 10% functional. Fasting on juice or water can help the liver deal with an overload. Milk thistle seeds eaten whole and raw have been scientifically shown to accelerate healing in the liver. Dandelion and its juice are also beneficial for the liver.

One of the best ways I have discovered to increase liver function quickly is to do the following flush:

Gall Bladder Flush

The gall bladder flush:
1. Fast 3 days on raw fresh apple juice (preferably made from sour green apples).
2. On Day 3, in the evening, suck on 5-7 cassia discs. Cassia is a wild pod-fruit possessing powerful laxative qualities (contact Nature's First Law at 888-RAW-FOOD to have cassia delivered to you).
3. At 3:00 pm on Day 4, at least two hours after your last drink, break the fast with 8 ounces (0.25 liters) of organic stone-crushed and cold-pressed olive oil drank straight.
4. Follow with 8 ounces (0.25 liters) of freshly squeezed lemon juice.
5. Rest the remainder of the day. Lie down on your right side. Stay warm. Place a castor pack on your abdomen over your liver.
6. During the evening of Day 4, suck on 5-7 cassia discs.

This will flush "gravel" out of the gall bladder and bile ducts which will be pushed out in the stool (usually on the morning of Day 5). The "stones" will be ovoid in shape and may range in size from smaller than a bell pepper seed to as large as a brazil nut. True stones consist of foreign cholesterol and starch (some stones may simply be saponified oil). Most people on a toxic diet have anywhere from 300-1500 "stones" of various sizes in their gall bladder and bile ducts. This flush dramatically increases liver function and bile flow as the bile ducts are a waste release area for the liver. Once cleared, the liver can detoxify itself and excrete its waste properly. Also, digestion will be enhanced.

The Two Selves

In his wonderful book, **The Master Key To Riches**, Napoleon Hill describes that every human being has two sides, two separate entities, two counterparts which become operative at birth. One is a negative sort of person who thinks and moves and lives in an atmosphere of doubt, fear, poverty, and ill health. This negative self expects failure and is seldom disappointed. It dwells on poverty, greed, superstition, fear, doubt worry, and physical sickness. The "other self" is a positive sort of person who thinks in dynamic, affirmative terms of wealth, sound health, love and friendship, personal achievement, creative vision, service to others, and who guides one unerringly to the attainment of those blessings.

I wonder if Napoleon Hill ever realized that these two mental selves have their physical equivalent? They have their physical basis in the foods we eat.

The average diet today consists of large amounts of animals (meat) and/or seeds (grains or rice), both of which are high in phosphorus and other acid-forming minerals. An overabundance of acid-forming minerals eventually causes an acid condition throughout the body, contributing to anxiety, edginess, irritability, and worry — all these are emotions associated with the "negative self."

Cooked animals and seeds leave residues behind which are difficult for the body to metabolize and detoxify. By eliminating these cooked foods, and increasing your intake of green-leafed vegetables and alkaline fruits (figs, oranges, papayas, etc.), you eliminate the physical basis for the "negative self."

After you detoxify your body; when you become a raw-foodist; when at last you reach the point of maximum weight loss; when your body has emptied itself of all toxins...that is when your outward appearance will alter. You will literally push out your old persona (your false body) and, as it is purged, you will momentarily take on that appearance. Some have called it: "the alternating faces of detoxification." It is one of the most stunning revelations one can experience. After that you will be a transformed person.

Rejuvenation

Then the body rebuilds. Your appearance will undergo a radical transformation. Your hair will be thicker and wilder. Facial lines may fade or even disappear. A chalky complexion will dissipate. The bone structure of your face may alter. You will be filled with a youthful vigor. You may appear younger and have people comment on this. You will radiate health and vitality. This entire change of your physiology will stand as proof that extraordinary transformations are possible.

When you begin eating only raw plant foods, when you start to delve deeply back into the plants and animals in Nature far away from civilization, you will see there are no longer familiar features in the world. Everything is new. Everything has never happened before. The world reveals itself and it is incredible.

Your own detoxification process will allow you to take on a wider vision of yourself and your potential.

When you cleanse yourself inside, you will surely find the outside cleansed and made perfect. You will unfold as if from a dull green bud into a brilliant flower. Imagine a neglected houseplant with brown leaves. If one changes the soil, provides it with the right lighting and water, sends positive energy to it, then it will dramatically change. So too, will an unhealthy person be changed into a healthy person through detoxification.

As you lighten the body of obstructions, a joy shall usher forth, such as you have never experienced in your life. You *will* laugh for no reason.

When one radiates health and vitality, one no longer draws on the vitality of other humans, animals, and plants. This is due to one's increased energy which diffuses from areas of greater concentration to areas of lesser concentration. As energy diffuses, it also creates a magnetism which manifests itself, in the form of charisma. A clean body is charismatic.

Action Steps:

1. Ask yourself the following question: How can I celebrate my life and enjoy the process of detoxification, while letting go of toxicity? As soon as your mind comes with the answer, write it down in your journal, and act on it immediately.

2. Decide in advance how you will deal with detoxification symptoms. Decide what level of detoxification will be too much for you to handle. Decide now what foods you will use to slow down the detoxification process. Write down your strategy in your journal.

3. In times of a healing crisis, maintain your poise, reread this lesson, and fully understand the physiology of detoxification.

4. Read Dr. Norman Walker's book: **Colon Health: The Key To A Vibrant Life.**

5. Call and set up a colon hydrotherapy appointment today. Check for listings in your local phone book or natural-food store.

Instant Transformation

What if your life was suddenly changed?
How would you feel if your destiny was one day — exchanged?

How long does each moment last?
How would your life be if you rewrote your past?

Could life be more than it seems?
What if you become something more — on the way to your dreams?

Can you undo the things you've done?
Just how and when is a new life begun?

Are such transformations true?
What if you awoke and everything was new?

What would you do or say?
What if your moment of transformation happened — today?

Lesson 11:
The Secret Revealed

Now that we know we should be eating a diet rich in raw plant foods: What do we do? How do we do it? How do we make the transition? How do we stay balanced? These questions and others will be answered in this and following lessons.

Since my partners and I founded Nature's First Law in April 1995, I have become one of the world's foremost promoters of The Raw-Food Diet. I have spoken to thousands of interested people on the telephone, at seminars, via e-mail, on radio, on television, and during one-on-one consultations. I have coached people over many years of eating raw plant foods. My company distributes nearly every book ever written on raw-food vegetarian diets. Doing this type of work has brought me into contact with many people in North America, Europe, and other parts of the globe, who have been successful with The Raw-Food Diet in the long-term. I do not know of another person who has communicated with as many successful 100% raw-foodists as I have. I know where people have gone right with raw-vegetarian diets, and I know where they have gone wrong.

Knowledge, we know, rests not upon truth alone, but also upon the understanding of error. Genesis 1:29 tells us to eat "herbs and fruits" but it does not tell us how much of each or which ones! I know where the gaps are in the knowledge; this book is designed to fill those gaps.

From studying both the successful and unsuccessful I have deduced a startling pattern which I have seen in every single person who is successful with a raw-vegetarian diet in the long-term. To me discovering this pattern was a revelation; it was like the Sun bursting through after 40 days of clouds and rain. This distinction improved my understanding of nutrition tremendously and tuned me up to an incredible level of health.

I discovered there are three essentials to The Raw-Food Diet (actually to any diet) or imbalances will occur. One can eat other foods, but these three elements must be there to achieve harmony. In every single long-term 100% raw-foodist I have encountered, I discovered the following dietary pattern:

1. Green-leafy vegetables
2. Sweet fruits
3. Fatty foods

If one of these food classes is missing in the diet for a significant period of time (ranging from a few weeks to several months), imbalances will occur. In fact, I have never discovered any raw-foodist to have gone more than 2 years with one of these food classes missing.

Every 100% raw-foodist who follows this pattern, whom I have met, has attained an extraordinary level of health and clarity. As raw-foodists tend to be more in tune with their diet and how it influences each facet of health, and also tend to experiment more with the effects of raw foods on the body, we may conclude that the collective wisdom which has attracted long-term raw-foodists into this dietary pattern brings forth a powerful insight for us all.

I have found this insight of the three food classes to be extremely insightful and useful in assisting thousands of people to improve and balance their diet, no matter what kind of diet they were following. I have found, even with people on standard diets, that if one of these three food classes is eaten in small quantities or is entirely missing in the diet, imbalances will occur within 2 years, and often much sooner.

Anyone who makes 80% or more of their diet consist of green-leafy vegetables, sweet fruits, and fatty foods (from raw plant sources) will begin to achieve a startling level of health.

These three food classes balance against each other in the Sunfood Triangle outlined below:

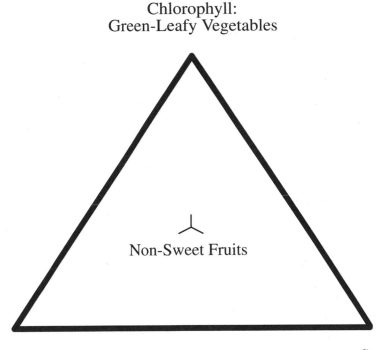

Chlorophyll:
Green-Leafy Vegetables

Non-Sweet Fruits

Fats:
Fatty Fruits, Nuts
Coconuts, Seeds

Sugars:
Sweet Fruits

The Sunfood Triangle

This is how it works: if one eats green-leafed vegetables, for example, then sweet fruits and fatty foods must be eaten in the same day to balance the body. If the green-leafed vegetables one is eating are very stimulating (i.e. kale), then stronger sweet fruits and fatty foods can be eaten to balance. If one is eating green-leafed vegetables that are not very stimulating (i.e. butterleaf lettuce), then less stimulating sweet fruits and fatty foods are all that is needed to balance.

Another example: If one eats avocados (a strong fat), then deeper green-leaves, along with stronger types of sweet fruits, may be eaten in the same day to balance.

Another example: If one eats bananas (a strong sugar), then heavier fats, such as nuts (which go well with bananas), may be eaten along with dark green-leafed vegetables in the same day.

Another example: If one eats cucumbers (a non-sweet fruit), then that individual will remain centered as non-sweet fruits are low in stimulation and are located at the center of The Sunfood Triangle.

For optimal results, all three food classes should be eaten each day (unless one is doing a fast or cleanse of some type). All three can be eaten at each meal, or two can be eaten at one meal, with a third eaten later, or all eaten separately throughout the day. Find out what works best for you and your digestion.

I have found that sweet fruits as the dominant food in the morning, green-leafed vegetables as the dominant food at lunch, and fats as the dominant food in the evening works rather well.

We must keep in mind that each body has its own biochemical individuality and the exact ratios of green foods (protein), sugar (carbohydrates), and fat differs from person to person. Through insights I have gained by working with Dr. Gabriel Cousens, I now help design exact diets for people by consultation. However, you can design your own diet, by following your intuition. A good place to start, unless one is going for a desired effect (see **Lesson 14: How To Use The Sunfood Triangle**), is to: eat 33.3% green-leafed vegetables, 33.3% fatty plant food, and 33.3% sweet fruits by dry weight (total food weight minus water). This puts one at the exact center of the triangle. For example:

<u>Daily Menu Item</u>:   <u>Dry Weight</u>:

Fats
0.33 lb. (0.23 kg) macadamia nuts (18% water) = 0.27 lb. (0.1 kg)
1 lb. (0.45 kg) avocados (75% water) = 0.25 lb. (0.14 kg)
Sugar
1.5 lbs. (0.68 kg) apples (84% water) = 0.24 lb. (0.11 kg)
2.5 lbs. (1.13 kg) oranges (87% water) = 0.26 lb. (0.12 kg)
Chlorophyll
1 lb. (0.45 kg) kale (65% water) = 0.35 lb. (0.16 kg)
2 lbs. (0.9 kg) lettuce (93% water) = 0.13 lb. (0.06 kg)
Non-Sweet fruits
1 lb. (0.45 kg) cucumbers = Not applicable
0.5 lb. (0.23 kg) tomatoes = Not applicable

From this example we can see how balanced this daily diet would be. All the dry weights balance out: fats at 0.52 lb. (0.24 kg), sugars at 0.50 lb. (0.23 kg), and chlorophyll at 0.48 lb. (0.22 kg).

If you would like to work out this type of analysis for certain meals, I have provided the following chart.

Chart: Water Content Of Fruits, Vegetables, And Nuts

<u>Food</u>:   <u>Water Content</u>:

Fruit:

Food	Water Content
Apples	84%
Apricots	87%
Avocados	75%
Bell Peppers	93%
Blackberries	82%
Cantaloupe	93%
Cherries	82%
Cucumbers	96%

Dates (fresh)	55%
Figs	79%
Grapes	79%
Grapefruits	91%
Honeydew Melon	94%
Huckleberries	78%
Lemons	85%
Lychees	82%
Mangos	83%
Mulberries	85%
Nectarines	80%
Okra	90%
Olives (Sun-ripened)	70%
Oranges	84%
Pears	83%
Persimmons (soft)	80%
Plums	84%
Prickly Pear	79%
Prunes (dried)	35%
Raspberries	83%
Strawberries	89%
Tangerines	87%
Tomatoes	94%
Watermelons	94%

Vegetables:

Asparagus	93%
Bok Choy	87%
Celery	93%
Endive	94%
Garlic Root	64%
Green Cabbage	90%
Kale	65%
Lettuce	94%
Onion Root	87%
Parsley	79%
Watercress	91%

Nuts & Seeds (unsoaked):

Almonds	26%
Brazil Nuts	15%
Coconut (young)	64%
Coconut (mature)	35%
Coconut water	92%
Macadamias	18%
Pine Nuts	15%
Sunflower Seeds	15%
Walnuts	25%

(Sources: Paul, A.A., Southgate, D.A.T., **McCance And Widdowson's The Composition Of Foods**, 4th Revised Edition, London: Her Majesty's Stationary Office, 1978; and various other references.)

Now I do not recommend that you break down every single daily menu as I have here to determine whether you are balancing chlorophyll, sugar, and fats properly! This example is simply to identify two simple relationships:

1. A small portion of nuts and seeds balances against a large portion of fruits and vegetables, because nuts and seeds are low-water content foods. (If nuts are freshly picked, or soaked in water, they can be eaten in larger portions, as they will have about twice the water content as is listed in the chart above.)

2. Green-leafed vegetables need to be eaten in significant quantities as they are actually high-water content foods.

The best path is always the simplest path. Balance the three classes in the easiest way possible, by intuition. If you feel low in greens, eat more. If you feel low in fat, eat more. If you feel you have overdone sugar, eat more fats and greens to balance. Just by knowing that these three classes are the essentials, you will have the tools to stay in balance.

Understand that if the quantities of one class are too low, one can go longer than a day, even for many days or weeks or months without requiring much of that food class — but eventually it will catch up. This helps us understand cravings. If one goes without sugar for several weeks, the desire can become great, and the body will grab for sugar however it can get it, raw (fruit) or even cooked (candy or cake). The same holds true for fat. If the body is deficient in fat, the craving will become overwhelming and one will grab for it, raw (avocados or nuts) or even cooked/pasteurized (cheese or ice cream).

Imbalances are caused by an excessive food stimulation away from the center of The Sunfood Triangle. Deficiencies can be caused by an excessive sugar stimulation which runs minerals out of the body. Frugal eating or fasting actually corrects deficiencies because it centers one on The Sunfood Triangle.

The fear of fruit (too much sugar), the fear of vegetables (too bitter), and the fear of fatty foods (too fattening) leaves one confused and with dietary health challenges. Motivational speaker Anthony Robbins provides a good metaphor for FEAR: False Evidence that Appears Real. Remember my earlier advice: Stop listening to anyone in any field who is not getting the results that you desire. By reading this lesson you have made the decision to dismiss any fears of fruits, green-leafed vegetables, or fats.

Chlorophyll, sugar, and fat are the three classes of foods which comprise humanity's natural dietary character. The eater of sweet fruits becomes a Sun-worshipping, zesty, clean type. Those who eat green vegetation take on the stoic calmness of that food class. The eater of plant fats becomes a stolid, beautiful being.

Chlorophyll

"If you're green on the inside, you're clean on the inside."
— Dr. Bernard Jensen

Green is good. Green is the very center of the rainbow. Green is centering.

Eat green-leafy vegetables for strength. Green leaves are transformed into the structure of the body.

Whether it is green herbs or big leafy vegetables, such as kale, green leaves must be a significant part of the diet. Green-leafy vegetables are our best and most reliable source of fiber.

Herbs have become quite popular in recent times. Green-leafed vegetables (lettuce, celery, parsley, cilantro, etc.) are truly herbs, but are so common, they are often overlooked for their healing and rejuvenating properties.

Chlorophyll is the pigment in plants within which photosynthesis takes place. Chlorophyll absorbs the vibrant Sun energy and transforms it into plant energy. This energy is transferred directly to you when you eat chlorophyll-rich foods, such as green-leafed vegetables.

Chlorophyll is the blood of plants, just as hemoglobin is the blood of the body; the only difference between the two molecules is that chlorophyll is centered on magnesium, while hemoglobin is centered on iron. Eating green-leafy food is a transfusion of Sun energy to blood energy in the arteries.

Green-leafed vegetables are overall the best source of iron; parsley and spinach are particularly high in iron. Greens heal anemia. (Other sources of iron include red-colored fruits, such as watermelon, berries, pomegranate, and red-flesh figs).

Green-leafed vegetables often do not taste as wonderful as fruits. But eating them nonetheless breaks associations of pleasure with eating, therefore decreasing the possibility of overeating. Green-leafed vegetables diminish the enjoyment in eating and act as a natural stop for us in the eating cycle.

Where does the cow get its calcium for its milk? From green grass of course. Now we are not grass eaters, but this analogy is instructive because it demonstrates that all the minerals a cow is constructed from are present in grass — in simple green grass!

Green-leafed vegetables are always the best source of heavy minerals: calcium, magnesium, etc. The alkaline minerals in greens balance the acid-forming minerals (sulfur, chlorine, and phosphorus) found in avocados, nuts, seeds, onions, garlic, etc.

Green-leafy vegetation is also an excellent detoxifier of the liver, especially wild green vegetation. Deep green and wild green vegetation binds with heavy metals and chemicals from recreational drugs and allows the body to wash them out as salts through the urine.

If green-leafed vegetables, which are high in oxalic acid, such as beet greens, chard, lamb's quarters, rhubarb, and/or spinach are cooked, then the heat-altered oxalic acid can combine with calcium in the body, interfere with iron absorption, and eventually (if eaten in large quantities over a long period of time) form stones in the kidneys. If eaten raw, the oxalates in these vegetables are normally metabolized properly by the body. If one feels kidney pains 3-6 hours after eating these vegetables (even if in the raw state), then they should be avoided.

Alkaloids

Alkaloids are bitter organic compounds which are derived from plants bearing seed. Aspirin, caffeine, cannabinoids (THC, THCV, CBD, CBC), cocaine, morphine, nicotine, etc. are all alkaloids. Alkaloids provide the heating quality in hot peppers. Peyote contains the most powerful alkaloids in the world. Drugs such as ecstasy, in their original plant derivation (from sassafras and nutmeg), contain alkaloids as their active agents.

Joshua Rainbow, a fruitarian activist, has described in his booklet **Biotrophic Protocol** that when alkaloids are introduced into a body with an acidic biochemistry, they neutralize the acid and eliminate acid-induced pain. Alkaloids create a high for a time as acids are neutralized and the blood is alkalized. The alkalizing of the blood tunes one into the human body's natural frequency and insights begin to be drawn in from infinite intelligence — that is until the body's acid-biochemistry begins reasserting itself mostly through the desire for acid-forming foods which "acid-up" the blood and diminish the alkaloid high. The insights diminish as one is tuned back into the static.

We can see from the effects of alkaloids on the body, why drugs, coffee, and the smoking of marijuana and tobacco, etc. are so popular. The typical body, acidified by a cooked animal-food diet, is actually alkalized or balanced by the alkaloids of these substances and achieves glimpses of higher consciousness.

By eating significantly more green-leafy vegetables, especially wild herbs, one will alkalize the body chemistry and be able to tap into the natural human frequency more easily and more often, without drugs and their side-effects. (Joshua Rainbow believed this could be done with fruits also, but fruits do not contain enough alkaline elements to produce the effect.) Placing green leaves in an acid body raises the consciousness as the body becomes more alkaline.

One can overcome coffee addictions (coffee is a cooked beverage as it is made by passing hot water through ground-up roasted seeds [beans] from the coffee fruit) by drinking fresh green-vegetable juice in the morning instead of coffee. This will stimulate an excellent bowel movement and give the body the alkaloid stimulation it desires.

I know some raw-foodists who smoke marijuana regularly. Even if all-raw, the habit of typically overeating sugar and fat and undereating green-leafed vegetables leads to a slightly acid and constricted body chemistry — leaving one tuned-out, just a bit. This condition is alleviated by smoking marijuana, hence the desire. The alkaloids in the marijuana smoke neutralize the acid condition, relax the body, and tune one into a higher knowledge. But smoking marijuana actually perpetuates the same biochemistry which created the desire for alkalinity (alkaloids) because smoking marijuana interferes with the ability of the blood to carry sugar.

The more you smoke, the more sugar the body desires. Also, the higher you go, the more acid-forming foods the body asks for (avocados, nuts, and seeds) to bring you down. This cycle is broken by eating significantly more green-leafed vegetables and wild herbs which alkalize the body, loosen the tissues, and open the mind.

To overcome the desire for cooked alkaloids, one should replace them by eating them raw and/or by eating more green-leafed vegetables and wild herbs. Raw green leaves have the same effect as alkaloid substances, however, their high lasts much longer. By repeatedly introducing significant amounts of green-leafed vegetables and wild herbs we raise the alkalinity of the body and loosen the constriction of body tissues.

Green leaves soothe the nerves and calm the body. Those with chronic back and muscle pains should be sure to eat plenty of green vegetables. Green leaves relieve pain. Green-leafy foods decrease the overall stress of the body and facilitate yoga practices. For those raw-foodists practicing yoga: eat more greens for better flexibility.

Consider that the number one cause of death in the western world is heart disease. The heart chakra is green. An abundance of green in the diet strengthens the heart.

Sprouts

In my classification, there are two different types of sprouts: seed/legume sprouts and green sprouts.

Seed/legume sprouts fall into the first stage of sprouting; these types of sprouts are protein-dominant foods. As the plant matures, it begins to form green leaves of one type or another; it has then become a green sprout and falls into the green-leafy vegetable category. So, for example, sprouted wheat is a seed sprout, but as it grows its green blades, and turns into wheatgrass, it becomes a green sprout.

Seed/legume sprouts include: sprouted sunflower seeds, sprouted wheat, quinoa sprouts, mung bean sprouts, lentil sprouts, pea sprouts, soaked peanuts, sprouted rice, etc. Seed sprouts are *not* essential in the diet. However, if they are eaten occasionally, they can be beneficial because high-quality seeds contain many trace minerals. Also, seed sprouts are therapeutic in the transition from cooked to raw food as they are very high in enzymes and help reverse and enzyme deficiency situation. If overeaten, seed sprouts will cause digestive distress.

Green sprouts include: wheatgrass, clover, sunflower greens, barley, radish sprouts, pea shoots, etc. Green sprouts are not as powerful as big green-leafy vegetables such as kale or collards, but they fit into the category of essential chlorophyll foods. Sunflower greens are the best sprouts of all; they are the "softest" and most nourishing for the body. Wheatgrass often comes from weak hybridized seed strains; quality counts and one should seek out the best quality seed stock available. Other grass seeds tend to be of a higher quality (kamut, rye, barley) than wheatgrass. Grass juice is an excellent transition and detoxification food (especially for overcoming heavy metal poisoning). Grass juice may be too harsh on a purified body and many long-term raw-foodists (5+ years) whom I have met rarely drink such juices.

Sugar

Eat natural sugar foods for intelligence. Cognition is dependent on blood sugar.

Our brains run exclusively on oxygen and glucose (or fruit sugar). That ought to give us a clue as to what our natural fuel is. Glucose is the fuel of our being.

The more (mentally and physically) active you are, the more fuel (sugar) you require. The less (mentally and physically) active you are, the less fuel (sugar) you require.

Sugar is the fuel of the human body, but it must be taken in the correct form. *Sugar in the diet should come from one primary source: sweet fruits with seeds.*

Refined and processed sugars (e.g. high fructose corn syrup, table sugar, brown sugar) are drugs. Natural sugars are also drugs when taken in excessively through hybridized foods. Refined and hybrid sugar slips past the liver like a slipping gear. The liver tries to recognize the sugar, but for the most part, it is unidentifiable and slippage occurs as unprocessed sugar enters the blood rapidly, causing a "high," or sugar rush which has been described by many people addicted to refined sugar or even by people hooked on carrot juice.

Obviously, refined and processed sugars should be released from the diet. But even amongst certain raw foods, there are some sugars that should be avoided. I definitely recommend against the prolonged daily intake of carrot or beet juice. Both carrots and beets are extremely hybridized foods. They may heal one to a certain degree (because they are raw plant foods), but once you reach a certain level of purity, the body begins to react to the sugar. I have seen many people on carrot juice cures begin to become unbalanced as they progressed in their cleansing. If used to sweeten juices, please do not use more than one carrot or one beet per 1 quart (1 liter) of juice. You are better off using apple or pear to sweeten vegetable juices. Cucumber softens the bitterness of vegetables and is an excellent base for vegetable juices.

I also recommend against seedless fruits such as: bananas, seedless grapes, seedless oranges, pineapple, seedless watermelon, etc. These foods, are genetically altered, artificial, and loaded with hybrid sugar (however, if these foods have their seeds they are okay). A more detailed discussion of hybrid foods will follow in **Lesson 16: Hybrid Food**.

Hybrid sugar, like refined sugar, can overstimulate the endocrine system, unless it is mitigated with fats and green-leafed vegetables, to "lessen the shock." The glands sense the body is loaded with food, but hybrid foods (especially commercial fruits and root vegetables) are fairly empty of trace nutrients and the body signals more hunger, which leads to an overeating of hybrid sweet fruit (seedless fruit). This overeating can be stopped by eating high-quality green-leafy vegetables, which have the trace elements.

A diet heavy in hybridized sweet fruit can lead to constipation, especially if the individual is not highly active. Because excess sugar spills off into the urine, excessive urination can occur when the sugar is not being immediately utilized (due to a lack of activity). Excessive urination leads to dehydration and a potassium overdose, behind which follows constipation. This process is accelerated if nuts are included in the diet (without greens) as nuts are more difficult to digest and slow digestion. If this process continues unabated, a minor diabetic condition will occur as the body is constantly urinating to spill off excess sugar.

Too much sugar in the blood calls forth alkaline minerals, such as calcium, from the bones and tissues to buffer the acidifying effects of too much sugar. These minerals are also lost with the urine. So, excessive stimulation of the body by sugars (including hybridized sweet fruit) can not only cause constipation, but can leach minerals from the body in the long term.

This condition is completely reversible through regular exercise, considerably decreasing the intake of sugary fruits, and by adding a large portion of dark green-leafy vegetables and a variety of raw plant fats to the diet (again reference The Sunfood Triangle). The best way to rehydrate the body is with green-vegetable juice. High-sodium foods, such as celery, are excellent to include to rehydrate the body and to relieve constipation as sodium counterbalances a potassium overdose (which could have contributed to constipation).

Refined and hybrid sugars in the form of sucrose ($C_{12}H_{22}O_{11}$) actually take water away from the body. In order to break sucrose ($C_{12}H_{22}O_{11}$) down into two molecules of glucose ($C_6H_{12}O_6$), a molecule of water (H_2O) is required. Thus, drinks or smoothies containing refined or hybrid sugar can actually make one thirstier. This is why I believe it is best to rehydrate the body with fresh green-leafy vegetable juice rather than with fruit juice. Celery/kale/cucumber juice is particularly excellent to rehydrate the body.

Excessive intake of refined and even hybridized sugar (those foods listed in the chart below with a typical glycemic index of 70 or above) can cause a hyperinsulinization of the blood. This can lead to drowsiness and fatigue.

The glycemic index is the rate at which sugar is absorbed into the blood. Consider the following glycemic index for certain foods (the higher the number, the greater the influx of sugar into the blood):

Chart: Glycemic Index

Maltose (sweetener)	152
Glucose (pure)	138
Baked Potato	135
Carrots (cooked)	127
Honey	126
Cornflakes Cereal	119
Rice Cakes	117
Pretzels	116
Jelly Beans	114
Waffle	109
Donut	108
French Fries	107
Commercial Beer	105
Corn Chips	105
Kaiser Roll	104
Mashed Potato	104
Cooked Millet	103
White Bagel	103
Dates	**103**
Watermelon (seedless)	**101**
Millet (cooked)	101
White Bread	100
Melba Toast	100
Whole-Wheat Bread	99
Shredded Wheat	97
Brown Rice	96
Croissant	96
Rye Bread	95
Green Pea Soup	94

Pineapple	**94**
Seedless Raisins	93
Cantaloupe	**93**
Black Bean Soup	92
Macaroni & Cheese	92
Beets (cooked)	88
Oatmeal	87
Ice Cream	87
Pizza (cheese)	86
Split Pea Soup	86
Carrots (juiced)	85
White Rice	83
Paw-Paw	83
Apricots	**82**
White Pita Bread	82
Corn (cooked)	81
Pastries	81
Potato (boiled)	81
Wild Rice (saskatchewan)	81
Seedless Bananas	**79**
Popcorn	79
Sweet Corn	**78**
Potato Chips	77
Kiwifruit	**75**
Beets	75
Baked Yams	74
Frozen Peas	74
Watermelons	**74**
Orange Juice	**74**
All Bran Cereal	73
Pumpernickel Bread	71
Baked Sweet Potatoes	70
Grapefruit Juice	**69**
Mangos	**69**
Baked Beans	69
Porridge Oats	68
Pineapple Juice	**66**
White Spaghetti	66
Mixed Grain Bread	64
Lentil Soup	63
Oranges	**62**
Grapes	**62**
Wheat Spaghetti	61
Green Peas (dried)	56
Kidney Beans	54

Tomato Soup	54
Apples	**53**
Yogurt	52
Whole Milk	49
Chickpeas	49
Pears	**47**
Skim Milk	46
Apricots (dried)	**44**
Soy Milk	43
Lentils (red)	43
Peaches	**40**
Grapefruits	**36**
Plums	**34**
Cherries	**32**
Nuts	16-32
Soybeans	20
Tomatoes	**16**

Glycemic Index: This index compares the total amount of glucose appearing in the bloodstream after eating a food with the total amount of glucose appearing in the bloodstream after eating the same amount of carbohydrate in the form of white bread (some researchers use glucose itself, which adjusts all numbers on the chart down by about 1/3). Fruits are shown in bold for clarity.

(Sources: Foster-Powell K., Brand Miller J. "International Tables of Glycemic Index," **The American Journal Of Clinical Nutrition**," 62:871s, 1995; Jenkins, D.J.A., "The Glycemic Response To Carbohydrate Foods," **Lancet** 2:388, 1981; Jenkins, D.J.A., "Glycemic Index Of Foods: A Physiological Basis For Carbohydrate Exchange," **The American Journal Of Clinical Nutrition**, 34:362-366, March 1981; and various other sources. Overall, these GI values are based on over 80 studies in the peer-reviewed literature.)

From this chart we can clearly understand which foods cause sugar problems. Cooked grains and cooked hybrid vegetables (beets, carrots, corn, potatoes) cause a greater sugar rush into the blood stream than fruit! Sugar imbalances (diabetes, hypoglycemia) are best addressed by removing refined sugars, cooked grains, and cooked or raw hybrid foods from the diet.

The chart makes evident the sugar imbalance that beer can cause. Alcoholics, in general, have a disrupted sugar metabolism, but they can find relief eating fruit as a replacement for alcohol. Regular fruit meals can keep the blood sugar levels balanced; assorted greens and plant fats can provide the B vitamins and trace minerals which are usually deficient in the alcohol consumer.

On The Sunfood Diet, those with hypoglycemia or diabetes can choose low-sugar fruits initially, then move to high-sugar fruits eventually. However, it is extremely important to mention that those with a sugar metabolism problem still need some sugar and that sugar should come from natural fruits (with seeds).

Fats

Eat raw plant fats for beauty. They make the skin and hair shine. Natural, raw fatty foods contain oils which lubricate the mucus linings and joints of the body. They help cushion and suspend tissues and organs. Raw plant fats keep everything clean and "well-oiled." Just as sugar is the fuel of the body, raw plant fat is the oil or lubricant of the body.

In this section, we are going to discover why a diet containing a sufficient quantity of raw plant fat is essential for good health.

In the intestines we find villi (small hair-like tissue structures containing capillaries) designed to absorb carbohydrates (fruits) and amino acids (green-leafy vegetables). We also find, upon the villi of the small intestines, lacteals (lymph channels), which absorb fats into the lymphatic system. The fat is conducted through the lymphatic vessels to the liver where the fat is prepared for distribution throughout the body.

All fats are made up of two substances: glycerin and fatty acids. The number and kinds of fatty acids attached to the glycerin molecule determine the fat type.

Some fatty acids are called "essential" because the body is not independently capable of manufacturing these substances at sufficient levels. Raw-food expert and co-founder of Excellence Inc., Annie Jubb, mentions in her seminars that population studies have shown that 100 out of 100 Americans are essential-fatty-acid deficient! The essential fatty acids are linoleic and linolenic fatty acids, both of which are found abundantly in fatty raw plant foods, especially in avocados, nuts, and seeds. The highly-touted omega 6 and omega 3 fatty-acid groups contain the essential fatty acids. Omega 6 and omega 3 fatty acids are found in an excellent ratio in flax seed oil.

Because of their unique biochemical structure, fats "cut" or disguise more potent substances. This is why milk is used in coffee. It is also why avocados go well with hot chiles. In Mexico they eat young coconut flesh (high-fat) with chiles and fresh lime juice. Fats tone down "hot" foods (such as ginger, garlic, chiles, etc.).

Fatty foods slow the release of sugars already in the digestive track. One can eat fruit in the morning with an avocado and have a longer time release of sugar, which allows one to experience a higher energy level longer.

Excellent foods containing raw plant fats and the essential fatty acids include: avocados, durians, Sun-ripened olives, young coconuts, nuts, seeds, olive oils, and seed oils.

Plant fats contain no cholesterol. Cholesterol is not found in the plant world. Every cell in the human body produces the amount of cholesterol that it needs. Animals and humans produce their own cholesterol. Infants are the only humans who need dietary cholesterol, which they get from their mother's milk, as they use it for healthy brain formation. All cholesterol problems are eliminated by removing animal foods from the diet.

Studies have found that a diet adequate in fat intake is essential for healthy bone formation and mineralization. Raw plant fats are the "delivery vehicle" for the minerals in green-leafy vegetables.

Raw plant fats insulate the nerve tissue and protect us from pollution and from the harshness of present-day civilization. Many raw-foodists I have met agree that they seem to rarely desire avocados or nuts while living in the woods far away from the urban centers; however, once they return to the harshness of cement, cars, and big buildings, the desire for avocados and nuts also increases.

Raw plant fats effectively increase the electric tension on the cell membranes, making them more permeable to oxygen and nutrients.

All the craze against fats applies specifically to cooked fats. Cooked fats (containing trans-fatty acids) are totally destructive to sound health: they interfere with cell respiration; they are a major source of damaging free radicals; they lack their associated enzyme lipase and thus are difficult to digest. Trans-fatty acids cause the powerhouse of each cell, the mitochondria, to swell and malfunction, becoming less capable of efficiently producing energy. Fats are always incorporated directly into the cell wall; when trans-fatty acids are incorporated into the cell wall, the cell begins to lose control over what substances are entering through the cell membrane. Salt, carcinogens, damaging free radicals, and chemicals begin to accumulate inside the cell. The cell becomes susceptible to ultraviolet radiation and cancer.

Cooked fats include any fatty substances that have been heated, hydrogenated, pasteurized, or excessively oxidized. To prevent oxidation from light, all oils purchased in stores should be in dark bottles; all seed oils should be purchased while still refrigerated or else they will oxidize and become rancid.

Cooked fats are thick, heavy, and have a deranged structure. They clog up the blood, arteries, and the lymphatic system. Because cooked fat is not miscible with water, is clogging, and is generally difficult for the body to process, metabolize, and eliminate, eating cooked fats causes the body to gain excessive weight.

In contrast, raw plant fats do not cause the body to gain excessive weight unnecessarily. In fact, as one transitions away from cooked food, s/he can actually lose weight eating a significant portion of raw plant fats. Eating raw plant fats can help a person lose weight as they contain their lipase enzymes which allow body fat to be burned. Lipase enzymes are typically missing in the excessive fat tissues of the body. Lipase enzymes, from raw plant fats and their oils, help metabolize cooked fat deposits which have stagnated and accumulated throughout the body. Each raw essential fatty acid replaces each cooked trans-fatty acid incorporated into the cell walls. Raw plant fats are easily recognized by the liver and distributed properly throughout the body.

Raw plant fats do not clog the blood with red blood cell and platelet aggregation as cooked fats do. Long-time raw-food nutritionist, Ross Horne of Australia, tells us in his wonderful book **Improving On Pritikin**: "To prove that the fat of avocados did not cause excessive levels of triglycerides in the blood and did not cause red cell and platelet aggregation and blood viscosity when the avocado was eaten raw, I had blood tests done which clearly demonstrated this..."

Raw plant fats have exactly the opposite effect of cooked fats. Raw plant fats are incredible: they are antioxidants, they insulate the nerves, they protect us from pollution, they moisturize the skin, and they ease digestion by lubricating the delicate mucus lining. There is no evidence that a high raw-fat diet produces anything but outstanding health, especially if it is raw plant fat.

Many people who start into raw diets and vegetarianism think they need protein to fill the empty space left by eliminating animal food; what they need and want is fat. Most people and nutritionists mistake the desire for fat for the desire for protein as they cannot distinguish the difference between the two. Fats are soft, heavy, and full; proteins are hard, abrasive, and empty. Protein will not fill the empty space when you stop eating cooked food.

Vegetarians and vegans typically attempt to fill the space for fat with cooked vegetables. Cooking densifies vegetation and gives the body the illusion of "fullness" and satiation that fat provides. Many non-raw-food vegans and vegetarians I have met, to me, look deficient in raw fat and overloaded on cooked vegetable starch. I have observed that a fat-deficient state coupled with sugar imbalances due to cooked starch can lead non-raw vegans and vegetarians back to animal foods to get fat for its own sake, and to get fat to slow the entry of sugar into the blood. For vegans and vegetarians, I recommend replacing cooked starch with cooked non-starchy vegetables (purple cabbage, cauliflower, broccoli, asparagus, artichoke), transitioning into The Raw-Food Diet, and including significantly more raw plant fat into the diet.

Cooked, densified non-starchy vegetables slow down the absorption of sugar into the blood stream like fats do. I think Arnold Ehret took advantage of this with his low-fat **Mucusless Diet Healing System**. His system of eating raw fruits and non-starchy vegetables cooked or raw with almost no fats is excellent for detoxification, but deficient in fat in the long term.

Fats are the bridge which carry you from a cooked-food diet to The Raw-Food Diet. Fats fill that empty space perfectly. They are exactly what the body requires. They satiate hunger.

The most digestible fats come from the oleaginous fruits (oily fruits) such as avocados and Sun-ripened olives. They have a high-water content and a simple structure, making them easy for the body to identify, metabolize, and assimilate.

Those with liver damage, or a weak liver, may need to moderate their intake of raw plant fats significantly when beginning The Sunfood Diet. Nuts may have to be bypassed and avocados and/or blended seeds used instead. You will need to tune into your body, to know when you have eaten more fat than your liver can handle (acne may result from an excessive fat intake). Usually, when the liver is working hard processing raw plant fats, the appetite will shut down.

Saturated, Monounsaturated, And Polyunsaturated Fats

Research by Dr. Howell in **Enzyme Nutrition** and Udo Erasmus in **Fats That Heal, Fats That Kill** indicates both saturated and unsaturated fats are greatly beneficial as long as they are raw. If the fats are cooked or oxidized, they are altered chemically and may be devoid of lipase (the fat-splitting enzyme) which can lead to health challenges.

There are three major types of fats: saturated, monounsaturated, and polyunsaturated fats. Typically all raw plant fats have some of all three; however, the ratio of each to the other differs for each food.

Saturated fats are more stable than unsaturated fats and the most resistant to alterations due to heat. The best saturated fats come from the inner soft white flesh of young coconuts (available in Asian markets in North America). Because coconut fat is more stable, I have found benefit in drinking the coconut water and leaving the husk at room temperature for 2 or 3 days before opening it up and spooning out the white flesh. Leaving the coconut out allows the associated fat enzyme, lipase, to begin breaking down the coconut flesh. After a few days of enzymatic breakdown, the coconut flesh generally contains more "energy" and is easier to digest.

Monounsaturated fats are found abundantly in avocados, Sun-ripened olives, olive oil, almonds, and most nuts and their oils. The slight electrical nature of monounsaturated fats allows them to split and bind with some toxins.

Polyunsaturated fats are dominant in the substance and oil of walnuts, sunflower, flax, hemp, sesame, and other seeds. Polyunsaturated fatty acids have a horse-shoe shape. Their strong electrical nature allows them to easily split, enabling them to bind with toxins and carry them out of the system. Because of their ability to bind with toxins, raw polyunsaturated fats are the most healing fats for the body. Polyunsaturated fats are highly sensitive and are the most subject to structural derangement through heating, hydrogenation, and oxidation. Deranged polyunsaturated fats are the most damaging fats for the body and should be totally avoided.

Fats And Longevity

Eat fatty raw plant foods for longevity. Living a long and vibrant life is a matter of minimizing free radical damage to the body through a diet rich in antioxidants.

A free radical is an electron-deficient molecule produced from oxygen and cooked fat in the body. In seeking to acquire another electron, a free radical is capable of combining with and destroying enzymes, amino acids, and other cellular elements.

Whole raw plant foods rich in polyunsaturated fat (walnuts, sunflower seeds, flax seeds, hemp seeds) always contain antioxidants, such as Vitamins E, C, carotene, and selenium. Other raw plant foods, such as citrus fruits, contain the antioxidant bioflavonoids. Deep green leaves contain the antioxidant beta-carotene. No antioxidant supplements are necessary.

We want to minimize oxidation in the body due to free radical damage. A high oxidation means that electrons are being stolen from the body by refined and cooked oils (corn oil, safflower oil, etc.). Raw plant fats have long chain fatty acids which help protect cell membranes from oxidation. Raw plant fats deactivate free radicals by giving them electrons.

Essential fatty acids have an abundance of electrons. The spare electrons in fats help sweep toxins along to the liver. In a healthy body, there are spare electrons and having spare electrons equates into achieving longevity.

Humans should live longer than any other mammal on Earth because humans can consciously control the amount and quality of food material entering the body. If the intake of this food is decreased to a pleasant frugal minimum (but still includes high-quality raw plant fats, which are antioxidants), then the obstructions and free radicals in the system will be decreased to a minimum. In this way, the system becomes abundant in electrons, is more efficient (well-oiled), and operates with less friction, thus maximizing longevity.

Animal Fats

Those eating animal fats to fulfill the dietary requirement for fats have part of the picture, but they simply have not had the spiritual awakening with which to abandon animal products, and the death, enslavement, and torture which accompanies them.

Raw animal fats are typically saturated, so they are not as strong in their cleansing abilities as monounsaturated or polyunsaturated fats, therefore they do not directly help detoxify the body.

Animal flesh fats are particularly dangerous because they bring negative energy upon the consumer from the animal's death and they contain stored toxins collected from the environment. Farmed animals eat pesticide and chemical-sprayed foods which end up stored in their fat cells. This gives the consumer a double dose of negativity. The same holds true for fish liver oil, which can contain all the toxins present in the fish. The liver is the detoxification center of the body, through which all the toxins must pass.

As far as raw milk products go, they are high-fat foods. Generally, raw goat's milk is of a higher quality than raw cow's milk because goats are a cleaner, more discerning animal — if they do not find the food they like, they will go hungry, whereas cows will start chomping anything green.

Many have lived long lives taking in raw milk, butter, and cheese to fulfill their fat requirements as Professor Hilton Hotema reported in his classic book **Man's Higher Consciousness**, but none I am aware of have ever gone late into life eating raw flesh for fat because the negative karma is too great and does come back to entrap the one who ingests such substances.

Raw organic dairy products may be used in transition to fulfill the fat category of The Sunfood Triangle for people with weak fat metabolisms. Raw organic dairy products may benefit raw-foodists who have become deficient in alkaline minerals (calcium, magnesium, etc.) from not consuming enough whole green-leafed vegetables and/or who are experiencing a lack of excellent intestinal flora. The karma of raw dairy products is neutral, if the milk is freely given. However, this is rarely the case today, and most dairy animals are enslaved, lead sad lives, and are finally killed for their flesh. Also, drinking the milk of another animal, especially after the weaning age, seems quite unnatural. Raw dairy is mucus-forming and, if taken, should be consumed moderately.

All pasteurized dairy products should be avoided. They contribute greatly to atherosclerosis, encouraging the plaque buildup in arteries that is epidemic throughout the population. The two countries with the highest rate of heart disease, the U.S. and Finland, are also the two countries with the highest consumption of pasteurized dairy products. (For more information on this subject, please read John Robbins' book **Diet For A New America**.)

Tree Nuts

Contrary to popular opinion, nuts are a fat-dominant food, not a protein-dominant food.

Nuts and seeds can comprise part of the daily diet, however, they should be eaten in reasonable quantities (a maximum of 0.33 pounds or 0.15 kg per day). Remember, they are negative karma foods. If overeaten, they should be balanced with green-leafed vegetables and juicy sweet fruits.

It is best to eat nuts moderately — ration them and do not eat more than you set aside for yourself. It is easy to overeat nuts and eat them too fast, especially if you purchase them unshelled. Every couple of months I like to rest my body from nuts for a week or two.

Because nuts are so concentrated, they should always be eaten with or just before a large meal of green-leafy vegetables.

Some of the best nuts include almonds, hazelnuts, macadamia, pecans, pistachio, walnuts, and pine nuts. Macadamia nuts are the best nuts of all because they have the most fat and the least protein of all nuts. However, macadamias can be mucus-forming unless eaten with a significant amount of green-leafed vegetables.

Cashews have a shell filled with a thick black resin that makes cracking the shells, for the most part, unmanageable. Thus, cashews are cooked out of their shells. Even if they are labeled "raw," they are actually cooked (I did not like finding this out when I first discovered raw foods, but I eventually got over it!).

Tree nuts are also potentially mucous formers. If you eat too many nuts, you may find that clear mucus will flow from your nose. This is because nuts are acid-forming in the body. A mucous discharge is a way for the body to dispel some acid-forming minerals and create a more alkaline internal environment. Eating the alkaline-forming green leaves counter-balances the acid-forming elements in nuts, eliminating mucous discharges.

If you eat nuts in moderation and eat nuts with green-leafed vegetables, then you need not worry about soaking or mucus formation. A strong digestive tract, strengthened by months and years of eating quality high-fiber green vegetables, is capable of digesting nuts with little difficulty.

Quantities should be kept to less than 2.0-2.5 pounds (0.9-1.2 kg) of nuts per week. I recommend nuts over seeds because they have a higher fat content. And nuts with the highest fat to protein ratio are best of all. If not eaten fresh from below the plant or tree, you might consider soaking nuts and seeds in water and/or sprouting them for 3-12 hours to disarm their enzyme inhibitors. Enzyme inhibitors keep nuts and seeds in their dormant state until conditions are right for growth. If eaten in the dormant state without green leaves to help along digestion, nuts and seeds can burden the pancreas and sit "heavy" in the stomach.

Seeds

My experience and research has revealed that the best seeds are those which contain the highest ratio of fat to protein (the highest fat and the least protein). A good edible seed should contain no more protein than 2 parts fat to 1 part protein (2:1 ratio). These include flax, pumpkin, sesame (tahini), sunflower, and especially young coconut (a coconut is actually a seed).

The seeds of grains and legumes (which are seed foods) are protein-dominant, not fat-dominant. I recommend against excessive protein-dominant seeds. Proteins are harsh on the body, fats are soft on the body.

Grains (especially hybridized, weak seeds) are less than excellent foods for humans. They do not metabolize cleanly, especially when cooked. Raw or cooked grains, such as oats, rice, and wheatberries, may leave a gummy residue behind that will clog up the tiny lymph and blood vessels if overeaten over a long period of time.

If grains are eaten, the best grains are quinoa and millet, which should be sprouted. They have a higher ratio of fat to protein than other grains, although they are still protein-dominant. Quinoa and millet are also closer to the wild state.

Raw legume sprouts, such as mung beans, kidney beans, lentils, and soy beans, can drain the body of water. If legumes are eaten, the best legumes are chickpeas and peanuts (if uncontaminated with fungus). Chickpeas should be sprouted. Peanuts should be soaked until plump before eating. Both chickpeas and peanuts have a higher ratio of fat to protein than other legumes, but chickpeas are still protein-dominant. Soy beans have a high ratio of fat to protein (1:2) so they are one of the better legumes, even if cooked. However, they are such hybridized foods (so far out of the natural wild state) that I do not endorse them or products made from them (soy milk, soy cheese, soy burgers, etc).

Protein

Perhaps the biggest misconception in the field of nutrition is the confusion between fat and protein. When someone says: "I need protein," what they really need and want is fat. Most people and nutritionists cannot distinguish between the desire for fat and protein. Many raw-food advocates have recommended nuts for protein, when in reality, the value of nuts is in their fat. People can give up steak much easier than cheese, because steak is mostly protein whereas cheese is mostly fat.

Protein is what we are; it is the structure of our physical body and each one of our cells. The protein theory essentially states that you need flesh protein to build flesh protein. If that were true, then gorillas should have to eat flesh to develop their incredibly muscular 400+ pound (180 kg) bodies.

Imagine a newborn human baby doubling its body weight in several months on a diet of breast milk. Most breast milk is less than 2% protein and even the heavier "hind-milk" is only about 10% protein. Breast milk itself, is a fat-dominant food.

The construction of proteins actually occurs from the free amino acids available to the body. The body has to break down all protein (if it can) into its constituent parts, the amino acids, before the material can be utilized. Protein is nothing more or less than a collection of amino acids. The protein structure consists of amino acids strung together like grapes on a vine.

Most protein-dominant foods (animal muscle, sprouted grains/legumes), whether raw or cooked, create obstructions inside the human body.

Mushrooms are protein-dominant, but are not very concentrated, thus they create few obstructions. Mushrooms are a fungus, not a true Sunfood. They should be eaten in moderation. Many wild mushrooms are toxic, and some are even deadly. Wild mushrooms should be avoided unless one is highly skilled in their identification.

Green-leafed vegetables are the true body builders. They are our true "protein food." They contain all the amino acids we require. Real strength and building material comes from green-leafed vegetables where the amino acids are found. If we look at the gorilla, zebra, giraffe, hippo, rhino, or elephant we find they build their enormous musculature on green-leafy vegetation.

Is there enough protein available in the all-raw diet? Consider the following analysis of Day 3, Wednesday, of the All-Raw Menu (Spring/Summer) (**Appendix B: The Sunfood Diet Weekly Guideline And Menu Plan**):

Item	Weight (lbs,)	Mass (g)	Protein/100 g	Protein
5 apples	1.8 lbs.	810 g	0.2 g	1.6 g
20 pecans	0.12 lb.	60 g	7.8 g	4.7 g
25 macadamia nuts	0.18 lb.	80 g	8.3 g	6.6 g
3 cucumbers	1.2 lbs.	550 g	0.6 g	3.3 g
3 large tomatoes	1.2 lbs.	550 g	0.9 g	5.0 g
1 zucchini	0.35 lb.	160 g	1.2 g	1.9 g
2 orange	0.80 lb.	360 g	1.3 g	4.7 g
Spinach	0.44 lb.	200 g	2.9 g	5.8 g
Lettuce (romaine)	0.44 lb.	200 g	1.6 g	3.2 g
Endive	0.44 lb.	200 g	1.7 g	3.4 g
Kale	0.44 lb.	200 g	3.3 g	6.6 g
Green cabbage	0.44 lb.	200 g	1.2 g	2.4 g
			Total Protein:	**49.2 g**

The World Health Organization has established a minimum daily requirement of 32 grams of protein for a 150 pound (68 kg) male. Women require slightly less protein than men, except when pregnant (then they require slightly more than men).

To satisfy the powerful meat and dairy interests in the United States, the U.S. Recommend Daily Allowance (RDA) presents an inflated protein recommendation of 0.8 grams of protein per kilogram of body weight. This is not a minimum daily requirement, but a "recommended" daily requirement that includes an added 30% "safety margin." Under the U.S. RDA, a 150 pound (68 kg) male is recommended to consume 54.4 g of protein per day.

As I have demonstrated, protein can be adequately supplied by raw plant foods. Animal protein is not necessary. The consumption of cooked animal protein has been statistically correlated with all the major diseases of civilization. As the cooked animal protein increases in the diet, the rate of disease increases in a one-to-one correlation (for more on this see John Robbins' book **Diet For A New America** and Gary Null's book **The Vegetarian Handbook**). Most of the diseases of civilization are actually caused by animal-protein poisoning because protein-dominant animal foods are acid-forming and not natural foods for humans to consume. Fat-dominant plant foods are far more important.

I have had individuals walk into my office with severe liver and kidney damage caused by the high-protein diet. Seeing lives trashed by incorrect nutritional advice and fanciful theories sends the message home: Please, stop listening to anyone in any field who is not getting the results you desire.

Consider the words of Morris Krok in his book **Diet, Health, And Living On Air**:

> "In the metabolism of fats, sugars, and starches, the waste which is left behind is carbon dioxide and water. This however is not the case with protein, which leaves as its end-products uric acid and urea, which, if retained in the system, are very harmful. Thus not only is protein not well utilized for bodily heat, but it is also a potential danger to the health of the liver and kidneys, and because of this, is the greatest factor in acidifying the entire membranous tract."

Dr. C. Samuel West describes in his book **The Golden Seven Plus One** that the primary cause of disease is undigested protein trapped in the intercellular fluid between the cells.

Acid-forming, protein-dominant foods (protein foods which are not green) are outside of the essentials which comprise The Sunfood Triangle.

Although I recommend against them, if acid-forming protein-dominant foods (animal muscle, sprouted grains/legumes) are eaten, they should always be combined with green-leafed vegetables. The alkaline greens neutralize the acidity of the protein food. The fiber in greens helps push everything through the digestive system properly.

For the best health, I recommend that the diet contain proteins (amino acids) in the form of green foods, but that it should consist of few acid-forming, protein-dominant foods. The diet should never consist of more than 10% acid-forming protein-dominant foods by weight.

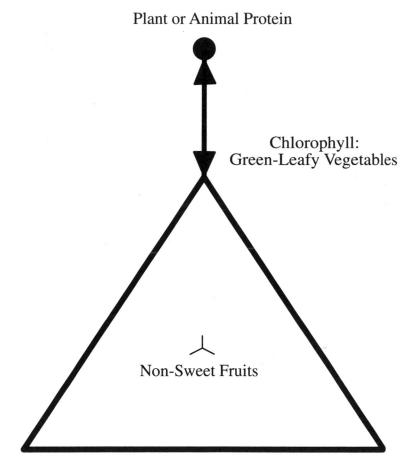

The Sunfood Triangle And Protein

The Center Point

Food, first and foremost, is a stimulant. We can do without one of these three classes of foods for a time, if we eat very little and do not stimulate our body too far in one direction. If we go too far in one direction, then the other foods should be brought in to pull us back. For example, if you eat too much sugar, you need fat and chlorophyll to pull you back. If you eat too much chlorophyll, you need fat and sugar to center you.

Many newcomers to raw foods and the Sunfood Diet tend to overeat dried fruit and nuts as a replacement for the heavier cooked foods. They are getting a strong dose of concentrated sugar and nut fat. These foods must be balanced by also overeating green-leafed vegetables, such as kale, or one will eventually be thrown off balance.

The least stimulating food on the human body is a low-sugar, high-water content, low-fat fruit, such as the cucumber.

Eating low-sugar, non-fatty fruits keeps us close to the center point. Non-sweet fruits are low stimulation foods. Some low-sugar fruits include:

Bell Pepper (not green)
Breadfruit (raw)
Cranberry
Cucumber
Dragon Fruit
Grapefruit
Jalapeno Pepper
Lemon
Lime
Noni
Okra
Pumpkin
Serrano Pepper
Summer Squashes
Tomatillo
Tomato
Zucchini

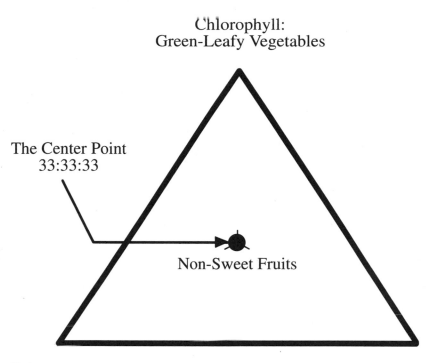

The Sunfood Triangle: The Center Point
Ratio Key: (Chlorophyll:Sugar:Fat)

Food definitely stimulates the body. You can demonstrate this on your-self, when you are tired, perhaps even sleepy, by eating any raw plant food and you will come wide awake. You may eat to stay awake if nec-essary.

Aside from eating a balance of foods, there are other ways we can become more centered. Deep breathing, exercise, laughter, sex, and yoga all help to return you to the center point.

Meditation returns one to the center point. I once spoke with a gentle-man who had met and spoken in depth with Fred Hirsch, the publisher of Arnold Ehret's **Mucusless Diet Healing System**. This gentleman described that Arnold Ehret's largely fruit diet was also accompanied by deep meditation, but this was purposely left out of the book, because meditation did not fit the western paradigm of mainstream thought. Meditation is greatly beneficial in centering the mind and body and facilitates the fulfillment of the fruit diet.

Consider that Arnold Ehret's fruitarian diet consisted considerably of apples and raisins with occasional green-leafed vegetables. Back in his time (the beginning of the 20th century), the hybrid foods (such as seedless raisins) available today, did not exist. Arnold Ehret ate apples (sugar) with raisins with seeds (fat) and green-leafed vegetables, which covers the three classes. Real raisins with seeds are a totally incredible food, especially for those living in northerly climates where grapes grow wildly. Raisins can be stored and eaten all through the winter.

Fasting also helps return us to the center point. Our spiritual powers are highest when fasting.

Ideal Foods

Good, fresh durian must be one of the most incredible edibles on Earth. Once, the editor of the Nature's First Law radical raw-food magazine **Just Eat An Apple**, Fred Patenaude, and I were passing by an Asian market in San Diego, we stopped in and, sure enough, they had fresh, ripe, durian! I bought the ripest durian available. In the car, Fred and I split the durian. It was ambrosia. The taste was so light, so subtle, so powerful that it immediately sent us into an altered state. While we ate, I told a story to Fred. Afterward, I looked over and Fred had not heard a word I said. He was in outer space. I could not reach him — he did not want to be reached. That is the power of the durian!

The durian fruit of southeast Asia contains incredible fat and sugar, putting us right at the midpoint between the two. Added with green-leafy foods, we can live on Durian alone, at least for some time. A raw-foodist once told me he believed durian and raw cannabis constituted humanity's most natural foods. I thought that was interesting.

We can live for some time on seeded grapes and/or natural seeded raisins. Seeded grapes and natural Sun-dried, vine-ripened raisins with seeds are some of the most incredible foods on Earth. They have the sugar and the fat (the grape seed). Add that to the grape leaves (green-leaves) which come with the grape plant and we could live on the grape plant alone for quite some time. In the future, I am going to conduct an experiment on myself when my grape vines (grown from seed) reach fruition. I am going to see how long I can go with my grape plants as my only nourishment.

Watermelon is one of the top foods on the planet. If you chew up some of the seeds for fat (which I have found to be quite an aphrodisiac), and take in the natural melon sugar, you again have a close to balanced picture. Add green-leafed vegetables in and you can go quite some time on those alone.

Apricots are a sweet fruit (sugar) with an edible kernel which tastes like an almond (fat). They also have the sugar and fat wrapped in one package. The Hunzas, one of the longest-lived tribes on Earth, are world-renowned for their diet of apricots. The apricot kernel contains specific compounds that work to repair the prostate. They should be immediately included into the diet of anyone experiencing prostate troubles. I know of several people who have healed themselves of prostate cancer naturally, and who swear by these kernels.

Young coconut is also one of the Earth's most perfect foods. With sweet water and soft spoon meat on the inside, few foods can compare. Again, green leaves are required to make a coconut diet work for you in the long-term. Also, coconuts are a seed and thus they have a negative karma charge, which should be balanced with positive or neutral karma foods.

Fruitarianism

The present-day fruitarian movement finds its philosophical roots in the scriptures (Genesis 1:29), the writings of spiritual masters, such as Sri Yukteswar in his book **The Holy Science**, in the writings of Professor Arnold Ehret, in the fascinating accomplishments and philosophy of Dr. Johnny Lovewisdom, in the writings of Morris Krok in **Fruit The Food And Medicine For Man**, and in the writings of T.C. Fry.

At this moment, the world's foremost promoter of the fruitarian diet is Rene Beresford of Australia. Rene is the editor of the worldwide **Fruitarian Network News**. For information about how to subscribe to this magazine, please see the **Publications** section at the end of this book. Rene has done a wonderful job of spreading positive energy into the world and attracting people to fruitarianism.

What exactly comprises a fruitarian diet has been the subject of much debate over the years. In this book, I believe I have finally settled the matter. For the record: a fruitarian is an eater of fruits (fatty, sweet, and non-sweet) and green-leafed vegetables.

The fruitarian diet lifestyle is a beautiful way to live, it is in total harmony with the philosophy of Ahimsa (a Sanskrit word that means causing no harm). However, as I have described, raw foods — especially fruits — carry with them a strong karma and energy. For that reason, they must be eaten in a balanced fashion. Too much hybridized sweet fruit will throw the body off balance. The fruitarian diet has to be done correctly. Specifically, green-leafed vegetables must be eaten as they contain heavier minerals, calming properties, fiber, and certain intangible items not available in fruits — all frugivorous (fruit eating) primates include green leaves in their diets; also, fats must be derived from avocados, durians, or olives instead of nuts if one is to remain within the fruitarian Ahimsa paradigm — eating nuts kills the plant embryo.

I do not recommend giving up green-leafed vegetables. If one goes too long on an all-fruit diet, the first thing that will happen is that s/he will go deficient in salt (sodium), the next thing that will occur is a deficiency in calcium. However, for those experimenting with a high-fruit diet, I recommend the following:
1. Eat no more than 33.3% high-sugar fruits, such as melons, mangos, peaches, etc.
2. Eat plenty of non-sweet fruits, such as cucumbers, tomatoes, etc.
3. Eat plenty of high calcium, alkaline-forming fruits, especially: figs, olives, oranges, panini (prickly pear), papaya, and rambutan.
4. Breathe in pure air.
5. Take in and swim in only pure water (containing no acid-forming minerals such as chlorine).
6. Avoid stress-inducing and acid-forming environments (e.g. cities).

7. Eat plenty of silicon-based foods: peppers, chiles, okra, etc. Silicon can be biologically transmuted into calcium by the liver (see **Biological Transmutations** by Kervran).

8. Avoid all nuts! (They are too acid-forming. One will be thrown off center by eating them if no greens are in the diet. Nuts must be balanced with greens).

9. Eat a sufficient quantity of olives. Olives have a naturally high sodium content (even when unsalted).

Keys to a high-fruit diet:

1. You must be active to burn up all the sugar (fuel) you are putting into your body.

2. You must be mentally positive.

3. You must be emotionally stable.

The Ideal Spiritual Diet Of Humankind

"And by the river upon the bank thereof, on this side and on that side, shall grow all trees for meat, whose leaf shall not fade, neither shall the fruit thereof be consumed: it shall bring forth new fruit according to his months, because their waters they issued out of the sanctuary: and the fruit thereof shall be for meat, and the leaf thereof for medicine." — **Ezekiel 47:12**

To elevate the spiritual powers, I promote a Live-Alkaline Fruit (LAF) Diet of green leaves and fruits for positive karma, avocados for fat (the acid-forming element required in the diet), wild green-leafed vegetables (the alkaline elements), and non-hybridized sweet fruits of a high alkaline content (i.e. blackberries, cherries, currants, figs, grapes, kumquats, lemons, limes, loganberries, mameys, mulberries, oranges, papayas, prickly pears, raspberries, sapodillas, and tangerines).

The Ancients, Longevity, And The Secret

The longevity of the biblical patriarchs is legendary.

One of the most startling discoveries I came across by suggestion of my friend Steve Adler was the "Bible Code" concept. It has been discovered that the first five books of the Bible, commonly known as the Torah, are encoded. What is interesting for us is the dietary law laid down in Genesis 1:29 — herbs and fruits. By analyzing Genesis 1:29 after understanding the Bible Code it was discovered that it contains, in code, the seed-bearing plants which existed in the Garden of Eden. The seven seed-bearing plants embedded in this verse are: barleygreen, wheat (grass), vine (grapes), dates, olives, figs, and pomegranates. The three food classes are there. For more on this fascinating subject, please see **Cracking The Bible Code** by Dr. Jeffrey Satinover.

Consider how the Bible Code discovery mirrors the 8 most important bioactive fruits of the ancient Essenes: grapes (vine), dates, olives, figs, pomegranates, apricots, carob, and small yellow apples. The Essenes are a religious group originally based in the Dead Sea region of Israel. They are historically known for their raw-vegetarian dietary philosophy, well-developed wisdom, and remarkable longevity. The Essenes are still around today — at the moment, the worldwide Essene Church is headed by raw-foodist Reverend David Owen (see **Organizations** at the end of this book).

The ancient Britons, according to Plutarch, only began to grow old at 210. Their food consisted almost exclusively of acorns, berries, and water. The ancient Greeks of the pre-heroic age lived on oranges and olives. We know from the food triangle I have deduced that wild green-leafy foods were included as well. The fat is there, as well as the fruit, and the green leaves. They all must be there.

Again we see such longevity in the Bulgarians, who are the longest-lived people in present-day Europe. They often reach ages exceeding 105 and even up to 125. Their simple diet consists of fruits (sugar), vegetables (chlorophyll), and sour milk or buttermilk (fat). They are a thin people typically weighing between 122 and 130 pounds (56 and 59 kilograms). This again goes to show the truth that the less weight you carry the longer you live — we have yet to discover an obese centenarian.

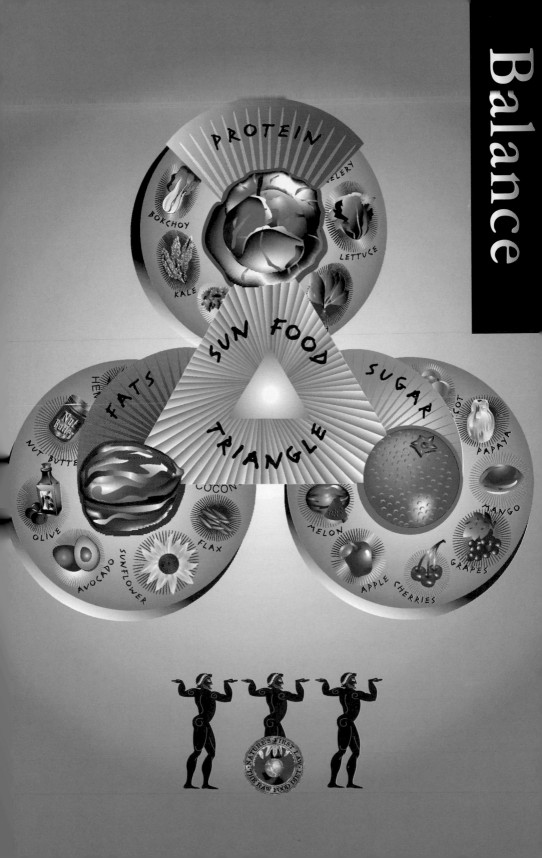

Action Steps:

1. Decide today to include significant portions of green-leafy vegetables, sweet fruits (with seeds), and raw plant fats in your diet. These food classes should constitute 80%+ of the diet.

2. Balance the three food classes against each other to achieve exceptional health!

Of Special Interest:

Consider **The Zone Diet**, a system enjoying popularity recently and see how its developer Dr. Barry Sears describes a balance of three food classes for optimal performance similar to The Sunfood Triangle. He describes that protein (amino acids), complex carbohydrates (sugar), and fat should be eaten in roughly equal proportions. Consider how this mirrors The Sunfood Triangle of green-leafy vegetables (amino acids), sweet fruit (sugar), and raw plant fats. **The Zone Diet** does make some sense, however, the challenge with it is that it is cooked, contains animal foods, and does not use organic foods!

Chart: 3 Food Classes And Their Benefits:

Green-leafy Vegetables, Benefits:
    Insure good, daily elimination.
    Chlorophyll, Nature's medicine
    Counteract acid-forming foods such as nuts, seeds, avocados,
        cooked foods, apple cider vinegar, proteins, animal
        products (not recommended).
    Counteract acid-forming air toxins such as carbon dioxide,
        carbon monoxide, sulfur, nitrous oxide, chlorine, etc.
        Greens are the lung cleansers.
    Deactivate, combine with, and help wash out heavy metals.
    Alkaline-forming foods. Greens make the blood alkaline.
    Best source of minerals (calcium, sodium, magnesium, trace
        minerals).

Balance the endocrine system (especially if wild greens are
     eaten).

Green-leaves naturally brush and clean the teeth.

Green-leaves naturally broom out the entire digestive tract as they
     pass through the body.

They ground the mind.

They calm the system.

They are karmically neutral.

Sweet Fruits, Benefits:

Glucose/Fructose/Sugar: Immediate energy.

Karma: A positive role in spreading fruiting plants and trees about
     brings us good luck.

Pleasure.

Captured nutrients from the Sun — Sunfood!

Cleansing food: Fruits are relentless cleansers and mucus
     dissolvers.

Fatty Foods, Benefits:

Antioxidants.

Insulate the nerves; protect the body against pollution.

Helps reverse heart disease and atherosclerosis because the lipase
     enzyme present in raw plant fats helps metabolize the
     cooked fat clogging the arteries and lymph system.

Replace trans-fatty acids which have hindered the respiration of
     each cell.

They are a stabilizing factor in raw diets.

They ground the body.

Long-term fuel.

They deliver minerals to the bones; they help with the
     assimilation of minerals, including calcium.

They help transport vitamins A, D, E, and K, along with other
nutrients, to the tissues.

Chart: 3 Food Classes And The Effects Of Overdose:

Symptoms Of A Chlorophyll Overdose:
  Spaciness.
  Laziness.
  The feeling of being too passive.
  Feelings of being too cold.

Symptoms Of A Sugar Overdose:
  Excessive urination.
  Light-headedness.
  Tooth sensitivity.
  Edginess.
  Constipation.
  Sores in the mouth (potassium overdose: eat sodium-residue
      foods, such as celery or seaweed, to relieve this condition).
  Black circles under the eyes.
  Grogginess.

Symptoms Of A Fat Overdose:
  Mucus elimination.
  Liver stagnation.
  Edginess.
  Sluggishness.
  Oily pores. Pimples.
  Constipation.
  Feelings of being too hot.
  Feelings of being "hung over"
  Strong body odor.

Chart: 3 Food Classes And Variety:

The Best Sugary Fruits Include:
  Apricots
  Berries of all types
  Black Sapote

Cherimoya
Cherries (wild are best!)
Crab Apples
Dates of all exotic types (avoid medjools for they are extremely
    hybridized).
Figs of all types (wild are best!)
Grapes with seeds
Jackfruit (quite a low-sugar fruit actually)
Loquat (they are close to the wild state)
Lychee
Mangos
Mangosteen
Melons with seeds
Mulberries
Oranges with seeds
Papayas
Passion Fruit
Pears (the wilder, the better)
Persimmons with seeds
Plums
Pomegranate (extremely strong fruit, resists hybridization)
Sapodilla
White Sapote
All wild sweet fruits

The Best Fatty Foods Include:
    Akee (a relative of the durian fruit; this fruit grows in West Africa
        and the West Indies)
    Avocados
    Borage seed oil
    Coconut butter (consume moderately)
    Durians
    Flax seed and its oil (cold pressed)
    Grape seeds
    Hemp seed and its oil (cold pressed)
    Nuts of all types (except cashews, which are cooked out of their

shell, even if labeled raw)
Nut butters (almond butter is excellent)
Olives and their oil (stone pressed if possible, cold pressed is also
    good)
Pumpkin seeds and their oil (cold pressed)
Sesame seeds
Sunflower seeds
Tahini (sesame butter)
Unhulled tahini (an alkaline fat, high in calcium)
Young coconuts (available in the US at Asian markets)

The Best Green-Leafed Vegetables Include:

Bok Choy
Celery (very important; an excellent source of sodium)
Cilantro
Crane's Bill
Collards
Dandelion
Dark Green Cabbage
Endive
Fennel (wild)
Kale (especially dinosaur kale)
Lamb's Quarters (Goose Foot)
Lettuce (all types)
Malva
Mustard (wild)
Parsley
Spinach
Spring Onions (green!)
Sunflower Greens
Wild Radish
All green herbs
All wild edible greens
Algaes (blue-green, chlorella, and spirulina; these are alkaline-green protein foods, they are not true leafy-vegetables; nevertheless they can be used in this category)

Lesson 12:
Transition Diet

"...for the temple of God is holy, which temple ye are."
— **I Corinthians 3:17**

"You don't become a raw-foodist, you already are one.
Your body is designed to process raw materials."
— Nature's First Law

First, we understand that The Sunfood Diet transforms you in three specific stages, all of which will elevate you to a new understanding of your inner potential:

1. Detoxification
2. Rejuvenation
3. Refinement

Second, we understand every life process is reversible. It might take from a few months to many years to make the transition back to the most fitting diet for the human being, but once we embark on the path, the benefits will be worth the effort.

Third, we must know that we are always in control. Success philosopher Napoleon Hill was well-known for his belief that the power of thought is the only thing over which any person has complete, unquestionable control.

Napoleon Hill was wrong. The power of thought is not the only thing which any person has complete, unquestionable control. Any individual has complete and unquestionable control also over their food choices! No one has ever accidentally eaten a meal in their whole life. Now that fact is truly astounding. It means, unequivocally, you may choose to give your body the very highest-quality foods and it will, in turn, give you the very highest-quality performance.

What To Eat

The Sunfood Diet is not about restriction, it is about abundance. Eat any kind of raw plant food you like in the quantities you like, keeping in mind the balance outlined in The Sunfood Triangle.

The Sunfood Diet requires green-leafed vegetables, sweet fruits, and fatty plant foods. But it can contain all kinds of raw plant foods: all fruits, herbs, vegetables of all types, sea vegetables, and nuts and seeds, all preferentially in their wild state and secondarily grown at home or organically from non-hybrid strains. As a transitional stage The Sunfood Diet incorporates cooked vegetables with a preference for more natural plant varieties. For example, choosing baked sweet potato or yam preferentially over the standard hybrid potato. This program is to be coupled by individually advised short and long fasts on vegetable juices and or water.

Organic Food

Let's begin the transition with organic food. Organic foods are not sprayed or grown with pesticides or fungicides. Pesticides and fungicides are chemicals specifically designed to kill living organisms. They should not be used on our pristine lands, put on our foods, or fed to our children.

Spend the extra money for organic food, you are worth it. That investment will come back to you multiplied a hundredfold. You will also be supporting the organic farmers and organic food distributors who need our financial assistance.

The famous 12 year Schuphan study tooted the nutritional superiority of organically grown foods. Among other things, Schuphan found:

1. Organic foods have far higher mineral and trace mineral contents, with the exception of sodium. Organic produce contains far more iron, potassium, magnesium, and calcium than conventional crops. (Most studies of this type demonstrate that organic foods have 2 to 10 times the mineral content of conventional foods — you really do get more value for the money).

2. Organic spinach contained 64-78% more vitamin C.

3. Organic savoy cabbage contained 76-91% more vitamin C.

4. Organic crops had a dry weight (after dehydration) of 69-96% more than conventional crops, demonstrating a higher food-value content.

In 1993, Bob Smith, a trace minerals laboratory analyst, began a small experiment. For two years he visited stores in Chicago and purchased 4 to 15 samples of both organic and commercial produce. He brought these samples back to his laboratory and tested them for trace elements. His conclusions were as follows:

1. Organically grown wheat had twice the calcium, four times more magnesium, five times more manganese, and thirteen times more selenium than the commercial wheat.

2. Organically grown corn had twenty times more calcium and manganese, and two to five times more copper, magnesium, molybdenum, selenium, and zinc.

3. Organically grown potatoes had two or more times the boron, selenium, silicon, strontium, and sulfur, and 60% more zinc.

4. Organically grown pears had two to nearly three times more chromium, iodine, manganese, molybdenum, silicon, and zinc.

Overall, organically-grown food exceeded commercial-grown crops significantly for twenty of the twenty-two beneficial trace minerals. Organic foods also had lower quantities of toxic trace elements, such as aluminum, lead, and mercury.

Pesticides are poison. According to data gathered from the Internet, the top 10 worst commercial fruits and vegetables based on lbs./acre or kg/hectare of pesticide used are:

Chart: Pesticides

	lbs./acre	kg/hectare
Strawberries	302	340
Dates	140	158
Carrots	119	134
Pears	112	126
Cabbage	102	115
Lemons	93	105
Grapes	91	102
Sweet Potatoes	88	99
Peaches	71	80
Nectarines	70	79

The lowest pesticide use was in the following:

	lbs./acre	kg/hectare
Figs	2	2
Avocados	2	2
Pecan	3	3
Garlic	3	3

Increasing Digestive Strength

The digestive organs act as one big muscle. If you have weak digestion, you can strengthen your digestive capacity by slowly increasing the raw green-leafy foods in your diet over time. To help breakdown the leaves and to ease digestion, soak green-leaves in olive oil for 2-3 hours before eating them. Chew your food well. One will automatically increase their digestive strength by introducing more and more raw foods at an appropriate pace, allowing the body to adjust.

After about 6 months on raw foods, once the eating disciplines are in place, it is a great idea to do a raw herbal cleanse such as EJUVA (please contact Nature's First Law at 888-RAW-FOOD for more information on how to acquire and conduct this cleanse). A cleanse will help strip out impacted mucus in the digestive tract, thus increasing digestive strength.

In my experiences working with people, I have found that their digestive energy increased when they stopped taking vitamin, mineral, and various other types of supplement pills, tinctures, and powders. My conclusion is that the long-term intake of supplements weakens digestion and can throw off the pH (acid/alkali balance) of the digestive organs.

Chinese oriental medicine claims that some people do not have enough "fire" in their constitution to thrive on raw foods. Anyone, however, can increase their fire to help digest raw foods. The best way to increase the fire in one's constitution is to Sunbathe. It is my experience that the more direct Sun energy the body receives, the greater is the digestive strength. Other ways to increase the fire in one's constitution is to practice vigorous exercise, deep breathing, and astanga yoga. In yoga we find the "breath of fire," which entails inhaling passively, exhaling in bursts through the nose as you pull the lower belly in, drawing up from the perineum.

Eating Healthy In Social Situations

What do you do when you go out to eat? Visit family? What about business lunches? Plan ahead. Bring 1-2 avocados and/or 1-2 apples with you. Order a salad, and mix the avocados and/or apples in with it. Generally, restaurants do not serve organic food, but we have to do the best we can in each circumstance. I have found that the best approach is to intelligently avoid the situation altogether. Do something different. Business people are tired of doing the "standard business lunch." Take them to a juice bar or, where possible, a raw food restaurant (see the **Raw-Food Restaurants** section at the back of this book)! Take them to a park. Without food in the way, you can conduct business quickly and efficiently — this will save you the expense and time in your day.

You have the most sophisticated computer in the world between your ears — use it! Leverage your mind to figure out a way to redirect family events and business lunches to fit your dietary health habits.

My experience as a raw-foodist has taught me a wonderful lesson: *The way people react to you and your diet has nothing to do with the diet itself, with other people, or with anything else; the way people react has everything to do with what is going on in your own mind!* Once your mind is set right, everything else will set right.

People have thousands of preconceived notions about vegetarian diets, but no preconceived ideas about eating raw foods! So you can say it is anything you want! Eating raw fruits and vegetables makes sense to most people, but eating tofu, seitan, or millet does sound strange to the average person.

When your attitude is positive and supportive towards other people and their food choices, they will not feel threatened by you, but will feel uplifted by you. Once we change, everything else changes around us.

Peer Pressure

Imagine if everybody smoked cigarettes and one day someone decided to stop. Imagine also, that as soon as the withdrawal symptoms began all the cigarette experts would get together and accost and attack anyone who did not smoke cigarettes for being nicotine deficient.

You are going to face peer pressure; it is part of the process. All great endeavors have their challenges, or they wouldn't be great!

When people offer you toxic food, they may be projecting upon you their own lack of information or fears. Let them know why you are making better choices. If they persist with negative behaviors towards you, and make you feel uncomfortable, then you should minimize or eliminate spending time with those people. Use these incidents of negativity to drive you to stay resolute with your own diet and spiritual path.

Eating While Traveling

Cucumbers, nuts, seeds for eating and sprouting, dried fruit, my all-raw superfood powder **Nature's First Food**, spirulina, blue-green algae, and grass powders for chlorophyll and minerals are beneficial to take with you while traveling. You may find that it is easy to be a Sunfoodist while traveling, especially in Europe and Mexico during the summer, because fresh fruit stands are abundant.

Water is another factor while traveling. Airplane travel dehydrates the body as airplane cabin air is extremely dry. Be sure to bring quality water with you while flying.

I once spoke to a Mormon missionary on the phone who had befriended a raw-foodist as they were both working to spread their message in a third-world country. On the phone, the missionary told me that the raw-foodist was known for cooking his water, instead of his food! The lesson I picked up from this conversation was valuable: if you are in a less-developed country with a questionable water supply, boil your water before drinking it to kill any parasites. Water-born parasites are a primary source of illness in less-developed countries.

Consider packing powdered cayenne with you on your travels. Powdered cayenne has been shown to protect against water-borne amoebic dysentery, a common ailment afflicting travelers in less-developed nations. Powdered cinnamon has also been shown to be very effective.

Eating while traveling requires planning ahead. Leverage your mind. You have built within you the intuitive ability to intelligently set goals and think ahead.

Contact Nature's First Law to pick up the book **Tofu Tollbooth** by Dar Williams, which is a state-by-state directory of over 1,000 natural-food stores in the United States and/or the book **Vegetarian Journal's Guide To Natural Foods Restaurants In The U.S. And Canada** which contains a listing of over 2,000 vegetarian-friendly restaurants, juice bars, and delicatessens. The Nature's First Law magazine, **Just Eat An Apple**, regularly updates readers on the status and location of all raw-food restaurants in the world. Also, review the **Raw-Food Restaurants** section at the back of this book.

How To Eat Raw In The City

Cities typically abound with chemicals and toxins. Because of all the toxicity in the air and water, we need to protect ourselves. I have found that densifying the body with more young coconuts and nuts protects the body from pollution. If we are totally purified on a raw-food diet containing little or no fats, pollution can filter into us (things move from areas of greater concentration to areas of lesser concentration). By eating nuts we provide a dense fat substance which moves into the lymph and thickens our tissues — this protects us. Nut fats also provide us with more antioxidants to protect against free radicals formed from city toxins.

I have also found protection in the city by eating significantly more ripe hot peppers. Every city contains ill people who are carrying within them large amounts of toxicity which may be breeding virulent bacteria. City life often brings us into direct physical contact with these people. Hot peppers are antibiotics which wipe out harmful bacteria, thus aiding our immune system. Hot peppers may be eaten with avocados or nuts to "cut" their heat. If hot peppers are too strong for you, you might want to add garlic, onions, or ginger to your diet while in the city.

Eating Food Naturally

Food tastes better when you eat it naturally. The taste is altered when utensils are used. Have you ever eaten juicy, ripe, organic watermelon without a knife, just with your hands? One time my cousin and health partner R.C. Dini and I decided to eat a ripe organic watermelon (I had grown in my backyard) without using a knife. We waited until it was ripe and soft enough for us to punch into the shell with our fists. Then, under a shiny afternoon Sun, we broke into the melon and began scooping out handful after handful of luscious melon. It was one of the most incredible eating experiences I have ever had. The melon tasted better. The seeds never got in the way, because when a watermelon is eaten naturally, the seeds slip through your fingers! Watermelon seeds only get in the way when the melon is eaten unnaturally with a knife! Those types of insights make life wonderful! Try eating a watermelon with your bare hands and you will agree with Nature's First Law's saying: "Watermelon is the top food on the planet."

Superior Food Combining

Natural Hygiene is philosophy that promotes entirely natural means to heal the body by using properly combined whole plant foods, exercise,

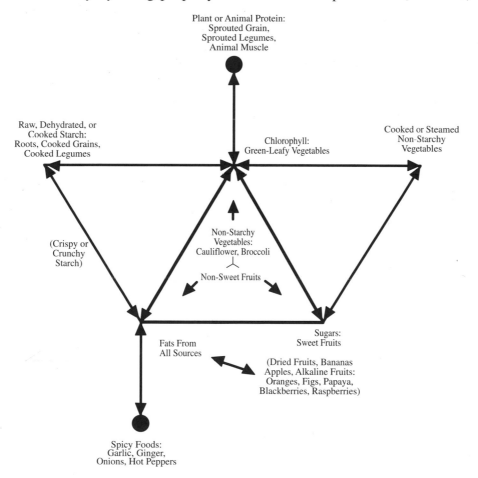

Superior Food Combining: Arrows indicate good combinations.

Sunshine, and rest. The principles of food combining espoused by Natural Hygiene in books such as the Diamond's **Fit For Life** and Herbert Shelton's **Food Combining Made Easy** work extremely well for the average cooked-food eater. They worked for me when I first applied them. These principles essentially demonstrate that cooked proteins (steak) and cooked carbohydrates (potatoes) should not be eaten together, and that all cooked foods should be eaten with a salad. They also demonstrate the vital point that only one type of concentrated (cooked) food should be eaten at a meal. Also, they suggest fruits should be eaten alone.

The challenge with the old food combining principles is that they are outdated and much has been learned since they were formulated decades ago. My new guidelines are not strict (but helpful!) — eating should be fun. Below, I have listed my suggestions for superior food combining:

1. If cooked or dehydrated foods are eaten, try to eat only one type per meal.

2. Fruit always digests best on an empty stomach. It is always best to eat sweet fruits in a mono-diet (one type of fruit per meal) unless they are hybridized (seedless or have weak seeds) in which case they should be combined with greens or even fats. Sweet fruits may be eaten with green-leafed vegetables.

3. The following fruits combine well with fat-dominant foods: dried fruits, bananas, apples, and alkaline fruits (citrus, figs, papaya, berries). Fat-dominant foods include: avocados, olives or their oil, nuts, seeds or their oil, coconuts, seeds, and raw dairy (not recommended). Combining sweet fruits and fats will allow the sugar from the sweet fruit to be time-released, providing more long-term energy.

4. If sweet fruits are eaten with cooked or steamed non-starchy vegetables (asparagus, cauliflower, broccoli), the fruit should be eaten first. Combining sweet fruits and non-starchy cooked vegetables will allow the sugar from the sweet fruit to be time-released, again providing more

long-term energy. Sweet fruits should otherwise not be mixed with cooked or dehydrated foods due to the potential for fermentation and gas.

5. Initially, stay with one type of sweet fruit at a time. One may eat multiple types of sweet fruit together as the digestive strength increases over weeks, months, and years of eating raw plant foods.

6. Green-leafed vegetables of different varieties may be mixed and eaten together.

7. Green-leafed vegetables should always be eaten with any cooked starches (bread, pasta, rice, cakes), except for crispy or crunchy starches (corn chips, potato chips, toast, popcorn), which should be eaten with fats (avocados, olives or their oil, young coconut, seed oils, etc.). Crispy or crunchy starch is very coarse and harsh on the soft tissues of the body. Fats soften the abrasive quality of these foods.

8. Foods dehydrated below 104 degrees Fahrenheit are great for transition and for an occasional treat because the enzymes are intact and they provide a bridge away from cooked food. Typical dehydrated foods should be eaten with green-leafy vegetables. Crispy dehydrated foods should be eaten with plant fats. When transitioning onto raw foods, I found benefit in squeezing lemon or lime juice on cooked foods and dehydrated foods. This adds flavor, enzymes, and alkalinity without contributing to fermentation of the food in digestion.

9. Cooked foods and dehydrated foods should not be mixed together as it may cause a clash, fermentation, and overall poor digestion. Again, only one concentrated food should be eaten per meal.

10. All plant or animal protein-dominant foods, such as sprouted grain, sprouted legumes, and animal muscle (not recommended) should be eaten with green-leafed vegetables to cut the acid-forming potential of those foods, and to add fiber. Meat and dairy products have no fiber.

11. Initially, stay with one type of fat per meal. Eventually, one may eat multiple types of raw fats together (e.g. avocados with nuts in a salad) as the digestive strength increases over weeks, months, and years of eating raw plant foods.

12. Spicy foods, such as hot peppers, garlic, onions, ginger, etc., are not toxic if they are amenable to you. Eat them with fats. I can eat ripe red jalapeno peppers one after the other while feeling only a slight heat. (And that is an important point, peppers must be *ripe* or they are toxic.)

13. Low-sugar fruits and raw non-starchy vegetables may be eaten together (e.g. okra and cauliflower). Different types of low-sugar fruits may be mixed together (e.g. cucumbers and tomatoes). Different types of non-starchy vegetables (e.g. asparagus and purple cabbage) may be mixed together.

14. Low-sugar fruits and raw non-starchy vegetables may be eaten alone (mono-diet), or with greens or fats. If sweet fruits are eaten with low-sugar fruits and/or non-starchy vegetables (asparagus, cauliflower, broccoli), the sweet fruits should be eaten first.

15. For purposes of food combining, seaweeds (dulse, nori) or algaes (blue-green, chlorella, spirulina) may be treated as green-leafed vegetables; however, they are not a replacement for green-leafed vegetables.

16. Raw fermented foods (e.g. seed cheeses or sauerkraut), which often appear in accelerated healing diets due to their high enzyme activity, may be eaten with green-leafed vegetables to calm their digestion. Seed cheeses can combine well with cooked and/or dehydrated crackers.

17. After some time of eating all raw plant foods you may find your digestion will have strengthened to the point where you can combine almost any foods within The Sunfood Triangle together without any adverse reactions. I have even combined watermelon, macadamia nuts, avocados, cucumbers, kale, and tomatoes at the same time without an adverse reaction!

18. The overall balance of your food intake should keep you within The Sunfood Triangle no matter what you are eating. For example, if you eat protein, eat it with greens, then eat fats and/or sweet fruits when the meal is totally digested to help pull you back within the triangle. If you eat cooked starch (sugar), you need more greens and fats to find a balance.

Transition Guidelines

1. Control and direct your thoughts. The more you think about yourself as you could be, rather than as you perceive you are, the more excited you will become about increasing your health. You will begin to see yourself as a radiant being. You will be convinced you can do it. One day you will succeed in performing something you previously thought of as quite impossible to accomplish. You may not even notice this extraordinary deed. But as you keep on performing impossible acts, or as impossible things keep on happening, you become aware that a sort of power is emerging.

2. What you do must be the product of your own conclusions. At some point on this dietary journey, you are going to have to have faith. Faith in the restoring power of natural foods. Faith in yourself and your own good judgment. No degree of success is possible without some degree of trust in our intuition and the unknown. This was laid out in Napoleon Hill's book **Think And Grow Rich**. In fact, he dedicated a whole chapter to faith, and I present you a lesson on faith as well.

3. Guard your mind against the negative influences of other people. Critically think through the free advice. Anything acquired without effort and without cost is generally not helpful. Seek out and listen to those who are getting the results you desire.

4. Transition smoothly away from the meat-based diet as calmly and as quickly as possible. People often first let go of red meat, then pork, then chicken, and then fish. This pattern works extremely well. Replace meat with avocados, nuts, and seeds. By transitioning from a cooked-meat diet

to a vegetarian diet, happier feelings, more vigorous health experiences, and positive emotions will arise more often.

5. Transition smoothly away from dairy foods by first letting go of eggs and milk, and then cheese. Move to raw organic milk or cheese if you feel it is necessary in transition. Replace dairy foods with green-leafed vegetables for calcium and avocados, nuts, and/or seeds for their excellent raw plant-fat content.

6. Continue to eat a large percentage of raw plant foods throughout your transition. Once you have let go of animal foods and have adopted a vegan diet, then you may find the transition to all raw foods easier.

7. The body feels a shake up and discomfort with a sudden change in diet. Counselors who have worked with drug addicts know that it can be dangerous to stop a drug habit too abruptly. The body can be shocked by being deprived of a certain poison, such as cocaine, especially when this drug's constant use has forced the body to adapt itself to the poison. A drug can actually become a physiological necessity one must wean away from. This same principle holds true with cooked food. Transition at your own pace, but continue moving forward. To be successful in anything, you must be willing to step outside of your comfort zone. Push the bounds of your potential. All successful people have this in common. You may realize your comfort zone was never really comfortable! Stabilize at 70% raw, then 80%, then 90%. A 100% raw plant-food diet is the real magic.

8. The ultimate diet and health success formula: "Increase raw, decrease cooked." It works every time.

9. Take massive raw-foods action. Start consistently putting significant amounts of high-quality raw plant foods into your body instead of cooked food. Just get the raw food into your body and everything else follows. Invest in a juicer. Drinking fresh vegetable juice daily (about 1/2 liter or more) is extremely important in the transition process and beyond. Drink slowly; mix the juice well with your saliva before swallowing. Drinking

fresh vegetable juice allows minerals to reach the blood and tissues quickly. Contact Nature's First Law to find out how to obtain the **highest-quality juicers** in the world:

(888) 729-3663 or (619) 596-7979
http://www.rawfood.com

10. Eat wild, home-grown, and/or organic food. Organic food is grown without pesticides and other dangerous chemicals, such as chemical fertilizers (see the section on **Organic Food** above). Eating pesticide-free food is extremely important for health.

11. For the ideal digestion and assimilation of fruits, maintain a mono-diet (one fruit at a time) whenever comfortable. If you do eat more than one type of fruit, give yourself 30-60 minutes between fruit types. Fruits may be combined, but the mono-diet does provide the best digestion. The mono-diet is based on the realization that when you eat any fruit in its original state, its taste changes at some point from pleasant to unpleasant. This means that when the organism has filled its need for that particular food, it no longer wants any more and the taste of the food changes. Pineapple, for example, gives a very strong taste change and can actually burn the mouth if one continues to eat past the signal. This is called an aliesthetictaste change.

12. For ideal digestion and assimilation, eat green-leafy vegetables with raw plant fats and eat raw plant fats with green-leafy vegetables.

13. Chew your food well (50 to 100 chews per mouthful). This is going to take some concentration. An East Indian proverb states: "Chew your food well for the stomach has no teeth." Another proverb states: "Drink your food, chew your juice." Remember, the entire premise behind digestion is to turn the food into a liquid so it may be absorbed.

14. Eating seasonal fruits and green-leafed vegetables is Nature's way of telling you what to eat and when. My health partner, Stephen Arlin,

stresses this point greatly. His book **Raw Power!** contains a comprehensive guide to seasonal produce availability.

15. Eat fruits which contain good, strong, viable seeds. Eat fruits in their perfectly ripe stage. A perfectly ripe jalapeno pepper is red. A perfectly ripe lime is yellow. A perfectly ripe eggplant is yellow.

16. Eat more sweet fruit if you are active. Eat more green-leafy vegetables if you are sedentary.

17. Be aware that cooked-food cravings present themselves when you are tired (at the end of a long day). Be prepared. Go to sleep early if necessary. Drink a glass of pure water with a twist of fresh lemon. Persist, break the cravings, and soon the desire disappears.

18. For ideal food use and assimilation: eat only when actual hunger exists. Avoid "emotional" or "boredom" eating.

19. Exercise is the key to metabolizing food. Food is best metabolized when the desire is created for it through exercise. Exercise creates a "draw" for nutrients within the blood and lymph systems. *To thrive on a raw-food diet, exercise is essential.*

20. Digestion is an art. Try eating while standing up. When you are sitting, your internal organs are pinched and digestion is hindered. Also, try fully squatting, instead of sitting, during a bowel movement elimination.

21. Make a practice of eating the foods that digest well for you.

22. Food itself is an anchor which accesses different emotional states. To break food addictions, identify which emotional state you are trying to reach and then discover a way to get there without food. Periods of food obsession will pass, just stay the course. Work through emotional addictions to food. You can do it.

23. Have a relative, friend, spouse, or lover do The Sunfood Diet with you. Support each other.

24. Get a job, career, or simply volunteer in either the diet, exercise, health, or success field! This will challenge you to walk your talk and keep pushing beyond former boundaries. It will bring you in contact with positive, supportive people. Introduce this book to new, positive acquaintances to help them along.

25. Consider donating all the cooked foods, pots, and pans in your home to charity. When you decide to make the "jump," go to local organic food stores, farmer's markets, or farms and purchase a massive amount of raw plant food — get a good variety — and let the fun begin.

26. Initially, experiment with the all-raw diet on a small scale. First go 100% raw for a day. Then extend that to a week, or a month. Set in advance a specific date and mark each successful day on a calendar. Understand that after you go 100% raw for 5-7 months straight, your body will resist any type of return to the previous cooked-food diet.

27. What is the method by which your body returns to its natural state? It is the pain/pleasure principle. As your body becomes more and more in tune with itself, the pain/pleasure principle takes over. Raw plant foods eventually become so pleasurable that other choices are no longer possible!

28. Meet other people excited about eating a raw plant-food diet. Hold regular raw-food potlucks. Place a raw-food potluck notice on the bulletin board of your local natural-foods market.

29. This book has been designed as a constant source of motivation. My desire is that the intensity of the emotion and the inspiration with which I live my life and which I have put into this book are passed along to you consistently. This book was created for you. Refer to it often. For support, reference our Internet web-site (http://www.rawfood.com) or e-mail

us (nature@rawfood.com). If you do not have a computer, Internet access is available at any public library.

30. Educate yourself. Saturate your mind (see **Lesson 25: Saturation Point**). Read, listen to audio tapes, watch video tapes about natural, raw plant-food nutrition. Discuss the idea with others. What you think about, comes about. If you would like to read other books on eating raw plant foods, browse our on-line Internet catalog:

http://www.rawfood.com/cgi-bin/order/index.cgi
Or contact Nature's First Law to receive a free copy.

Cooked Starches

Cooked starches (breads, pastas, cakes, rice, corn chips, potato chips, baked potatoes, popcorn, cookies) are typically the last cooked foods to go for most people as they transition into raw foods. This is because cooked starch is the most addictive and the most blood-sugar-altering food. LifeFood nutritionist Dr. David Jubb has pointed out that starch does not appear in foods growing wildly, starch develops as foods are genetically cross-bred and hybridized (see **Lesson 16: Hybrid Food**).

A diet heavy in cooked starch over many decades can cause arteriosclerosis, hardening of the blood vessels, ossification of the tissues and joints, skin thickening, and premature aging. As Professor Arnold Ehret pointed out, the reason a cooked-meat eater might live longer than a starch-eating vegetarian is because the first produces less obstructions than the starchy overeater; but the meat-eater's later diseases are always more dangerous because of the accumulated poisons, pus, and uric acid found in the meats.

To help overcome addictions to cooked starch, one can switch to dehydrated starchy foods. Every little discipline adds upon every other. Another useful tool is to combine sweet fruits and fats together in a meal. For example, oranges can be eaten with avocado or apples with nuts.

This simulates the gradual sugar release from the breakdown of complex carbohydrates (cooked starch) in digestion.

Dehydrated Food

Dehydrated foods (foods heated below 104 degrees Fahrenheit) are an excellent tool to help succeed with the raw-food approach. Dehydrated foods still have the enzymes intact and my experience has been that they do not dampen the raw-food "high." However, I rarely eat dehydrated foods and I imagine they could alter the raw-food "high" if overeaten regularly. Many raw-food recipe books describe how to make dehydrated foods. I recommend **Living In The Raw**, **The Raw Gourmet**, and **RAW: The Uncook Book**.

Frozen Food

Generally, freezing food destroys anywhere from 30% to 66% of the enzymes in the food. Freezing is not as damaging as cooking. My own experiences and experiments have demonstrated that freezing alters the water in food and causes slow or constipated digestion if frozen food (even if defrosted) is eaten in excessive quantities. Water expands when frozen. The delicate fibrous structures inside all fruits and vegetables are damaged as water expands during the freezing process.

Some raw plant foods are more tolerant of freezing than others. Durians, for example, tolerate freezing well. Berries are tolerant of the freezing process. Nuts and seeds are more tolerant of freezing temperatures as they have a low-water content.

Overeating

Every Sunfoodist grows through periods of eating large quantities of raw plant foods, especially during the transition and beyond. This is part of overcoming cooked-food cravings and releasing emotions. I recommend that you tune in to the aliesthetic taste change, progressively simplify your diet, face sunken emotions when they come up, and enjoy the process of becoming healthier, happier, and more joyful.

My personal feeling is that occasionally overeating raw plant foods is okay! You still get the results and the spiritual connection. A gorilla might eat 60 pounds (27 kilograms) of fruits and vegetables a day! Considering that a gorilla weighs 3 times as much as the average person, we may deduce that eating 1/3 of a gorillas fare would not be overeating. 1/3 of 60 pounds is 20 pounds of fruits and vegetables! Nobody can eat 20 pounds (9 kilograms) of raw fruits and vegetables every single day.

If you overeat one type of food, such as sweet fruit, remember The Sunfood Triangle: balance by eating more fats and green-leafed vegetables. Many new Sunfoodists overeat dried fruit and nuts; this is okay, as long as it is balanced by green-leafed vegetables (see The Sunfood Triangle). Also, it is better to overeat avocados than nuts, as avocados are more digestible.

Something to keep in mind: a raw-foodist once gave me a great piece of knowledge, he said, "Any food is addictive, if you eat too much of it." *Switch your common foods around occasionally.* Also, sometimes skip a meal and just drink water. Drinking water helps to alleviate hunger.

Eating more high-quality green-leafy vegetables and less sweet fruit stops you from overeating. This demonstrates that overeating is often caused more by a desire for minerals, and less by the desire for calories.

The best way to overcome the desire for eating is to be so busy striving for and achieving goals that no time is left to eat!

Enjoy your new diet. Once you feel capable, begin experimenting with eating less, until you feel comfortable with less food. Refine your diet with time — be patient. The saying goes: "Eat a little, that way, you'll be around long enough to eat a lot." Systematic undereating slows the aging process.

Flatulence

When one begins The Sunfood Diet, fermentations may occur which form gas and flatulence in the intestinal tract. This may have several causes which are listed below:

1. When Sunfoods reach plaque encrusted intestines (impacted with mucus and hardened fecal matter), they will not digest properly and a fermentation will occur. To alleviate this situation, one should have a series of 5 to 8 colonics conducted by a registered colon hydrotherapist and also undertake an herbal cleanse such as EJUVA (please call Nature's First Law at 888-RAW-FOOD for more details on this cleanse).

2. Foods are being combined haphazardly in less than ideal combinations. It is best to eat one type of food at a time, waiting twenty minutes to an hour to consume the next item.

3. Foods which are difficult to digest, such as bean sprouts, wheatberry sprouts, or soaked oats, are eaten in large quantities without being mixed with a sufficiently large quantity of green-leafed vegetables.

4. Overeating apples and pears (or their juices). These foods contain large quantities of pectin and other bowel cleansing compounds which can increase flatulence.

5. Undereating sodium-residue foods — especially greens (kale, celery, dandelion, spinach). These foods cool the intestines. When the intestines are heated by too much potassium or sulfur-residue foods, flatulence results.

If one repeatedly experiences gas and fermentation from eating sweet fruit as a mono-diet, this could be a sign of a candida infection. If this is your situation, please review **Lesson 13: How To Use The Sunfood Triangle** under the section **Eating To Overcome Candida**.

Natural healers know that snake bites are dangerous, not only because of the venom, but also due to the fermentation they cause in the tissues. Ice on a snake bite will halt fermentation (and also decrease circulation to slow the spread of the venom). To stop digestive fermentation, place a cool object or ice-pack on the diaphragm, or get into cold water. Sucking on ice cubes for 15 minutes may also be helpful.

Better Choices

Choose positive friends over negative relatives.

Choose wine over beer. Wine is raw! Wine is simply the product of grape fermentation. Beer is brewed (cooked)! I have experienced that an occasional glass of wine does not break or hinder the Sunfood "high." Beer, however, always snapped the spell and I gave that up years ago. Choose organic wine containing no added sulfites.

Choose dandelion over iceberg lettuce. Commercial iceberg lettuce contains very little nutrition. Dandelion is a wild food which contains a full complement of minerals.

Choose yams over potatoes. Potatoes are genetically weak, hybridized foods. Yams are closer to the wild state; they contain far better nutrition.

Choose raw corn over corn chips. Have you ever eaten raw corn? We call it the "raw corn revelation." Even though it is a hybrid food, a little white sweet corn in the summer time is beautiful during the transition process.

Choose ocean water or dulse seaweed over salt. Taste ocean water or dulse seaweed with lime, with tomato, with avocado! If any sprinkled salt is to be used, consider using highly-mineralized celtic sea salt.

Choose dried fruit over candy. Dried fruit is filled with natural sugar which the body can recognize. Candy contains refined sugar which the body does not recognize and which acts as a powerful behavioral drug. Eat green-leafed vegetables with or following dried fruit to clean the teeth.

Choose dates over honey. Because most farm bees are cruelly treated and have their honey (food) taken away and replaced with sugar-water and antibiotics, I do not recommend honey. However, those with problems with bread addiction may find relief by spreading raw organic cruelty-free honey on their bread. The enzymes (amylase in honey) will begin to predigest the bread starch.

Choose dates and almonds over chocolate. To conquer addictions to chocolate, replace chocolate with dates which have had their pits removed and a raw almond inserted. I had an encounter recently at one of my seminars with a woman to whom I recommended this months before. She had such success eating date-almond balls instead of chocolate that she actually decided to adopt The Sunfood Diet!

Choose dried prunes over dates. If you feel dates are too sugary or too strong, switch to dried prunes. If dates are eaten, they should be eaten in the fall and winter when they are in season. As far as dried fruit is concerned (while you are in the transition stage), prunes are a better choice than dates.

Choose dried figs over raisins. Raisins are great, if they have seeds! Without seeds they are hybrids (seedless). Dried figs are full of crunchy little seeds that compliment the taste and encourage thorough chewing.

Action Steps:

1. Enjoy your food without fear or anxiety. As long as you are eating the food and it is entering your body, allow it to be fully enjoyed and metabolized! Eat your food naturally — relax. How relaxed are your face, stomach, and hands while you eat?

2. Immediately act upon the transition guidelines outlined in this lesson. How can you adopt the transition principles into your lifestyle today and enjoy the process?

3. Use the Superior Food Combining chart daily. Photocopy the chart and post it in your kitchen or dining area.

4. If you are not able to get organic fruits and vegetables, what do you do?

> 1. Ask for organic food at your local store.
>
> 2. Order organic foods to be delivered by mail to your home (see the **Resources** section at the end of this book).
>
> 3. Start your own garden. If you do not have a yard, ask a friend if you can grow a garden in her/his yard.
>
> 4. Search for local organic growers. Perhaps you can volunteer your services in exchange for food?
>
> 5. Start your own organic farm!
>
> 6. Write a letter to your local politicians, newspapers, and other media outlets, telling them how you feel about the difficulties of finding non-poisoned food in your area.
>
> 7. Eat wild foods.
>
> 8. Plant fruiting plants and trees wherever you legally can and enjoy the harvest each year.
>
> 9. Consider moving to a better location where higher-quality foods are available.

Lesson 13:
How To Use The Sunfood Triangle

The charts provided in this lesson become applicable when 80-100% of your food intake consists of green-leafy vegetables, sweet fruits, and fatty foods. By balancing these three food classes against each other in different ratios, we can achieve different effects. If we eat more greens, and less sweet fruits and fats, we will get one effect. If we eat more sweet fruits, and less greens and fats, we will get another effect. Basically, we can move the center of The Sunfood Triangle around to achieve different results.

Many of the suggestions provided in this lesson are temporary measures. We do need a good, healthy amount of all three food classes in our diet. In some sections below, I recommend a certain food class may be limited, or totally eliminated, from the diet. *This is a temporary measure only!* For example, if we are **Eating For Spirituality** we would remove fat from the diet. We will eventually need fat in the diet; however, this is a temporary suggestion to achieve a specific result.

The diagrams in this lesson are keyed to following dry weight ratio of the three food classes — chlorophyll:sugar:fat.

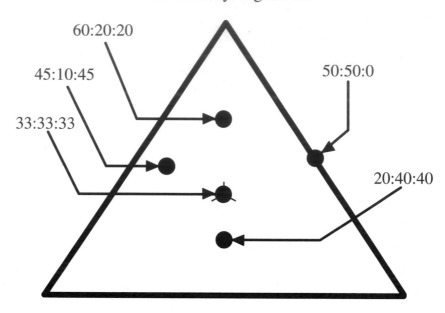

Chlorophyll:
Green-Leafy Vegetables

Fats:
Fatty Fruits, Nuts
Coconuts, Seeds

Sugars:
Sweet Fruits

The Sunfood Triangle: Moving The Center Point
Ratio Key: (Chlorophyll:Sugar:Fat)

Eating For Weight Loss

A diet of raw plant food easily takes off those unwanted pounds. Any cooked foods eaten should be properly combined. This means that cooked starch (complex carbohydrates) should not be combined with cooked protein (meat), and any cooked foods should be eaten with a large green-leafy salad.

Specifically target and minimize cooked fats (heated oils, pasteurized milk and cheese, cooked eggs, and fat-dominant meats, such as bacon) and cooked starch (bread, pasta, cakes, cookies) in the diet as they both put on the extra pounds. Pizza, which contains a high dosage of cooked starch and cooked fat, is particularly fattening. Cooked fats, devoid of lipase (the fat-splitting enzyme), accumulate in the body as they are difficult to metabolize and this results in weight gain (raw fats, such as avocados, can actually help one lose weight as they contain lipase — which the body can use to help metabolize stores of cooked fats). Cooked starch is essentially sugar, and if this sugar is not used as fuel, or urinated away by the body, it is converted to fat.

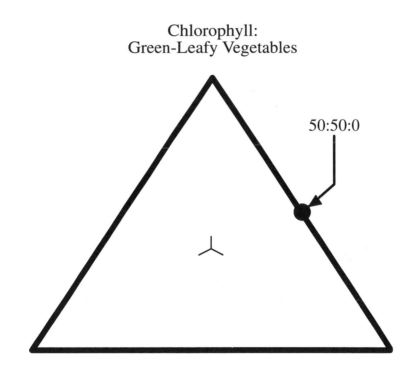

Chlorophyll:
Green-Leafy Vegetables

50:50:0

Fats:
Fatty Fruits, Nuts
Coconuts, Seeds

Sugars:
Sweet Fruits

To Lose Weight center at 50:50:0
Ratio Key: Chlorophyll: Sugar: Fat

The best strategy is to eat the raw fruits and vegetables that you like the best. As you progress, you will gradually decrease the amount of cooked food that you are eating, and you will develop a taste for different raw, healthy fruits and vegetables. R.C. Dini, co-author of the book **Nature's First Law: The Raw-Food Diet**, whom I have mentioned throughout these pages, lost 156 pounds (70 kg) eating raw plant foods! In 3 years he dropped from 300 lbs. to 144 lbs. (135 kg to 65 kg). That is a dramatic life transformation! As he learned, weight loss is easy when it is done intelligently and naturally with raw plant foods.

If one simply remains within The Sunfood Triangle regime at an all-raw level, the body will take off the necessary weight over time. However, if one is looking to accelerate weight loss, then one should cut fats out of the diet (or at least minimize them) until you have reached your desired weight. Nuts, in particular, should be eliminated from the diet for weight loss.

Eating For Weight Gain

How many obese animals do we see in Nature? Animals carry exactly the weight they need and no more. Every animal in Nature is at a perfect weight without exception. What is considered a normal weight by civilization's standards is actually an artificial weight created by a cooked-food diet. Your natural weight might be 5-10 pounds (2.3 to 4.5 kg) lighter than what is recommended in the charts. However, these charts are not always accurate as people differ in bone size, bone and tissue density, musculature, etc.

Initially, when you adopt The Sunfood Diet, you will most likely lose weight as your body detoxifies wastes it has accumulated over a lifetime. This is a necessary process. Don't worry about it, embrace it. First and foremost, allow your body to detoxify.

The inability to gain weight when eating raw plant foods may be caused by cooked-food transgressions. Eating cooked starch (bread, cookies, pasta, rice, etc.) actually promotes weight loss when one is significantly purified and has been eating 95%+ raw food for more than 6 months. When the body is at that level of purification, digesting cooked starch drains living water and vital energy, leaving one sallow.

The inability to gain weight when eating raw plant foods may also be due to an encrusted intestinal tract, which hinders food absorption and causes emaciation. Encrusted mucus on the intestinal wall will eventually be dislodged over time if one eats exclusively raw foods and green salads daily. However, the process may be accelerated by a series of 6-10 colon irrigations (colonics), and an herbal cleanse program (available from Nature's First Law. See the **Organizations** and **Resources** sections at the end of this book).

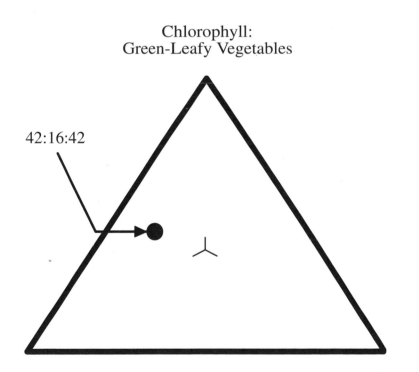

Chlorophyll:
Green-Leafy Vegetables

42:16:42

Fats:
Fatty Fruits, Nuts
Coconuts, Seeds

Sugars:
Sweet Fruits

To Gain Weight center at 42:16:42
Ratio Key: (Chlorophyll:Sugar:Fat)

The inability to gain weight when eating raw plant foods may also be due to parasitic infections which may cause emaciation. If you suspect that you have a parasitic infection, I recommend that you "burn" them out with daily meals containing one or more of the following: garlic, onions, hot peppers, ginger, and spicy wild greens (wild mustard is excellent). High-quality herbal remedies will be effective against parasites.

Once the body is significantly detoxified, which may take anywhere from 4 months to 2 years, depending on the toxicity of the body beforehand, then you can gain all the healthy weight you desire. I recommend you do so in the method shown in the previous diagram.

The secret to gaining strength and weight by eating a raw plant-food diet is to eat green-leafed vegetables and plant fats...together — and fewer sweet fruits. More non-sweet fruits may be included as well. My own experience proved this true. I found it worked for thousands of others I have counseled. Test for yourself and see.

Think of the gorilla: pound per pound the strongest land mammal. The gorilla possesses a fantastic musculature and is capable of bench pressing 4,000 pounds (more than 1800 kg). In his wonderful book, **L'Homme, Le Singe, Et Le Paradis** (Humans, Primates, and Paradise), Albert Mosseri describes:

(Translation) "The gorilla is not interested in eating so-called protein foods. How can they develop all that muscle mass, weighing many hundreds of pounds, eating only green vegetables and fruits? This fact is of great importance."

Since gorillas eat nearly 80% green-leafed vegetation and have a similar digestive physiology to the human body, the lesson here is that eating plenty of green-leafed vegetation increases strength and muscle mass.

All the building blocks necessary to construct and energize your body are present in plants. Out of the 22 amino acids found in the body, 8 must be derived from food. The body is capable of recycling and manufacturing the other 14 amino acids by itself. All 8 essential amino acids are packaged in abundance in raw plant foods, especially green leaves.

Raw plant fats are "fatty." They are heavy. They will put just the right amount of fat on your body to give you excellent proportions and a good shape. They also add weight indirectly by providing fuel for working the muscles to build muscle mass. However, eating more fats alone will not cause weight gain, greens must be added. Fats help the body assimilate the amino acids and minerals from greens.

My personal meal formula for gaining weight consists of a salad containing the following three foods:
   a. Tomatoes (Non-sweet fruits with a high water-content)
   b. Macadamia nuts (High-fat nuts)
   c. Kale leaves (Dense in minerals, amino acids, and protein)

I have eaten this mixture for lunch and dinner on many occasions. After several years on The Raw-Food Diet, my weight stabilized at 150 pounds (68 kg). This salad combination, in conjunction with vigorous exercise, helped me gain 18 pounds (8.2 kg) and reach 168 pounds (76 kg) in a span of two years while maintaining my all-raw diet and a body-fat level of 9.4%. I am 6 feet tall (190 cm).

Another good weight gain combination I have enjoyed is eating avocados with the Nature's First Law olives and chasing them with green juice.

The heaviest tissues in your body are muscle, fat, and bone in that order. It has been estimated that 50% of your body weight is muscle!

Consistent exercise is also important for gaining weight. Engage in rigorous exercise; work and enlarge your muscles; increase your muscle mass by doing more resistant, anaerobic exercise.

Also, consider the wise words of the Greek historian Herodotus: "Exposure to the Sun is highly necessary in persons whose health needs restoring and who have need of putting on weight." The ancient Greeks and Romans knew the Sun feeds the muscles. For males, the Sun's rays on the skin and the genital organs stimulate the production of testosterone which increases muscle size and sexual potency. The muscles receive an increased amount of blood flow when they are exposed to Sunlight. This helps to provide nutrients to build strength.

Slowing the metabolism will allow one to increase their weight. There is great value in avoiding frequent snacks. The way to gain weight on The Sunfood Diet is to eat more food, less often! The more often you eat, the quicker your metabolism runs, and the more weight you will lose. The less often you eat, the slower will be your metabolism, and the more weight you will gain or retain. Also and again, to gain weight one must eat more green-leafy foods and fats and eat less sweet fruits, as described above.

People who are of an ayurvedic vata constitution (typically a person who tends to be thin already) will find great weight gain value in blending salads to create soups (see Sequoia's Calcium Soup in the **Recipes** section of this book for more information on blended raw soups). Blending food adds more caloric value and increases the mineral density of foods, both of which have a balancing effect for a vata constitution.

For the best possible information on body-building and weight gain on a raw plant-food diet, read raw-food body-builder, Stephen Arlin's new book **Raw Power!** His book outlines many great strategies on gaining healthy weight and super-strength. It includes five weekly work-out programs, a raw-food recipe section for gaining weight and building muscle, and a seasonal produce availability chart. Stephen is 6'2" and currently weighs 225 pounds (102 kilograms) eating all-raw plant foods. Listen to someone who is getting the results you desire!

Feeding Healthy Children

The most beautiful children I have met or seen have been children raised on raw plant foods. They are alert, content, happy, and eager to explore life. The world's most famous childcare specialist Dr. Benjamin Spock recommended, in the final seventh edition of his famous book **Baby And Child Care**, breast-feeding until solid foods were introduced. He specifically recommended a vegetarian diet at that point and, beyond age two, a vegan diet with an emphasis on raw plant foods. Dr. Spock's own vegetarian diet had "given him a new lease on life." He wanted the seventh edition of his book to be in the forefront of linking animal foods and disease.

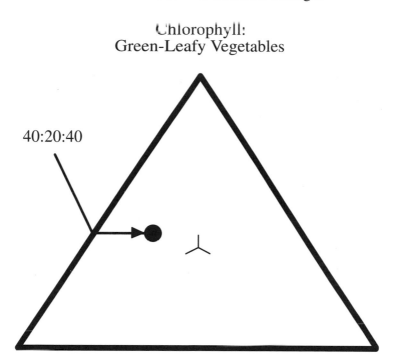

Chlorophyll:
Green-Leafy Vegetables

40:20:40

Fats:
Fatty Fruits, Nuts
Coconuts, Seeds

Sugars:
Sweet Fruits

To Feed Children center at 40:20:40
Ratio Key: (Chlorophyll:Sugar:Fat)

Children naturally gravitate towards sweet, bright-colored fruits. Parents must keep in mind that children also need fat and chlorophyll-rich foods. Calcium is extremely important for growing children, and if not coming from the mother's breast milk, it must be in the diet in the form of green-leaves and/or green juices in sufficient quantities.

If your children have trouble eating green-leafed vegetables, try mixing apples or pears with green-vegetable juice — all freshly made. Try feeding your children **Sequoia's Calcium Soup** found in **Appendix C: Sunfood Recipes** at the back of this book. Also, lead by example. Children do what you do, not what you say (as I am sure you have already discovered!).

Pregnant mothers should also balance their Sunfood Diet with more greens and fats with lots of variety to feed the growing baby. Foods with plenty of trace minerals (edible wild plants, flower pollen, seeds, etc.) should be included in the diet of children and pregnant mothers.

For more information on breastfeeding, natural childbirth, mother-child bonding, and raw-food parenting, please read Hygeia Halfmoon's beautiful book **Primal Mothering In A Modern World**. Also, **The Continuum Concept** is another classic book on natural child care.

Eating For The Elderly

Imagine that the entire digestive tract from the mouth all the way through the body is one big muscle. Over a lifetime of eating cooked foods lacking in fiber, vitamins, minerals, amino acids, various nutrients, and enzymes, the digestive "muscle" becomes weakened. A weak "muscle" may not be able to handle a large quantity of nutrient-rich, fiber-rich fresh fruits and green leaves immediately. Therefore, it is best to ease a more mature digestive system on to raw plant foods in a manner which allows strengthening and progress without shocking the system. I have found this principle of comfortable transition particular applicable to those over the age of 40 on macrobiotic diets who are switching over to raw foods.

By consistently eating fiber-rich foods (such as green-leafed vegetables) and chewing them very well before swallowing, the digestive "muscle" will be strengthened and cleaned over time.

Elderly people are typically not as active as the younger generation, therefore I recommend less sweet fruit in their diet. The soft, comforting fruit fats (especially avocado) help soothe the more mature digestive system.

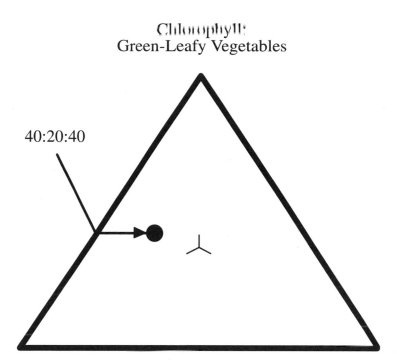

Chlorophyll:
Green-Leafy Vegetables

40:20:40

Fats:
Fatty Fruits, Nuts
Coconuts, Seeds

Sugars:
Sweet Fruits

The Elderly can center at 40:20:40
Ratio Key: (Chlorophyll:Sugar:Fat)
Eating For Detoxification

By eating a diet of 100% raw plant foods, you will automatically detox-ify and heal disease conditions.

To accelerate detoxification and healing, we remove fat from the diet. Juicing and blending foods saves the body digestive energy channeling more energy for healing and detoxification. Dr. Norman Walker recom-mended a sugar food (carrot, beet, apples) and green-leafed vegetables in nearly all his curative juice recipes. He did not quite understand the prob-lems with hybrid foods (foods were not as hybridized in his day as they are now), but he did understand the power of juice fasting! He understood the detoxification power of chlorophyll foods and natural sugar foods with no fatty foods included.

If you are doing an extended juice fast (15 days +), you may want to include small portions of cold-pressed olive or flax oil in with your drinks to provide the body with necessary fat.

My colleague Roe Gallo, a fruitarian and natural healer, has a working theory that one should continue on a juice fast cleansing program until all excessive body fat is eliminated. She believes, as do I, that body fat is where most of the body's poisons are stored. In her book **Perfect Body** she presents testimonies of her clients whom she has helped heal of major illnesses, including breast cancer, through juice fasting.

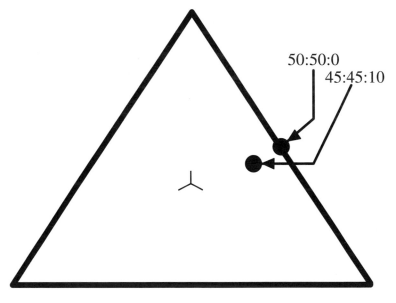

Chlorophyll:
Green-Leafy Vegetables

50:50:0
45:45:10

Fats: Sugars:
Fatty Fruits, Nuts   Sweet Fruits
Coconuts, Seeds

For Detoxification center from 45:45:10 to 50:50:0
Ratio Key: (Chlorophyll:Sugar:Fat)

Eating To Overcome Hypoglycemia And Diabetes

Eating animal foods typically weakens the system to the point where hypoglycemia and diabetes manifest, but (aside from the obviously dangerous white sugar and high fructose corn syrup) cooked hybridized plant starch is the real culprit. Hypoglycemia and diabetes are caused by eating cooked hybrid starchy foods the worst of which includes: white or wheat breads, beer, cooked corn of all types, stewed carrots, refined (beet) sugar, baked potatoes, white rice, french fries, cookies, potato chips, etc. All these food types contain hybrid sugars the liver does not fully recognize and cannot regulate. These sugars send the glycemic index of the blood shooting sky-high causing either too much or too little insulin to be secreted by the pancreas (reference the Glycemic Index Chart in **Lesson 11: The Secret Revealed**).

Hypoglycemia is a condition where too much insulin is secreted into the blood by the pancreas to control blood sugar. Too much insulin in the blood causes blood sugar to drop too rapidly causing mood swings and erratic behavior. Avocados contain a seven-carbon sugar that depresses insulin production, which make them an excellent choice for people with hypoglycemia.

Diabetes (type II) is one-step beyond hypoglycemia, when too little insulin is secreted into the blood. This is an eliminatory process of unused and/or unassimilable sugars, with the pancreas for a time stopping its secretions of insulin so the cells can unload their stocks of undesirable sugars into the bloodstream, and from there send the sugars into the urine to be eliminated. By stepping in at the critical moment and blocking this purge, injected chemical insulin forces the body to live with unacceptable sugars it can hardly tolerate, without being able to dismiss them.

To restore a healthy pancreatic condition, find the center in The Sunfood Triangle. Use good sweet fruits (with seeds) to boost the blood sugar when you feel it is dropping. Fats can be used to thicken up the blood if blood sugars rise too quickly. Green-leaves and especially fresh green vegetable juice eventually provide the body with the alkaline protein and minerals it needs to restore itself to a healthy metabolism.

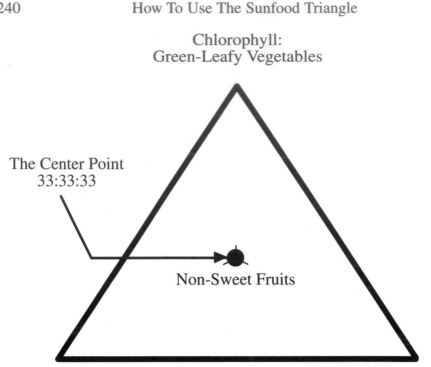

Chlorophyll:
Green-Leafy Vegetables

The Center Point
33:33:33

Non-Sweet Fruits

Fats:
Fatty Fruits, Nuts
Coconuts, Seeds

Sugars:
Sweet Fruits

The Sunfood Triangle: The Center Point
Ratio Key: (Chlorophyll:Sugar:Fat)

If you are on insulin injections, please contact a naturopathic doctor to devise a plan to wean yourself from insulin.

It takes years to heal a diabetic condition, but it can be healed by staying the path. When I was on **The Dating Game**, I met one of the show producers backstage. We started talking about raw foods. She told me her roommate had diabetes and was just beginning to get interested in raw-food nutrition. I called her roommate and we became fast friends. After about 8 months of detoxification and natural foods, while working with a Natural Hygiene practitioner in the Los Angeles area, she was able to stop taking insulin for the first time in 8 years!

My young friend Sergei Boutenko was diagnosed with juvenile onset diabetes at age 9. This was after he collapsed into a near coma from bingoing on Halloween candy. The doctors said he would have to go on insulin for the rest of his life. His mother, Victoria, became determined and set out to find a better way. She asked everybody! Finally, in line one day (two weeks after Sergei's collapse) at the local natural food store, she randomly asked the woman in front of her if she knew anything about helping a child with juvenile onset diabetes. The woman told Victoria she had to get the child on The Raw-Food Diet immediately, and recommended some books by Ann Wigmore. Sergei went raw immediately, his whole family soon followed suit. Within two months he was completely back to normal.

Sergei first visited me in January 1998. He spent a week at my house helping me with business and just having fun (he's now 14 years old). Sergei, his sisters, and parents travel around the United States and Canada catering raw-foods events and teaching people the incredible benefits of The Raw-Food Diet. To have them host an event for you, please contact the Nature's First Law office.

Eating To Overcome Candida

Candida is a fungal parasite that excretes toxic waste that can get into the bloodstream and cause symptoms of bloating, clouded thinking, depression, diarrhea, exhaustion, halitosis (bad breath), menstrual pains, thrush, unclear memory recall, yeast vaginitis, etc.

Diets high in cooked-starches (bread, baked potato, cakes, cookies, pasta) and diets loaded with refined or hybridized (seedless) fruit sugars both feed candida. When all this sugar is added into a body whose levels of good intestinal bacteria (probiotics) are low and whose tissues have become acidic due to a prolonged lack of alkaline mineral salts (which come from vegetables) in the diet, then candida proliferates.

Those suffering from candida typically have had a long history of antibiotic use. This eliminates much of the good intestinal bacteria and also allows candida to spread. High doses of healthy intestinal probiotics that will implant and colonize the intestines are required to overcome candida.

Chlorophyll:
Green-Leafy Vegetables

50:0:50

Fats:
Fatty Fruits, Nuts
Coconuts, Seeds

Sugars:
Sweet Fruits

To Overcome Candida, center at 50:0:50
Ratio Key: (Chlorophyll:Sugar:Fat)

Systemic yeast infections (candidiasis) find growth potential in a damp, musty condition in the body. The very first recommendation I give to those with candida is to get more direct Sunlight on the skin. Candida is a yeast and then a fungus when its rhizoids (long roots) penetrate the tissue mucosa and bridge the boundary between the internal body and digestive tract. Yeasts and fungi are destroyed by direct Sunlight. Those with candida must get their naked body into the Sun as much as they can. Candida can thrive only in a dark, moldy environment.

When cooked starch and refined or hybridized fruit sugars are removed from the diet, when the body tissues become more alkaline, when good flora begins to proliferate, and when the dark, moldy environment is eliminated, candida automatically comes under control.

For all my clients with candida, I recommend a specific diet of raw vegetables (mostly greens or non-sweet vegetables such as nopales or jicama...no potatoes, beets, or carrots), green juices, occasional soaked nuts and seeds, young coconut, raw coconut butter (oil), a wide-variety of low-sugar fruits, and one to two sweet fruits a day (if they need it or feel comfortable with it).

Excellent low-sugar fruits include:
    Avocado (fatty fruit, excellent)
    Bell Pepper (not green; green peppers are harsh and unripe)
    Bitter Melon
    Breadfruit (raw)
    Cranberry
    Cucumber (very healing)
    Grapefruit
    Lemon (may irritate the candida sufferer)
    Lime (may irritate the candida sufferer)
    Noni
    Okra (very healing)
    Olives (not from a can., Call Nature's First Law for the best)
    Pumpkin
    Sour apples
    Squash
    Tomatillo
    Tomato
    Zucchini

A food that provides particularly excellent benefits is raw coconut butter (oil). Coconut oil is easily digested and is excellent for people who have trouble digesting fats. Coconut oil consists of 48% lauric acid, a substance that exhibits anti-microbial, anti-bacterial, and anti-fungal properties. All of these characteristics help to combat a candida overgrowth. (Cold-pressed Fijian coconut oil is now available from Nature's First Law, call 888-RAW-FOOD.)

One can find great benefit eating no sweet fruit for several weeks or months and simultaneously dosing up on probiotics (good intestinal flora) and soil-based organisms (the intestinal microbes should always reflect the soil microbes). The best combination of probiotics and soil organisms in a matrix of raw-alkaline nutritionally-packed superfoods can be found in a product designed to my specifications by HealthForce founder, Jamey Dina, N.D., called **Nature's First Food** (please see the **Resources** section at the end of this book or call 888-RAW-FOOD for more information about this product).

Sprouted grain can yield a slight quantity of usable sugar. When fasting from sugar for long periods, the little bit of sugar from sprouted grain can be beneficial and will not foster candida growth. Sprouted grains must be of a high-quality or heirloom seed stock. A good daily salad while on a sugar fast is below:

Candida Salad
Kale
Lettuce
Parsley
Avocado
Flax oil
Sprouted barley, sprouted rye

However, in the long term, when the desire for real sugar appears it must be addressed with high-quality, seeded sweet fruit and not cooked starch. Some sweet food must be eaten or the body will go off balance eventually. One to two pieces of non-hybridized fruit (0.4 pound or 0.2 kg) each day should be fine. Fermentation of the fruit from too many combinations must be avoided. If cooked foods are eaten, they should be non-starchy vegetables (i.e. broccoli, cauliflower, asparagus, etc.).

One may cautiously return to eating more sugary fruits in the diet once the body is cleansed and the candida symptoms have disappeared.

I recommend following a cleansing and intestinal rebuilding program either before or after a sugar fast such as the FITVA program offered by Nature's First Law. Important guidelines for herbal cleansing while overcoming candida:

1. Do not have fruit juice if you have candida, especially while on an herbal cleanse. Use only vegetable juice or water for the psyllium shakes.

2. Take a high-quality probiotic formula, such as **Nature's First Food**, at least 1 hour before bedtime throughout all the cleansing steps, 1/2 hour after each set of herbs and 1/2 hour after each meal.

3. Take ample amounts of the probiotic bifidobacterium infantis through rectal implants (either through enemas or have your colon hydrotherapist implant you). Bifidobacterium infantis is found in breast-fed infants, and is probably the most basic of all intestinal bacteria in the human species. Be sure to have your colon hydrotherapist provide you with an implant of bifidus bacteria following each session.

There is a psychology necessary to heal chronic candida. Candida is associated with subconscious self-destructive feelings of rejection and a lack of self-worth. Negative, self destructive thoughts destroy good bacteria in the intestinal tract allowing candida to proliferate. Positive, self-confident thoughts help good bacteria proliferate in the intestines.

An emotional cleansing is required to overcome chronic candida. Be aware that unresolved issues usually involve parents or past lovers. While healing candida (and while moving into raw foods in general) one should seek out counselors, friends, books, and/or audiotapes which can assist with emotional releases.

In review, a candida condition can be remedied by the elimination of cooked starch and antibiotics, lots of Sunshine on the skin, a sugar fast, adequate dosages of **Nature's First Food**, a rebuilding program with colon cleansing, emotional cleansing, and the important dietary changes mentioned above.

Some additional recommendations: Those with candida should keep a clean house; musty homes are bad for the candida sufferer. Panty hose should not be worn; they trap moisture and lead to yeast vaginitis. All body orifices should be allowed to breathe.

Eating For Mental Clarity

To achieve the maximum clarity of mind, fast or eat only one type of juicy, sweet fruit for several days.

Two or three days of only sweet fruit (not overdone) will heighten your mental clarity. Your brain runs on glucose exclusively, which is best derived from sweet fruit. In fact, several parts of this book were written while I was on a 6-day watermelon fast.

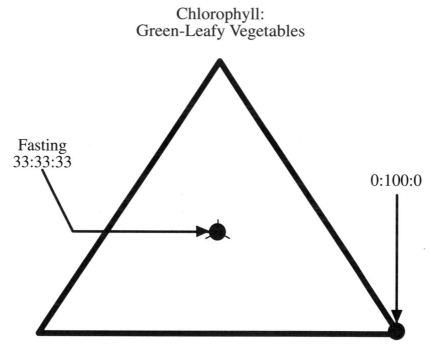

Chlorophyll:
Green-Leafy Vegetables

Fasting
33:33:33

0:100:0

Fats:
Fatty Fruits, Nuts
Coconuts, Seeds

Sugars:
Sweet Fruits

For Mental Clarity center at 33:33:33 by fasting
Or center at 0:100:0 by eating sweet fruit moderately
Ratio Key: (Chlorophyll:Sugar:Fat)

Fasting on water places one right at the center of The Sunfood Triangle — perfect balance. Fasting intensifies thoughts and wishes. After you fast on water for several days, your mind will become so clear it will astonish you. Remember, one should only undertake a water fast when the body is in balance and the blood is clean.

While fasting, stored glycogen (super-densified glucose) is released from the liver and from within the cells to fuel the body. As one purifies their diet over a long period of time, the cells and liver will accumulate stores of glycogen, allowing one to fast longer and longer without a major blood sugar drop. In his book **The Golden Seven Plus One**, Dr. C. Samuel West reports that each unit of glycogen contains 27,000 units of glucose — all of which can be released at once!

Eating For Athletics And Endurance

I advise athletes to stay right in the center of the triangle by increasing all 3 food classes equally. This provides more calories to burn for endurance. More sweet fruit, more fat, more green-leafed vegetables. Instead of "carbo-loading" (loading up on cooked starch, such as pasta, bread, and baked potatoes), the athlete should be loading up on raw plant fats (avocados, young coconuts, nuts, and/or seeds) for several days leading up to the event. From my experience surfing, I have noted that tree nuts, in particular, provide excellent endurance fuel. Sweet fruits should be eaten regularly throughout competition to keep the blood sugar up. If the blood sugar bottoms out, the athlete can lose mental poise and quickly experience fatigue. Chewing green-leafed vegetables can be time consuming for an athlete, so juices may be substituted for salad for athletes during peak training periods.

I have worked with several world-class athletes and they have found great benefit from my green drink formulation. It consists of: kale, celery, and cucumber put through a juicer. The kale provides the heavy minerals necessary to nourish the muscles (its alkaline elements neutralize lactic acid build-up); celery replaces the sodium lost through perspiration; cucumber provides excellent fluids and soluble fiber.

Another excellent drink for athletes is coconut water, which is the highest source of electrolytes found in Nature. Electrolytes are electrically-conductive charged minerals in solution that, once in the digestive system, directly nourish the tissues.

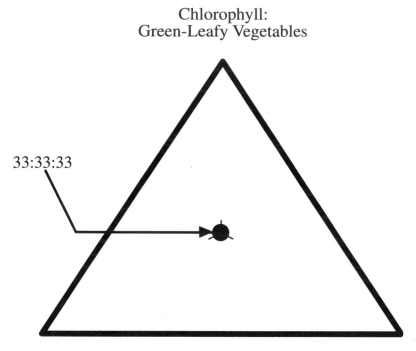

Chlorophyll:
Green-Leafy Vegetables

33:33:33

Fats:
Fatty Fruits, Nuts
Coconuts, Seeds

Sugars:
Sweet Fruits

For Athletics and Endurance center at 33:33:33
Ratio Key: (Chlorophyll:Sugar:Fat)

Eating To Warm The Body

"Nevertheless, the calorific value of foods definitely exists.
A number of years ago when I swam during the winter, I
found that on a diet consisting mainly of salads and fruits,

the body would take a minute or more to warm up and withstand the cold water. However, the reaction would be almost instantaneous when nuts, dried fruits, and cereals were added to the diet. Adding these foods enabled me to stay longer in the cold water."
— Morris Krok, **Fruit The Food And Medicine For Man**

The feeling of coldness when one begins a Sunfood Diet is typically caused by a thickening of the blood during detoxification episodes; this decreases circulation. It is also caused by an increased blood flow to the internal organs, which are finally given a chance to heal, and a corresponding decreased blood flow to the extremities.

As was demonstrated earlier in **Lesson 1: The Principle Of Life Transformation**, life change comes from the inside out. This is also true with the internal structure of the body. The most vital, central organs heal and transform first (so the blood focuses there first). The musculature and the outer perimeter of the body are the last to heal.

After you persist through the transition and detox — through the feeling of coldness — you will discover that your resistance to both cold and hot weather will increase by eating raw plant foods.

A doe in the forest survives the harshest winters on a diet of simple grass. She has no cooking pot or stove.

Eating hot food can actually *decrease* your resistance to cold weather in the same way that a hot shower decreases your resistance to the cold. Just as a cold shower increases your resistance to cold weather, "cold" raw food also increases your resistance to cold weather.

To keep the body warm, consider eating food which is at room temperature. Cold refrigerated food will cool the body. Perhaps you can adjust your refrigerator to the warmest temperature it will allow.

Serving raw soups in warmed up ceramic bowls may be helpful to

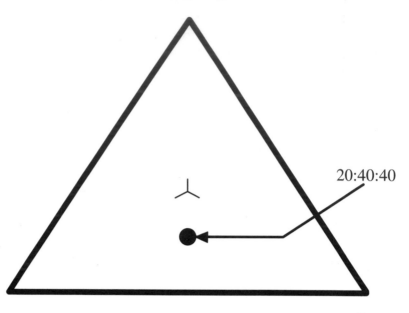

Chlorophyll:
Green-Leafy Vegetables

20:40:40

Fats:
Fatty Fruits, Nuts
Coconuts, Seeds

Sugars:
Sweet Fruits

To Warm the body center at 20:40:40
Ratio Key: (Chlorophyll:Sugar:Fat)

make the transition. Warm water with a twist of lemon juice may also be helpful. To test if the water is too hot, you should be able to keep a finger in it for 4 seconds without discomfort.

We can eat certain types of food to warm the system.

Fats warm the system. Fats contain the same elements as the carbohydrates, but the hydrogen is present in a much larger quantity, and this results in more heat being produced by its break-down and digestion.

Potassium-rich foods are warming foods. Some nuts, such as

macadamias, have a high level of potassium, as do seeds, such as sun-flower seeds. Most fruits are rich in potassium. Some of the most warm-ing, highest-potassium fruits are: avocados, dates, durians, persimmons (with seeds), prunes, pumpkin, raisins (with seeds), and sun-dried apri-cots. You will also notice that these fruits correspond to what is available in the fall and winter.

Sulfur-residue foods warm the body. Sulfur-residue foods include: cru-ciferous vegetables, garlic, and onions. Durian has a high sulfur and potassium-yield. In Asia, one who overeats durian is often said to have "hot eyes."

Eat a meal that is high in fats, potassium, and/or sulfur and you will notice a heating reaction within 45 minutes as the food begins to digest. This reaction will become more pronounced over time as one becomes more purified by eating a raw-food diet.

Eating To Cool The Body

"The life force flows through the body, and by acting on the resis-tance offered by food, generates heat and energy as a by-product."
— Dugald Semple

We can do four things to cool the body nutritionally:
1. Fast. When you fast, your body temperature lowers.
2. Eat cold, refrigerated, or frozen food.
3. Eat only green-leafy vegetables. Green-leafy vegetables do not pro-duce much heat as they pass through the human digestive system.
4. Eat high-sodium foods. Sodium-rich foods are cooling foods. Dark green-leafy vegetables, such as kale, dandelion, and spinach, are extremely cooling. Celery is an excellent summer-time cooling food. Seaweed, such as kelp, is also cooling. Coconut water has a sodium yield and is a great cooling cocktail on hot, humid days.

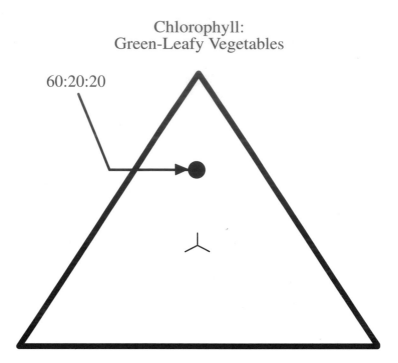

Chlorophyll:
Green-Leafy Vegetables

60:20:20

Fats:
Fatty Fruits, Nuts
Coconuts, Seeds

Sugars:
Sweet Fruits

To Cool the body center at 60:20:20
Ratio Key: (Chlorophyll:Sugar:Fat)

Eating To Ground The Body

Grounding occurs due to minerals. The more minerals in the food, the more grounded you feel...the more minerals, the more "ground" — literally! Generally, fatty foods and green leaves are the highest source of minerals. So, to ground the body, one would balance there.

Eating For Spirituality

"All philosophy in two words — sustain but abstain."
— Epictetus

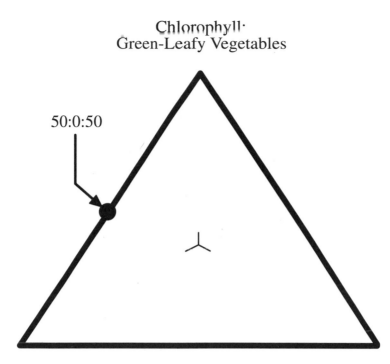

Chlorophyll·
Green-Leafy Vegetables

50:0:50

Fats:
Fatty Fruits, Nuts
Coconuts, Seeds

Sugars:
Sweet Fruits

To Ground the body center at 50:0:50
Ratio Key: (Chlorophyll:Sugar:Fat)

   Dr. Johnny Lovewisdom taught me the spiritual value of avoiding fats for a selected period of time with his Vitarian Diet. Dr. Lovewisdom himself attempted to completely eliminate fats from his diet by swearing off all avocados, nuts, and seeds (see his book **Spiritualizing Dietetics: Vitarianism**). He eventually ended up including goat's milk (pure fat) in his diet (see Viktoras Kulvinskas' book **Life In The 21st Century**) — which justifies the conclusion that fats are essential. We have already seen the value of a momentary period of a fatless diet for detoxification. When you strip away all the internal insulation created by fats, after all improper foods have been removed, then you tune directly into the cosmic spiritual energy which pervades all things. This is the Vitarian Diet, which contains few fats, and only fruits and vegetables of a high-water content.

My friend Joshua Rainbow told me one day on the phone that he became so sensitive on the Vitarian Diet that simply turning into the wind became an ecstatic experience.

Because the desire for fat (and its insulation) increases the closer one is to civilization (pollution), this type of spiritual diet is heightened when one is living in Nature — far away from toxicity.

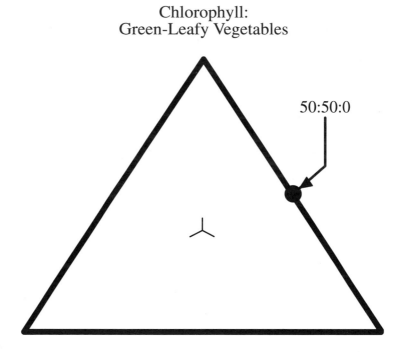

Chlorophyll:
Green-Leafy Vegetables

50:50:0

Fats:
Fatty Fruits, Nuts
Coconuts, Seeds

Sugars:
Sweet Fruits

For Spiritual Clarity center at 50:50:0
Ratio Key: (Chlorophyll: Sugar: Fat)

Lesson 14:
Sapoty Brook's CaPNaK Chart

One of the most interesting books I have read since becoming a raw-foodist is Sapoty Brook's **Eco-Eating** (a book Nature's First Law now imports from Australia and distributes in North America.)

Sapoty Brook is a long-time raw-foodist who developed a remarkable chart based on the concept of balancing the dominant minerals in foods: Calcium (Ca), Phosphorus (P), Sodium (Na), and Potassium (K), for optimal performance.

The CaPNaK chart is one of the best in existence. It objectively replaces some of the subjective classifications of foods coming from macrobiotics. Its value for us consists in the knowledge of which foods are acid-forming (phosphorus dominant) and alkaline-forming (calcium dominant) and which foods are yin (potassium dominant) and yang (sodium dominant), based on their minerals.

I have found Sapoty Brook's chart tremendously beneficial. I present the chart to you because I think his concepts, along with my Sunfood Triangle, provide an excellent understanding of how to use foods to stimulate the body to achieve certain effects or to balance.

Sapoty Brook's deductions are as follows:
That you must eat a healthy balance of foods so that the dominant four minerals (Ca, P, Na, or K) all balance against each other. Perfect balance would put you right in the center of the chart. You can move this balance

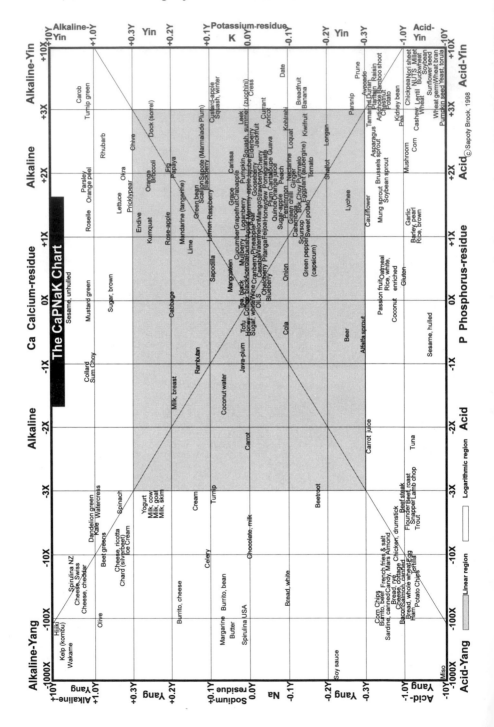

The CaPNaK Chart

© Sapoty Brook, 1998

Food Index

Acerola 1X 0.0Y
Alfalfa Sprout -1X -0.3Y
Almond See NUTS 10X -1.0Y
Apple 1X 0.0Y
Apricot 3X -0.1Y
Artichoke 3X -0.3Y
Asparagus 3X -0.3Y
Avocado 3X -0.3Y
Bacon -100X -1.0Y
Bamboo Shoot 10X -0.3Y
Banana 3X -0.1Y
Barley, Pearl 1X -1.0Y
Bean See Green Bean
Beef Steak -3X -1.0Y
Beef, Roast -3X -1.0Y
Beer -1X -0.3Y
Beet Green -10X 1.0Y
Beetroot -3X -0.2Y
Blackberry 2X 0.1Y
Blueberry 0X 0.0Y
Bok Choy 2X -0.1Y
Brazil Nut See NUTS 10X 10X -10.0Y
Bread, Rye -100X -1.0Y
Bread, White -100X -0.1Y
Bread, Whole Wheat -100X -1.0Y
Breadfruit 3X -0.1Y
Broccoli 3X 0.3Y
Brussels Sprout 2X -0.3Y
Buckwheat 10X -1.0Y
Burrito, Bean -100X 0.1Y
Burrito, Beef -100X -0.3Y
Burrito, Cheese -100X 0.2Y
Butter -100X 0.0Y
Cabbage 0X 0.2Y
Candy, Mars Almond -10X -1.0Y
Cantaloupe Melon 2X -0.1Y
Capsicum See Green Pepper
Carambola 1X -0.1Y
Carissa 2X 0.0Y
Carob 3X 1.0Y
Carrot -2X 0.0Y
Carrot Juice -2X -0.3Y
Casaba Melon 1X 0.0Y
Cashew 3X -10.0Y
Cauliflower 1X -0.3Y

Celery -10X 0.1Y
Chard (Silverbeet) -10X 0.3Y
Cheese, Cheddar -100X 1.0Y
Cheese, Cottage -'00X -1.0Y
Cheese, Ricotta -10X 0.3Y
Cheese, Swiss -10X 10.0Y
Cherimoya Insufficient Data
Cherry 2X 0.0Y
Chestnut 3X -1.0Y
Chicken Drumstick -10X -1.0Y
Chickpea 3X -1.0Y
Chilli See Green Chilli
Chive 3X 0.3Y
Chocolate, Milk -10X 0.0Y
Coconut 0X -1.0Y
Coconut Water -2X 0.1Y
Coffee, Black 0X 0.0Y
Cola 0X -0.1Y
Collard -1X 1.0Y
Corn 2X -1.0Y
Corn Chips -100X -1.0Y
Crabapple 2X 0.0Y
Cranberry 1X 0.0Y
Cream -3X 0.1Y
Cress 3X 0.0Y
Cucumber 1X 0.0Y
Currant 3X 0.0Y
Custard-Apple 3X 0.1Y
Dandelion Green -3X 1.0Y
Date 10X -0.1Y
Dock (Sorrel) 3X 0.3Y
Durian 3X -0.3Y
Egg -10X -1.0Y
Eggplant (Aubergine) 2X -0.1Y
Elderberry 2X 0.0Y
Endive 1X 0.3Y
Feijoa 1X 0.3Y
Fig 2X 0.2Y
Flounder -10X -1.0Y
French Fries & Salt -10X -1.0Y
Gai Choy See Mustard Green
Garlic 1X -1.0Y
Ginger 2X -0.1Y
Gluten 0X -1.0Y
Gooseberry 2X 0.0Y
Grape 2X 0.0Y
Grapefruit 1X 0.0Y

Green Bean 2X 0.1Y
Green Chilli 1X -0.1Y
Green Pepper (Capsicum) 1X -1.0Y
Guava 2X -0.1Y
Ham -100X -1.0Y
Hazelnut See NUTS 10X -1.0Y
Hijiki -100X 10.0Y
Honey 0X 0.0Y
Honeydew Melon 2X 0.0Y
Ice Cream -10X 0.3Y
Jackfruit 3X 0.0Y
Java-Plum -1X 0.0Y
Jujube 2X -1.0Y
Kale -10X 1.0Y
Kelp (Kombu) -100X 10.0Y
Kidney Bean 3X -1.0Y
Kiwifruit 3X -0.1Y
Kohlrabi 3X -0.1Y
Kumquat 1X 0.3Y
Lamb Chop -3X -1.0Y
Leek 3X 0.0Y
Lemon 1X 0.1Y
Lentil 3X - 0.1Y
Lettuce 2X 0.3Y
Lime 1X 0.2Y
Loganberry 1X 0.0Y
Longan 3X -0.2Y
Loquat 3X -0.1Y
Lychee 2X -0.3Y
Mammy-Apple -1X 0.CY
Mandarine (Tangerine) 1X 0.2Y
Mango 1X 0.0Y
Mangosteen 0X 0.0Y
Margarine -100X 0.1Y
Milk, Breast -1X 0.2Y
Milk, Cow -3X 0.3Y
Milk, Goat -3X 0.2Y
Milk, Skim -3X 0.2Y
Millet 10X -1.0Y
Miso -1,000X -10.0Y
Mulberry 1X 0.0Y
Mung Sprout 2X -0.3Y
Mushroom 2X -1.0Y
Mustard Green 0X 1.0Y
Nectarine 2X -0.1Y
Nori Sheet 10X -1.0Y
Oatmeal 1X -0.3Y

Oheloberry 0X 0.0Y
Okra 2X 0.3Y
Olive Oil See OILS 0X 0.0Y
Olives, Canned -100X 1.0Y
Onion 0X -0.1Y
Orange 2X 0.3Y
Orange Juice 2X -0.1Y
Orange Peel 2X 1.0Y
Papaya 2X 0.2Y
Parsley 2X 1.0Y
Parsnip 3X -0.3Y
Passion-Fruit 0X -1.0Y
Pea 3X -1.0Y
Peach 2X -0.1Y
Peanut See NUTS 10X -10.0Y
Pear 1X 0.0Y
Pecan See NUTS 10X -1.0Y
Persimmon 1X -0.1Y
Pine Nut See NUTS 10X -10.0Y
Pineapple 1X 0.0Y
Pistachio See NUTS 10X -10.0Y
Pitanga 1X 0.0Y
Plantain 3X -0.3Y
Plum 2X -0.1Y
Pomegranate 2X -0.1Y
Potato 3X -0.3Y
Potato Chips -100X -1.0Y
Potato, Sweet 1X -0.1Y
Pricklypear 2X 0.3Y
Prune 10X -0.3Y
Pummelo 2X -0.1Y
Pumpkin 2X 0.0Y
Pumpkin Seed (Pepita) 10X -10.0Y
Quince 1X -0.1Y
Radish 1X 0.0Y
Raisin, Seedless 10X -0.3Y
Rambutan -1X 0.1Y
Raspberry 2X 0.1Y
Rhubarb 2X 1.0Y
Rice, Brown 1X -1.0Y
Rice, White Enriched 0X -1.0Y
Rockmelon See Cantaloupe
Rose-Apple 1X 0.2Y
Roselle 1X 1.0Y
Salmon, Canned -100X -1.0Y
Sapodilla 0X 0.1Y
Sapote (Marmalade Plum) 2X 0.1Y

Sapote, Black Insufficient Data
Sapote, White Insufficient Data
Sapote, Yellow Insufficient Data
Sardine, Canned -100X 1.0Y
Scallion (Spring Onion) 2X 0.1Y
Sesame, Hulled -1X -10.0Y
Sesame, Unhulled 0X 10.0Y
Shallot 2X -0.2Y
Snapper -3X -1.0Y
Sorrel See Dock
Soursop 1X -0.1Y
Soy Sauce -1,000X -0.2Y
Soybean 10X -10.0Y
Soybean Sprout 2X -0.3Y
Spinach -3X 0.3Y
Spirulina NZ -100X 10.0Y
Spirulina USA -100X 0.0Y
Squash, Summer (Zucchini) 2X 0.0Y
Squash, Winter 3X 0.1Y
Strawberry 2X -0.1Y
Sugar, Brown 0X 1.0Y
Sugar, White 0X 0.0Y
Sugar-Apple 1X -0.1Y
Sum Choy -1X 1.0Y
Sunflower Oil See OILS 0X 0.0Y
Sunflower Seed 10X -10.0Y
Tamarind 3X -0.3Y
Tangerine See Mandarine
Tea, Black 0X 0.0Y
Tofu 0X 0.0Y
Tomato 2X -0.1Y
Tortilla -10X -1.0Y
Trout -3X -1.0Y
Tuna -2X -1.0Y
Turnip -3X 0.1Y
Turnip Green 3X 1.0Y
Wakame -1,000X 10.0Y
Walnut See NUTS 3X -1.0Y
Watercress -3X 1.0Y
Watermelon 1X -1.0Y
Wheat 3X -10.0Y
Wheat Bran 10X -10.0Y
Wheat Germ 10X -10.0Y
Wine 0X 0.0Y
Yeast, Torula 10X -10.0Y
Yogurt -3X 0.1Y
Zucchini See Squash, Summer

around, producing different types of effects and stimulations. For instance, if you eat foods high in sodium and phosphorus (cooked animal foods), you need to balance that stimulation out with foods high in calcium and potassium (fruits and green vegetables) — this is right in line with the food combining principles Natural Hygiene has taught for decades. If you eat foods high in potassium and phosphorus (avocados and bananas), you tend to crave foods high in calcium and sodium (spinach and kale).

The chart exposes some of the raw-food myths. In general, most fruits are slightly acid-forming, not alkaline-forming. Almonds, we see, are phosphorus-dominant foods, and are not an excellent source of calcium. Carrot juice, long-recommended for its alkalinity, is also found to be phosphorus dominant and thus acid-forming to a certain degree.

Also, the chart helps us to understand cravings. I have known many new fruitarians eating too much potassium-rich foods without balancing with sodium-rich foods, such as kale or seaweed. They typically end up craving and eating salty cooked foods, such as corn chips or potato chips. Cravings for cooked foods may actually be cravings for minerals.

The importance of organic sodium, in particular, is evidenced by the chart. I have worked with many people who have spent years eating a low-sodium raw-food diet; they have found that their digestion improved and endurance increased when they added more sodium-residue foods (kale, celery, dulse) into their diet.

Calcium, phosphorus, sodium, and potassium are not the only minerals in foods. Other alkalizing minerals include magnesium, iron, and silica. Other acid-forming minerals include chlorine and sulfur. These are usually secondary and tertiary minerals in foods. Sapoty Brook's chart is still very accurate, because foods high in magnesium (such as olives) are usually high in calcium; foods high in chlorine (such as avocados) are usually high in phosphorus too.

To clear any confusion: Many alkaline fruits contain citric and other acids; thus, they will have an acid pH reaction in digestion, but because of their high content of alkaline-forming minerals (calcium, magnesium),

Sapoty Brook's CaPNaK Chart

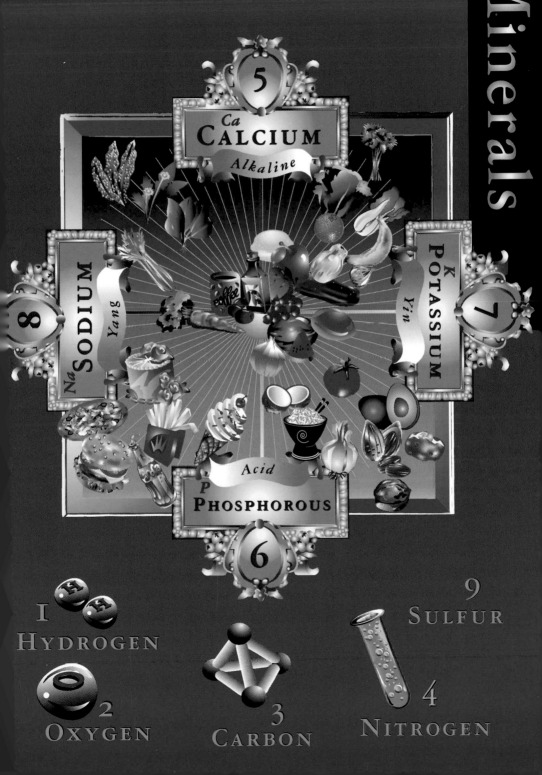

Minerals

their reactions can be alkaline in the body tissues. Thus, they usually alkalize the body and neutralize the acid-forming mineral residues. However, if one is already deficient in alkaline minerals, citric acid will not be broken down properly and thus citrus fruits will be acidic because the alkaline minerals within the food cannot be accessed properly.

Ripe hot peppers are not directly and accurately identified in the chart. By experience, I classify them as alkaline fruits. They are acid in digestion (like citrus fruits), but alkaline in the tissues if broken down properly. I have found they balance against phosphorus foods, such as avocados and nuts.

The fact that Brook includes animal foods and cooked foods in his chart does not mean I endorse their use. But the chart is included to help people make the transition into a raw plant-food regime while feeling balanced and healthy.

The philosopher Spencer wrote that perfect correspondence always prevails in Nature — one thing is always balanced by another. You will find by incorporating The Sunfood Triangle in conjunction with the CaPNaK Chart that a great balancing occurs and an incredible health arises.

Not all foods are listed in the CaPNaK chart. If you would like a book with the pertinent information on natural foods to see where they fit into the chart, I recommend the book, **Whole Foods Companion**, which Nature's First Law distributes. It is written by my friend Diane Onstad, whom I first met while doing research at the Price-Pottenger Nutrition Foundation many years ago. It is a wonderful book, and the best I have seen in the field.

Action Steps:

1. Review the CaPNaK chart.
2. Memorize the locations of your favorite foods.
3. Use the chart to balance the minerals in your diet.

Lesson 15:
Hybrid Food

Some philosophers, such as the great writer, translator, and thinker Edmond Bordeaux Szekely, believed humans were once a frugivorous creature, but have been altered due to centuries of unnatural feeding. However, it is not humanity's biological form which has changed, it is the food itself, which has been altered and hybridized.

When the earliest humans first began cultivating crops and fruit trees, they unwittingly also began to protect these crops and fruit trees from natural selection (which, as we have seen in **Lesson 9: Origins**, does occur within a species, but cannot create a species). The cultivated crops were cross-bred for better taste, longer durability, stronger skins, etc., yet at the same time were growing genetically weaker as the unfittest strains were allowed to survive as long as they "tasted better" or "lasted longer." Eventually, certain crops and fruit trees were grown for so long in protective environments (away from wild Nature) that they no longer had sufficient "genetic energy" to survive in wild Nature untended. These foods I have termed "hybrid foods."

Hybrid foods are foods which will not grow in Nature. My colleague, Dr. David Jubb, tells us that hybrid foods are "missing vital electrics." They are foods which must be nurtured and protected by humans or else they will be overcome by birds, insects, worms, fungi, and bacteria.

Most fruits sold in large supermarkets are cross-bred and hybridized to some degree, but are still excellent foods; often they are still capable of reverting back to a wild or semi-wild state. Fruits, such as avocados, cherimoyas, jalapeno peppers, and tomatoes are great examples of these. As a general guideline, fruits which have been hybridized too far include all seedless fruits or fruits with non-viable seeds. These fruits should be avoided, because they are genetically altered and weak.

Also, grafted trees produce awkward fruit, often without seeds. Grafting is a process whereby one variety of fruit tree is united to another variety of the same fruit tree. Many varieties of orange trees are actually two trees in one. The root stock is of a totally different variety than the stem and branches. Again, focus on the seeds, if they do not exist, or are not viable, then avoid those foods.

Genesis 1:29 actually warns of the danger of hybrid foods. The verse advises us to eat only herbs *bearing seed* and fruits *bearing seed*!

Seedless foods are so hybridized they can no longer reproduce. The inability of hybrids to reproduce stems from a deficiency in the procreative cells. Hybrids can lack a double set of chromosomes in their reproductive cells, and this leads to the inability to produce viable seeds.

Common hybrid fruits include: seedless apples, bananas, several date varieties (especially medjools), kiwis (their black seeds are not viable), seedless pineapples, seedless citrus fruits, seedless grapes (raisins), seedless persimmons, and seedless watermelons.

The standard bananas we all know are excessively hybridized foods. I was raised on bananas and this was difficult for me to accept! The black "seeds" found in the common banana are not seeds at all, but are non-viable remnants of what should be hard, pellet-sized seeds. I transitioned away from bananas by eating fewer and fewer until I finally let them go.

Hybrid fruit is not only unnaturally high in sugar, but is also "off" in its mineral ratios. I have noticed that I can eat super-sweet wild berries in massive abundance and get no unusual reaction or high at all. I have also noticed that if I eat a mildly sweet hybrid fruit I get a "weird" reaction from just a small amount   seedless grapes send me into "la-la" land (sugar high).

Hybrid foods are devoid of the proper mineral balance all wild foods contain. Excessive hybrid fruit consumption leads to mineral deficiencies. It is not only that hybrid fruits and sweet/starchy vegetables (carrots, beets, potatoes) themselves are unbalanced in minerals, it is that an overconsumption of hybrid sweet fruit and sweet/starchy vegetables causes the body to bring heavy minerals from the bones into the blood to buffer the hybrid sugar, which is not completely recognized and dealt with by the liver and pancreas. The minerals and the sugar are then spilled off into the urine. So, in the long-term, hybrid sweet fruit and sweet/starchy vegetables can actually overstimulate you, causing you to lose minerals.

Common hybrid vegetables include: beets, carrots, corn, and potatoes.

Most of the vegetation people eat is not found growing wildly in Nature. The fields in which they grow are protected from natural forces. The natural insects are poisoned with pesticides, the soil microbes are poisoned with fertilizers. Crops grown chemically are artificial — their cultivation is unnatural.

Common hybrid nuts and seeds include: cashews, oats, rice, and wheat.

Common brown, white, and "wild" rice are hybrids. Commercial "soft" wheat is a hybrid plant.

Common, controversial alfalfa sprouts (often criticised for containing toxins) are hybrid foods. Clover sprouts are a better, more natural choice and should be chosen over alfalfa.

Most commercially available legumes are hybrids. I once grew lentils from seeds. Only one out of hundreds grew to fruition. When I harvested the lentils from that one plant, each lentil displayed an amazingly beautiful design on the seed surface — totally unlike the dull orange/brown lentils available from the store. Amazingly, the lentil plant had reverted back to its natural state!

Most primitive peoples, and all wild primates, eat foods from at least 100 varieties of plants. The majority of the world's population now, on civilization's various diets, consume only 13 varieties of plants: bananas, beans, beets (beet-derived sugar), corn, oranges, potatoes, rice, wheat, soy beans, sugar cane, sweet potato, cassava, and coconut. The first 9 of these 13 listed are such hybridized foods that they are either seedless or produce seeds incapable of surviving independently in Nature. Due to the deficiencies of nutrients in hybrid foods, this situation presents an enormous health challenge for the world; and yet, it also presents a tremendous opportunity to improve the health of the world.

People become addicted to bread, corn chips, french fries, baked potatoes, and even carrot juice, because these foods come from hybridized plants that contain an addictive quantity of sugar and a low-level of minerals.

I have noticed that hybrid foods are attacked by different forms of fungi than wild food. Hybrid foods are much more susceptible to early decay. For example, I can have extremely hybridized yellow seedless grapefruits outside in my back patio in the Sun alongside seeded ruby red grapefruits. The ruby reds will last months out there as they ripen to perfection (citrus ripens best in the sun, on the ground), however, the yellow seedless grapefruits will be overcome by bright to dark green mold outlined by white. You will never see this type of mold attack a wild fruit.

From these types of observations, I can see clearly now how hybrid fruit, for example, can feed fungal conditions in the body, such as candida. Whereas non-hybrid or wild fruit would not lead to such a condition.

How To Make Hybrids Work For You

Hybrid foods are everywhere and most of us still need to eat something! It is possible for you to make hybrid foods work for you. The effects of hybrid foods on the body are usually not felt physically or consciously until one is significantly purified after many months and years on a pure Sunfood Diet.

Remember: start where you are now! When I started on raw foods I was probably eating 90% hybridized food! I did just great, but I learned over time to fine tune my diet and body to achieve an extraordinary level of health.

You can live on hybridized food, but you cannot thrive on hybridized food. Hybrid fruits and vegetables may be eaten in small amounts. Mixing bananas with fat (avocados, nuts, olives) lessens the hybrid effect of that fruit on the system. Eating more green-leafed vegetables and avocados, nuts, or olives with hybrid sweet fruits or vegetables will decrease their effect on the blood sugar and increase the utility of elements in the food. Hybrid grains and legumes should be sprouted, never cooked, to lessen their detrimental effect; as long as they are raw, the body can draw nutrients from them and can deal with them.

Even if hybridized, whenever possible eat food grown locally, indigenously under the Sun, under totally organic conditions.

Eat food that is in season. I have noticed that I can eat dates in abundance (up to 30 in a day if I am extremely active) when they are in season (fall and winter), but when I eat them out of season, they give me a strange reaction similar to the feeling of eating too much hybrid fruit and I cannot even eat two or three dates.

Action Steps:

1. Identify the hybridized foods (raw or cooked) in your diet. Decide to replace these foods with more natural foods as soon, and as often, as possible.

2. The solution to hybridized food? Grow your own food from heirloom seeds (contact **Seeds Of Change** seed bank at the address in the back of the book). Better yet, eat wild plants and fruits.

Lesson 16:
Wild Food

"In the first age food came by wishing and
grew from Earth without tending."
— **Ramayana**

"Electric foods are the most important component
of healing. They make the body alkaline. These are
all foods that are able to grow in the wild."
— Annie & Dr. David Jubb,
Colloidal Biology & Secrets Of An Alkaline Body

The basis of natural nutrition is 100% wild, raw plant food. Author and raw-food nutritionist Franz Konz of Germany calls it "original food." It has been the original food here since the beginning of time.

Wild food connects you immediately to the land. Eating wild food growing in your area acclimates you to the environment. I used to suffer from all kinds of allergies: hay fever, pollen, feline, etc. I completely conquered all allergies by undertaking The Sunfood Diet and by eating wild indigenous food. People who are allergic to the pollens of local plants can eliminate these allergies by eating local wild leaves, flowers, and fruits and acclimating themselves to the environment. Many people never eat anything growing locally or wildly in their life! This is not the lifestyle for which we were designed.

Wild food is a revelation. When you eat wild food you will discover how hybridized and domesticated standard food really is.

As long as you are eating wild raw plant food, you never have to think about nutrients again. Wild raw plant foods have everything the body needs to fulfill all of its nutritional desires.

Brian Clement, director of Hippocrates Health Institute in West Palm Beach, Florida, has reported that, based on his research, wild greens have the highest energy frequency of any food. I have experienced their energy first-hand by eating plenty of wild green salads. They send me into a new plane of thought. Evenings after eating such meals are filled with incredible clarity of thought and electricity.

A raw-foodist I was speaking with on the phone one day relayed a very important point: seaweeds and sea vegetables of all kinds have never been cultivated. They are still in their wild unaltered form! They fit within the wild raw plant-food category, and are high in trace minerals. This is an important factor in a world where many are suffering from endemic mineral deficiencies brought about by consuming medicines, pills, and cooked foods which drain the vital energy.

Wild Fruit

Wild food is Sunfood — food grown in abundance under the Sun, not under artificial conditions of any type. It is food as the Earth has given it to us in its original state.

Store-bought fruitarianism is not workable in the long-term. My health partner, R.C. Dini, continuously inspires people to seek out perfectly ripe fruit. Perfectly ripe fruit picked fresh, "from the tree right to me," is an unmatched experience.

Wild fruit is high in minerals, and often lower in sugar than commercial fruit. It is less stimulating and thus is closer to the center point of The Sunfood Triangle.

Wild fruits are the sustenance of the immortals. Fruit has tremendous spiritual power. The more natural (nonhybridized) the fruit is, the greater its spiritual value.

Common fruits which are close to the wild state and/or are extremely viable when grown from seed include: avocados, cherimoyas, crab apples, guavas, heavily-seeded citrus fruits, jackfruits, mangos, most melons, most peppers or chiles, papayas, peaches, tomatoes, tomatilloes, olives, white sapotes, and others.

A good quality citrus fruit should contain 14-15 seeds, even if the fruit is small in size. The more seeds in citrus, the better. The less seeds in citrus, the more hybridized is the strain. Keep citrus fruits in Sunlight or on the windowsill so they remain at their maximum nutritive value and quality. The riper and more Sun-exposed the citrus fruit, the sweeter and less acid are its contents.

Common vegetables which are close to the wild state and/or are extremely viable when grown from seed include: dandelion, garlic, kale, lamb's quarters, malva, mint, mustard, onions, watercress, wintercress, and others.

One of my favorite wild foods is malva (mallow). Malva seems to love growing on the outskirts of civilization — in canyons, back alleys, and back yards. Malva is one of those phenomenal greens which tastes incredible eaten alone. In the winter I typically start off the morning with fruit, then eat malva only for lunch, and have a salad with some raw plant fats for dinner.

Common nuts and seeds which are close to the wild state and/or are extremely viable when grown from seed include: coconut, macadamia, quinoa, and sunflower.

Every locale you find yourself in possesses wild foods with which to eat and live. Get out and explore your local canyons, fields, forests, hills, mountains, etc. My organization, Nature's First Law, distributes a book entitled **Edible Wild Plants: A North American Field Guide** by Elias & Dykeman. It is certainly the best I have seen. Take it with you on your hikes and identify your local edible greenery.

In his writings, the herbalist Earl Mindell has confirmed my experience. He has described that less than 1% of all plants are poisonous to eat.

The power of wild foods cannot be underestimated. Eating wild plant foods reconnects you with Nature in a most profound way. One time I was out hiking in a canyon near my home. On the way, I encountered several children ranging in age from seven to ten. We started talking and soon agreed that I would show them all the edible, interesting, and poisonous plants growing in the area. We had an extraordinary time together. After several hours, all the children had gone home except one. The two of us were hiking up a hill through brush on our way to a field of young dandelion when we almost walked into a coyote. The coyote looked at us and bolted away. The young child's eyes were wide open. Although earlier he had told me he had seen coyotes, I knew after that incident he had not — at least not like this. These moments are priceless, and this moment all came about in the fun of foraging for wild food.

The goal is to eat as naturally as possible. The more wild and natural your food, the more wild and natural you will become! Wild plant foods make you strong and robust and put you "in tune" with your local natural environment.

If you cannot get wild food, or it is impractical, please eat organic. You deserve it. You are worth it! You and your family are worth more than anything on Earth; give your family the best fuel possible. The organic farmers also deserve your support for not spraying pesticides (poisons) on the Earth. If you have to pay twice as much or more for organic food, do it! It is an investment in yourself (which always comes back multiplied). Organic food has more vitality, minerals, and value than commercial food. In my experience it is totally worth paying even three to four times as much money for organic food.

Vitamin B12

Vitamin B12 (cobalamin) represents a family of compounds that contain cobalt. Vitamin B12 helps maintain the myelin sheaths that insulate the nerve fibers from each other. Problems with vitamin B12 absorption and assimilation can result in nerve degeneration. A vitamin B12 deficiency, when in conjunction with a folate deficiency (due to a lack of green-leafy vegetables), can also cause pernicious anemia.

Although animal and dairy products are a source of vitamin B12, the natural soil microbes and bacteria found on wild food, unwashed garden plants, and also those supplied by plant fermentation, are typically adequate to supply the body with vitamin B12 needs. The natural microbes and bacteria in the soil need to be duplicated and colonize in our intestinal tract for optimal absorption of nutrients and elimination of waste without excessive fermentation or internal putrefaction. Vitamin B12 is produced by these natural microbes and bacteria as they colonize the intestines.

A problem with the formation of Vitamin B12 occurs when there is a sterilization which happens between the picking of the fruit or vegetable and the moment it reaches your mouth. Sterile environments are unnatural. The soil microbes and bacteria which grow on raw fruits and vegetables need to be duplicated in the intestinal tract for the proper assimilation of vitamin B12 to take place. Dr. Victor Herbert described in the **American Journal Of Clinical Nutrition** (1988, volume 48, p. 852-858) the experiences of Dr. James Halsted who traveled to Persia to study a colony of Iranian vegans who did not experience any vitamin B12 deficiencies. He found that their naturally fertilized vegetables were eaten without being carefully washed. He discovered that strict vegetarians who do not practice thorough hand washing or vegetable cleaning may be untroubled by a vitamin B12 deficiency.

Studies have shown that those eating a typical diet of animal products actually require more vitamin B12 than those who do not eat animal products. This is because the typical diet leads to digestive atrophy. Because vitamin B12 is peptide bound in animal products and must be enzymatically cleaved from the peptide bonds to be absorbed, a weakening of all gastric acid and gastric enzyme secretions (due to a cooked-food diet) causes an inability to efficiently extract vitamin B12 from external food. Raw-food vegans, who have more powerful digestion, actually get more vitamin B12 by reabsorption from the bile (liver secretions into the duodenum) than they do from external food.

The vitamin B12 standards recommended based on studies of the average cooked-food consumer are 0.0000001 ounces (3-4 micrograms) per day. Studies by Dr. Victor Herbert reported in the **American Journal Of Clinical Nutrition** (1988, volume 48, p. 852-858) demonstrate that only 0.000000035 ounces (1 microgram) of vitamin B12 are required per day. This is enough to produce a "beautiful hematologic response." These minimum vitamin B12 requirements are inadequate to explain the needs of raw-food vegans who require even less vitamin B12 due to excellent gastric strength, enzymatic activity, and a high ability to recycle vitamin B12. We may conclude that, as raw-food vegans, we need very little vitamin B12.

Dr. Gabriel Cousens, a long-term raw-food vegetarian, has included an excellent discussion of vitamin B12 in his book **Conscious Eating**. Dr. Cousens feels that a vitamin B12 deficiency, which is extremely rare, is typically caused by a lack of absorption in the intestinal tract, rather than a dietary lack of the vitamin. He states that vegetarian and meat-eating pregnant and lactating women alike seem to be susceptible to a vitamin B12 deficiency. He states that macrobioticists and fruitarians may also be susceptible. I have found that individuals who have damaged their digestive system with a high-protein diet are susceptible as well.

My own experience working with people who I have discovered were vitamin B12 deficient corroborates Dr. Cousen's hypothesis of poor absorption, but I have narrowed it down to a more specific cause: poor or absent intestinal flora.

Sugar, as I have mentioned, is an antibiotic. So a long-term high-sugar diet, whether the sugar is coming from refined sources or hybridized fruit, can damage or wipe out the intestinal flora.

Cooking also destroys microbes. A highly-sterilized cooked-vegan diet (macrobiotics) may not provide the intestines with enough excellent flora.

To insure an excellent quality of vitamin B12, be sure to eat some unwashed garden plants — more is better. Leave foods unwashed that were grown wildly, homegrown, or picked by you from an organic farm. Store-bought food is much different, it should be washed because it can be loaded with mold, pollution, and toxins.

Getting some soil microbes into your body is very important. Consider the words of Annie & Dr. David Jubb in **Colloidal Biology & Secrets Of An Alkaline Body**: "You can receive help virtually overnight for: seizures, diabetes, arthritis, pneumonia, Parkinson's disease, and immune challenges by simply ingesting some soil-born organisms. People have lived in such a sterile antiseptic environment that these necessary symbiotic organisms have been less than present in their diet...By ingesting soil-born organisms, you maintain an enormous reservoir of un-coded antibodies ready to transform specific pathogens...Iron metabolic challenges are solved by living the way Nature intended, occasionally eating a little dirt..."

I eat plenty of unwashed wild food to supply good bacteria for my intestinal flora. However, I have met many long term raw-foodists (20+ years all-raw) who do not eat unwashed food and who are very healthy. They do eat seaweed and/or spirulina (2-3 teaspoons a day), however, which contain vitamin B12 analogues. Also, they do occasionally eat fermented foods, such as raw sauerkraut, which does supply the digestive system with good intestinal flora to manufacture B12. Instructions for creating fermented live-food dishes may be found in **The Raw Truth: The Art Of Loving Foods** raw-food recipe book by Jeremy Safron and Renee Underkoffler.

Sapoty Brook, in his book **Eco-Eating**, feels that a vegan diet does not supply enough vitamin B12 for the body. However, my experience of meeting vegans and raw-food vegans who have been following those diets for 20+ years proves otherwise. If one's health is excellent, there is little chance of a vitamin B12 deficiency. A vitamin B12 deficiency is usually (but not always) symptomatic of a larger problem (poor absorption, poor or absent flora, also a lack of Sunlight) manifested in pale skin, emaciation, and extreme fatigue.

When I lived in Santa Barbara my friends and I would surf the beaches there. Since the beaches there are loaded with pockets of tar and oil, lots of tar would bubble up into the ocean water and get on our wetsuits and surfboards. It was such a hassle to clean and worry about, that one day I said, "I've had it, I'm through. I am no longer going to even worry about this anymore." And you know what? It was never a problem again. It is my opinion, that the vitamin B12 hype is used most often to scare people away from wonderful vegetarian and vegan diets. If you were to put the vitamin B12 issue out of your mind, and follow the action steps below, you might be surprised to find that it disappears from your consciousness never to be heard from again.

Action Steps:

1. Read **Edible Wild Plants: A North American Field Guide**. Take the book with you on hikes through Nature. Begin identifying the wild edible plants growing in your area. Begin experimenting with eating some of the wild foods you identify.

2. For excellent intestinal flora and vitamin B12 assimilation, include one or more of the following in your daily diet:
   a. Unwashed garden plants.
   b. Wild plants.
   c. Seaweeds (e.g. dulse, nori, etc.).
   d. Roots, such as burdock root, have been shown to contain levels

of B12, absorbed from soil organisms up to 0.5 millimeters into the outer skin.

e. **Nature's First Food**, the best probiotic superfood on the market today.

f. Spirulina or blue-green algae (2-3 teaspoons).

g. Occasional fermented foods (e.g. raw sauerkraut) when appropriate.

3. If the options in (2) are not available at the moment, taking a vegan-quality vitamin B12 supplement daily may be appropriate, especially if one is pregnant and/or nursing.

4. If you feel your intestinal flora and food absorption are not excellent, consider regularly including our product **Nature's First Food** in your diet. This product produces excellent colonies of good flora in the intestines. These colonies help synthesize nutrients, they counteract pathogenic microbes, and they improve the overall internal environment. **Nature's First Food** is available from Nature's First Law. I especially recommend probiotics like **Nature's First Food** in the diet for those with a history of prolonged antibiotic or other drug use.

5. To learn more, read Dr. Gabriel Cousens' writings on vitamin B12 in his book **Conscious Eating**.

Lesson 17:
My Personal Diet

Words alone cannot describe the level of health I have been privileged to attain eating a 100% raw plant-food diet. All that comes to mind is that I feel an immense gratitude. I feel incredibly fortunate to have even found or discovered the type of health information I have included in this book. I feel honored to be able to share this information with others.

When I went raw, I began to study the simple things, like my fingers and toes. I marveled at their dexterity and the functions they served. I became very aware of all my bodily systems: respiratory, circulatory, cardiac, glandular, and digestive. I was awestruck at the efficiency of our human organs. How could I ever have taken my body for granted? How could anyone? It was like being a billionaire and not realizing that you are rich. I thought about the less tangible things like sleep cycles, dreams, and the true nature of Life. I was filled with a new-found reverence for all living things.

I think about things differently now. My outlook on life is something I would describe as glorious. Life is so grand, so incredible, so full of amazement! What can match the grasp of a child's hand in your own, the crisp flavor of a fresh-picked apple, the kiss of a friend or lover, the smell of a spring breeze, the Sunlight penetrating your naked body, the inspiration of highly-emotional music, the feel of sand beneath bare feet, the flow of ocean water through your hair in the mid-summer?

When I initially embarked on the raw path, I was faced with overcoming addictions to bread and corn chips. I was losing a lot of weight. My face was changing and I did not look my best. In the midst of this, a wave of peer pressure from friends, family, and relatives descended upon me. But I persevered. Throughout the process two thoughts were dominant in my mind: Jim Rohn's saying, "For every disciplined effort there is a multiple reward," and Andrew Carnegie's saying, "Anything worth having is worth working for."

I kept pushing forward, reading and learning. I began to find that I was transforming in a most profound way and other people were noticing it. I found that many would take the time to listen to what I had to say. I found I was attracting certain people who were acting upon the raw-food information. I stopped trying to convince doubting friends and family and started teaching this diet system to people with dreams.

I found I had to walk my talk. To really make others healthy I had to become incredibly healthy myself. Many of the spiritual books I have read advise that addictions should not be fought, that they dissolve away when the mind is right. This may be good advice for some, but it did not work for me. I had to fight and conquer cooked-food addictions. And I succeeded, and so can you.

I feel incredibly fortunate for having created the opportunity to communicate The Raw Plant-Food Diet message through mass media (radio, television, magazines, newspapers, and the Internet). Over the years, I have had the incredible privilege of meeting and communicating with thousands of raw-foodists the world over. The Internet and e-mail have allowed communication and networking on this subject to reach a remarkable level. The time for this information to reach a worldwide audience has come.

Through my seminars, books, videotapes, and audiotapes I am helping, along with all other raw-foodists, to chart uncharted territory. I believe I am helping to do for nutrition what Roger Bannister did for running when he broke the four-minute mile barrier. Bannister overcame all the doubters and pessimists. What was once considered impossible became possible. The year after Bannister broke the four-minute mile, 37 other runners broke the four-minute mile. And many thousands have done it since.   Did human physiology change? No. What changed were the beliefs about human physiology!

Remember: if one person can achieve the unachievable, then what is possible forever changes.

The Sunfood Diet, when balanced correctly with The Sunfood Triangle, is the healthiest diet for eternal, resonating beauty. This is such an incredible secret! I feel The Sunfood Diet turned me into a lovely being, alive in each recess, capable of understanding every feeling, soothed, and healed of past injuries. It taught me that excellent health is essential to truly enjoying every moment of life.

Perhaps I was predestined to be a raw-foodist. My ethnic heritage comes from Persia where there is a long history of raw-foodism and veganism. In fact, in the Persian language (Farsi) there is a specific term for a raw-foodist: Khom Gia Khori (raw plant eater). This term is about as popular in Persia as the word "vegan" in the United States.

My diet may at first seem limited compared to the standard fast-food diet called "moderation," but the way I eat is actually filled with great pleasure, because I have developed the capacity to enjoy the simplest foods...and so can you.

In my personal life, the longer I have eaten raw, the more I find I prefer to eat alone, standing up, in a meditational state, listening to success tapes or reading books. I love to eat simply.

I am often asked what I eat. I might eat the following in a typical day:
1. 2 avocados, 30-40 ripe olives, and/or 25-30 macadamia nuts
2. 1 papaya, or 1 melon, or 20-30 figs (if in season)
3. 2 pounds of kale and/or wild green food from my gardens or the canyons near my house.

4. 4-5 pieces of citrus fruit, apples, or another juicy fruit in season (peaches, plums, nectarines, mangos, etc.).
5. 2-4 ripe hot peppers (usually jalapeno or habanero)
6. 2-4 strips of dulse seaweed

I typically eat two large meals a day: one at 11:00 am, the other at 7:00 pm. This works wonderfully for me. I may snack between these meals on fruits or greens.

I love to eat green-leafy vegetables (I chew them like gum sometimes if I am bored!). I have found that bitter green foods are very healing. When you cultivate a taste for bitter food, you will see a marked improvement in your health.

Ripe hot peppers are one of my favorite foods. For centuries, herbalists have told us of the beneficial effects of hot "cayenne" peppers in healing heart conditions for centuries. Hot peppers are also great for stimulating the digestive tract and for "burning" out parasites in the intestines. These foods are natural antibiotics and they contain an excellent quantity of sulfur, "the beauty mineral," which creates smooth skin, glossy hair, and hard nails. From both my experience and the experience of other long-time raw-foodists, I definitely disagree with the Natural Hygiene philosophy of including no hot peppers and other spicy raw foods in the diet.

I do not eat raw-food recipes often — a recipe for me is usually for disaster! But they are excellent transition tools and fun for family and parties! There are dozens of raw-food recipe books available. There are several raw-food restaurants in North America (see the **Raw-Food Restaurants** section at the end of this book). There are also chefs who specialize in "uncooking."

I also do not take supplements of any kind (vitamin pills, mineral tablets, colloidal mineral tinctures, enzyme capsules, protein powders, grass powders, etc.). Many commercial supplements are lifeless and overwhelm and confuse the body with too many concentrated extracts. In my opinion, one is better off investing her/his hard-earned money into higher quality organic foods. Any nutrient in any supplement can be found in any local garden.

If you feel too restricted eating exactly what I recommend, you can always take up the fall-back position: eat a wider variety of raw plant foods: fruits, vegetables, herbs, nuts, seeds, sprouts, sea vegetables, raw plant-food recipes, etc. Remember, the initial goal here is to eat as much raw plant food as we can adjust into our diet.

Water

I am often asked what I do for water. I typically do not drink much water, as the raw foods I eat already contain a sufficient quantity of water. I do have distilled water delivered to my home in glass bottles. I fill glass containers with the distilled water and leave them in the Sun on my porch. Distilled water is unstructured water, its pattern is chaotic. Once the water is placed outside for a few hours to a day, it begins to take on structure again. The water will actually metamorphosize; bubbles will appear in the glass container on the inner surface. After that, the taste changes and the water becomes more revitalizing.

Squirting fresh lemon or lime juice into distilled water will give it structure. Also, placing freshly-picked green herbs in the water will pro-vide it with structure.

Whenever possible, avoid water bottled in plastic. Plastic leaches into water and mimics estrogen (the female sex hormone) inside the body. The best commercially available water, in my opinion, is Evian in glass bot-tles.

Gardening

By eating raw plant foods, I believe you will become deeply interested in gardening as I have. Gardening cultivates an intimate connection between you, the plants, the Sun, and the Earth. Gardening nourishes us twice: once by the exercise involved in creating the garden and again when we eat the food. In my own life, my garden continues to show me new ways to experience the Earth.

Growing plants compels us to eat our food in its natural, raw state, because of all the energy we have put into harvesting the food. It compels us to compost our food scraps and to improve the soil each year. Growing our own food decreases pollution because we do not participate in the transportation pollution incurred by shipping food.

In the great outdoors you can never grow bored nor weary, but will remain content and joyful. "All my ills my garden spade," wrote Emerson. The most contented and happy people are those who breathe in the rich vapors of their home garden. I know that is where I feel best.

The essence of my entire message is found in growing gardens, living as close to Nature as possible, and in making friends with the animals. It is in doing those things that all may be learned. I am reminded of the maxim, "Before a person may govern a city, s/he must first be able to govern a garden." I find gardening one of life's greatest pleasures and watching fruit trees grow from seed to maturity one of the secrets of longevity.

Action Steps:

1. My challenge for this lesson is for you to begin bringing plants into your life. Start with simple house plants, sprouting trays, a greenhouse, and/or a backyard garden.

2. Eating raw plant food is the way to live in total harmony with the Earth. What if you took all the fruit and vegetable remnants left over from what you ate and, instead of throwing them away, you used them to fertilize your plants?

3. Make your home beautiful. The abode of the Sunfoodist is rich and luxuriant; it is filled in one place with exotic fruit trees and garden herbs — all fertilized by the compost of a plentiful Sunfood lifestyle. It is recognized as a special place of massive abundance.

Lesson 18:
100% Raw

"The Paradisical diet is not only sufficient, but it brings you higher and higher, into physical and mental conditions never before experienced."
— Professor Arnold Ehret

"The greatest value of The Raw-Food Diet is its transformative value. To a great extent, when you take up The Raw-Food Diet, you become a new and different and better person. You don't just stay the same old person only a little healthier. You become, to a great extent, a new being with new interests, a new philosophy and outlook on life, new goals and new desires. You become more of your essence, your true natural self. You become a person who is more a part of the one great life of Nature and less of the confused human world. You become less 'of the World' and more 'of the Earth.'"
— Joe Alexander, **Blatant Raw-Foodist Propaganda**

"For every disciplined effort, there is a multiple reward."
— Jim Rohn, success philosopher

The major transition to the raw side begins when one eats 100% raw plant food. Eating 100% raw allows one to master all the lessons necessary to achieve an absolutely extraordinary level of health.

Is 100% raw extreme? If you want extreme improvements in your life, you need to start taking extreme actions. Remember: life is extreme. It's life or death. This is no dress rehearsal; this is the real thing. People are dying. The major diseases in America are related to the way people eat. People are looking for the answers. People are sick and tired of being lied to (figuratively and literally). The world is actually bathing in pollution and it can be changed by simple fundamental changes. Permit this challenge: get out on a limb, you will discover that is where all the fruit is!

Anything that would tend to limit your greatest gift — the power to think and reason clearly — should be eliminated above all things. Any quantity of cooked, or otherwise unhealthy food, clouds the mind to some degree and leaves a residue of debris in the body which dampens the electrical circuitry in the brain.

The time is upon us to become more discerning in our food choices. The threat of pesticides, the danger of animal products, soil demineralization, and genetic engineering can no longer be ignored. Yesterday's cooked-food diet won't cut it today. The standard cooked-food diet is a gamble, we never know what is truly in the food.

Do not look at this process as starting a new diet with all the implied limitations. This is not about denial. 99.99% of all the food on Earth is raw plant food! This diet is the ultimate freedom. There is such a variety of raw plant foods on this Earth it is astonishing. Have you ever tried a: black sapote, cherimoya, durian, eggfruit, elderberry, galia melon, habanero pepper, jackfruit, lemonade berry, loquat, lychee, mamey, mountain apple, pomegranate, prickly pear, sapodilla, suriname cherry, or white sapote? Have you ever tried: butterleaf lettuce, chicory, dandelion, dinosaur kale, fennel, lamb's quarters, lemon grass, miner's lettuce, nopales, sorrel, watercress, wild mustard, wild onion, or wintercress? Obviously I have only just touched on some of the variety of edible plants that are out there. You could try a new fruit and vegetable every single day for the rest of your life and not even come remotely close to trying them all!! There is too much abundance!!

A 100% raw-Sunfood diet is the ultimate high. People are intelligent and they understand that they should be feeling great all the time. The depressing effects of cooked foods and animal products are a major reason why people resort to intoxicating liquors and drugs.

The question of going 100% raw is a question of persistence and spiritual maturity. Fruitarian Roe Gallo says, "You can't be healthy if you're miserable." Have the maturity to adjust your lifestyle to accommodate your diet while enjoying the process. I often tell my seminar listeners, "The old habits die hard, but they do die!"

It may be best to stabilize at 70% raw, then 80% raw, and continue on from there. We want to avoid the "yo-yo effect" — doing 100% raw and then binge eating and then returning to 100% raw. Set a level of raw-food consumption which is appropriate and realistic for you now.

When you reach a stable level of 95% raw, it will be fantastic. You may experience that the body eventually starts to push towards letting go of all cooked foods in the diet, and this is in the natural course of things. After many years on a high-raw, but not all-raw diet, the body becomes more refined and goes into an immediate "detox mode" as soon as any cooked food is ingested, leaving one functioning at less than optimal capacity.

If you follow 95% of the diet, you do receive 95% of the amazing results. After you follow 100% of the diet, you get 1,000% of the results. Make a commitment which requires you to surpass your physical and emotional obstacles. Refuse to consider any other option except your goal of vibrant health!

A 100% raw plant food diet is a wonderful goal. I know many people who have been eating 100% raw foods for 5, 10, 20, 30, even 40 years and longer and who have attained an incredible level of health and vitality.

I did not go 100% raw foods immediately. I went 95% raw overnight and then gradually weaned myself off the last 5%. However, I have met a few people who have gone all-raw overnight — it may be possible for you if you have eaten an excellent diet for many years and are ready for it.

In general, I have found it is better to give people shorter range goals, such as going one month 100% raw. It is best to have them envision that goal, than to have them envision going a lifetime without cooked food. Once the initial pattern is established, then they can duplicate that pattern — it becomes a blueprint for success.

As I mentioned in **Lesson 12: Transition Diet**, the key to transitioning to raw food is to experiment on a small scale. First, set a goal to go raw for three days, then expand that to a week the next time, then a month; keep expanding all the time. Write your raw goals down, and commit to them. Then see, after achieving your goals, how much further you can go.

What is fascinating is that the temptations of cooked food begin to lose their strength. The former "pleasures" associated with cooked food will automatically reverse as one continues to step outside of the old comfort zone into the raw realm. It is not that one has to discipline oneself forever to stay away from the "pleasures" of cooked food, it is that one is no longer attracted to those foods. They become seen as lifeless foods devoid of any nutritional and spiritual strength.

The best time to begin is always right now. Teddy Roosevelt's most famous saying was: "Do what you can, with what you have, where you are." The best place on Earth, the greatest opportunity in the world, is right where you happen to be right now. You are sitting on your own fortune — your own "Acres of Diamonds."

Let's make the change now! Your life is too important to allow your diet to fall to a point where it finally takes your desire for survival to overcome your appetite for "poor" foods.

There are many things you do now which would have seemed difficult to you ten years ago. Those things themselves did not change, but your idea of yourself changed. What if you were to think things differently today?

It is going to take courage. Where there is no joy there can be no courage; and without courage all other virtues are meaningless. Enjoy the process and let Nature take its course. Nature's smile is for the joyful, the courageous, the disciplined, and the all-daring.

Complacency is the great enemy of possibility. Just keep taking action. Focus all your energy, not on fighting the old, but on building the new habits.

It is going to take a view to the long-term. The ability to think long-term, to be long-sighted, depends on the ability to delay gratification. The ability to delay gratification determines how much spiritual power we have over our physical body. Delaying gratification is a sign of wisdom and maturity. By delaying cooked-food gratification you start making incredible strides.

Self-discipline has been defined as the ability to make yourself do what you should do, when you should do it, whether you feel like doing it or not.

To become a 100% raw-foodist, you must have the desire. You must be willing to pay the price. The price may be much or it may be little, but you must condition your mind to pay it (and pay it gladly!), regardless of the cost. Remember Andrew Carnegie's saying, "Anything worth having is worth working for." Once you have been 100% raw for a time (6 months or more), and you have cleaned the cooked-food residue out of your body, it becomes easy.

It is time for you to cross the border; to sail out into an unknown sea; to commit to reaching a 100% raw-food diet. As you'll see, you will not fall off the edge of the world! You will have to overcome the stormy seas of negativity and the waves of peer pressure, the perilous storms of accusation and the scurvy-ridden sailors of mediocrity, the glide down the wave-crests into the wave-valleys of detoxification, but afterwards it all will appear before you a new land, a land transformed into a paradise, a land explored thus far by only the curious and the brave! You may well discover the timeless truth that when you change, the world changes automatically. You will look through different eyes. You will be transformed into a new being! Commit! There is no strength in compromise.

When you let go of cooked food, life becomes even more exciting. After many years of eating exclusively raw foods, your mindset will become more resolute, flexible, clear, free of doubt; your body will become lithe, supple, sensitive, and filled with energy.

Eventually, you will reach a point where you are able to do all you need to do in the external world (social food visits with friends, business luncheons, etc.), yet have no inner conflicts since you will have attained a new consciousness.

The insights that a 100% raw plant-food diet gives you are powerful. Statements are made with great certainty, and one does not know how it happened. Uncanny events become common place.

I woke up after napping in my backyard one day with a bird bouncing around my head and face. We just looked at each other. When you go all-raw, the animals do not look at you as something strange anymore, you do not carry the obvious smell of civilization's foods. You become more of the continuum of life — one with the animals. What price can you put on a unified connection with Nature? It is priceless. That is what a 100% raw plant-food diet will give you.

Action Steps:

1. Many raw-foodists ask me why people do not go 100% raw. 100% raw does present challenges. These challenges may be overcome through persistence, effort, and discipline. I have discovered the following 10 reasons why people do not go 100% raw:

1. They are not ready, their body and mind has not adjusted. Their favorite cooked foods still taste better than their favorite raw foods. With time, the taste buds will change, the body will acclimate to new, cleaner foods, and progress towards 100% raw will become easier. Everyone should transition at a pace that is outside their comfort zone, but not in their shock zone.

2. They don't realize the importance of eating 100% raw plant foods and the magic in it. They require more education on the subject.

3. They simply are not serious. They talk, but never do. They want to make an improvement in their life, but they are not willing to make the necessary effort.

4. They don't know how, they are confused by conflicting opinions on diet. They don't understand the idea of eating 100% raw plant food.

5. They haven't accepted 100% responsibility for their lives and their health, happiness, and longevity.

6. They don't feel they are worthy enough to be extraordinarily healthy. They don't feel they deserve it.

7. They don't go 100% raw because of the fear of rejection. They fear their friends and family will reject them and their new lifestyle and/or that the opposite sex will reject them.

8. They fear the unknown. Eating 100% raw is the unknown for most people, and for that reason, they fear it instead of embrace it! Eventually, we have nowhere to go, but into the unknown. Which do you prefer? A known hell or a strange heaven? The way you are going now is leading down a specific path — a destiny. One day you will arrive...the question is where?

9. They get unbalanced because they do not exercise and/or eat a healthy combination of green-leafy vegetables, sweet fruits, and fatty foods. Thus they return back to familiar low-energy food habits.

10. The inability to face their suppressed emotional issues when they arise. One of the major challenges I have seen in people going 100% raw is facing suppressed emotional trauma. A 100% raw plant-food diet presents your emotional issues to you — it brings them right to your consciousness. These issues often involve one or both parents. To win through, one must have the courage to face these emotional issues squarely and release them. Holding on to 10% "comfort foods" in the diet will slow the emotional traumas from arising too rapidly.

Get out your journal. Do any of these ten reasons apply to you and why? How will you overcome these challenges? Record the answers in writing in your journal.

Remember: Going 100% raw is great, but it is also beautiful to give a 100% effort. Decide what works for you in your lifestyle.

Lesson 19:
Mineral Trade-Out

Vitamins are never an issue when eating raw plant foods. All raw plant foods, even if not of an excellent quality, are abundant in all the vitamins we need to thrive. For instance, the B vitamins may be found in deep-green leafy vegetables and nuts. Vitamin B12 was addressed in **Lesson 16: Wild Food**. Vitamin C is found in many fruits, especially citrus fruits and peppers of all kinds. The best source of vitamin E is the avocado.

This lesson is about minerals, because it has been my experience, in studying raw-food nutrition, that minerals are far more important than vitamins.

Colloids are the mineral building blocks of the body. A colloid is a mineral suspended in solution with energy. They are extremely small and resist the pull of gravity. They conduct electricity throughout the body.

The Sun evaporates water from the leaves of plants, concentrating the protoplasm solution. Thus, due to osmosis (the movement of water from an area of greater concentration to an area of lesser concentration), water containing minerals in solution is pulled up from the roots into the leaves of the plant. In this way the protoplasm is continuously concentrated and the leaves become loaded with colloidal minerals suspended with Sun energy. Each plant mines a different spectrum of minerals from the soil and provides a different nutrition to the body. Calcium (lime), however, is the primary leaf mineral. Interestingly, calcium also makes up about 50% of the mineral matter of the human body and is found in all bodily tissues, but chiefly in the bones, teeth, and the muscles. The importance of leaf minerals for the human body cannot be overstated. When we consume plant leaves we are provided with fresh colloidal minerals with which to construct our bodies.

We can see the colloidal leaf minerals precipitate out of freshly-made green juices if we allow the juice to sit and lose energy. As a juice loses energy (zeta potential), it begins to change from an alkaline medium to an acid medium; it no longer has the energy to hold minerals in suspension. This is what happens to the blood as it acidifies from poor nutrition. The blood no longer has the energy to hold minerals in solution and thus they precipitate out in all the wrong places, such as the muscle tissue, joints, bones, etc. causing arthritis, weakness, bone spurs, etc.

Arthritis occurs when the blood's acidity is high. High blood acidity means low blood energy and low blood solubility. During this state, minerals are not held in solution and thus precipitate improperly. Arthritis is typically the result of a meat-based diet. Meat, raw or cooked, is extremely acidic, thus, meat lowers the blood's energy, causing improper mineral precipitation.

Arthritis is definitely linked with an overabundance of cooked, acid-forming elements in the body (from meat), and also it is linked to irritants introduced into the body by eating cooked nightshade plants (tomato sauce, french fries, baked potatoes, fried eggplant, tobacco smoke, etc.). For those with an exacerbated arthritic condition I recommend against eating any meat, and to avoid all nightshades (chiles, eggplants, peppers, potatoes, tobacco, tomatilloes, tomatoes), even if eaten raw. I have noticed with some of my clients that sensitivities to cooked nightshades continue even when nightshades are eaten raw.

Osteoporosis also occurs when the blood's acidity is high due to an excess of acid-forming foods in the diet. Remember: the quality of the food entering the body directs the quality of the blood and lymph. To balance an acid condition in the blood, the body must draw alkaline minerals from the bones. Dairy products are acid-forming once the body no longer has the enzymes and vital energy necessary to metabolize them. An acid-forming diet, over the long term, will leach minerals from the bones, leading to osteoporosis. To reverse an osteoporosis condition, please reference **Lesson 14: Sapoty Brook's CaPNaK Chart**. Use the CaPNaK Chart to consistently introduce significantly more calcium-residue foods into your diet, such as lettuce, kale, collards, oranges, figs, broccoli, etc. In conjunction with nutrition, weight-bearing exercise is extremely important for healing osteoporosis. I have seen, on this Sunfood program coupled with exercise, up to a 22% increase in bone density over a two-year period.

Trade-Out

After eating Sunfoods under the Sun for a sufficient period of time, the body begins removing everything that is improper. This process will continue for several years until you become a rejuvenated being. As you continue eating raw, you will eventually replace every cell and restructure every tissue using the high-quality minerals, nutrients, and positive energy that you are putting in your body.

After a sufficient period of eating Sunfoods at a 100% level (usually between 1-3 years), the body will begin to purge acids and replace the heavier minerals. If one is eating a diet high in sweet fruit with no green-leafy vegetables, mineral trade-out may occur sooner (usually 1 year). This is when the teeth problems arise in fruitarians, which is indicative of the body purging acids and also indicative of a lack of minerals in the body, especially calcium, magnesium, and silicon. At the point of mineral trade-out, one needs to take in at least 2.5 pounds (1.1 kg) of green-leafed vegetables daily (one-third eaten, two-thirds juiced) and simultaneously cut down on eating hybridized sweet fruit. Once you make it past the period of mineral trade-out, which usually lasts about 6 months, you will have reached the "point of no return." After that point your body will reject dead foods powerfully. You will be locked into a greatly increased health level, which is unimaginable compared to the way you once lived.

Mineral trade-out signals to you that a deep cleaning and healing of the body tissues is taking place. It means your body has really gotten to the core tissues for replacement.

The lesson of mineral trade-out is to eat highly-mineralized fruit grown in highly-mineralized soil.

When you eat, always go for the highest-quality, highest mineral-content foods available to you. Unfortunately, most commercial fruit trees are short-lived and are shallow feeders. The fuller and richer the taste of the fruit, the more minerals it contains. The roots of wild fruit trees go down from 10 to 25 feet (3.0 to 7.5 meters) where there has been no soil depletion. The nut trees, that live for decades, send roots 40 to 50 feet (12 to 15 meters) deep to mine the Earth. Planting fruit and nut trees will help remineralize the Earth because they pull minerals from down deep and deposit them on the surface in the form of falling leaves, fruits, and nuts creating a fertile bed for gardening vegetables. (See **Chart: Tree Mineralization** on page 77.)

Remineralization

The yield, strength, and mineral content of raw plant foods — whether they are commercial, organic, or wild — is improved by remineralization. Remineralization is the process of loading the soil with crushed and pulverized rocks which restore the full spectrum of mineral elements. The soil microbes, earthworms, and plant roots are directly nourished by an abundance of soil minerals.

The research is in with soil expert and 22+ year 100% raw-foodist Don Weaver. Don Weaver has demonstrated conclusively in the book, **The Survival Of Civilization**, which he co-authored with John Hamaker, that plants and trees depend far more on the soil and its mineral content than they depend on climate to produce high quality leaves and fruits.

Insects always infest trees and other plants (as pathogens invade people) which are weakened by malnutrition and no longer have resistance to their natural enemies. The hybridized commercial crops grown today in weak demineralized soils are heavily sprayed with pesticides to keep the insects from overrunning the whole show.

John Hamaker writes:

"This question of the proper feeding of the soil is the crux of the whole food situation, for if the soil starves so does the plant and so do we. We cannot have healthy human beings without healthy food crops, and these depend entirely upon the healthy feeding of the soil."

"High yields depend on loading the soil with both a large surface area of available minerals and organic matter."

"Examine a stone, other than limestone, in the soil. Crack it open. Under a very drab demineralized exterior 'skin' you will see the minerals. That skin represents the depth which the microorganisms have been able to penetrate the crystal structure of the stone."

When the rock is ground to dust, more "skin" is exposed to feed the soil microbes.

The best fertilizer for trees and plants is crushed rock. When rock is pulverized, exponentially more of its surface area is exposed and more minerals are available to the micro-organisms in the soil. In one pound (0.45 kg) of finely ground gravel you have about 10 acres (4 hectares) of surface area for the microorganisms to feed on.

The mineralized rock dust you mix in with your plant soil will eventually show up as a major difference in the size, taste quality, and texture of the food grown therefrom. Any rock dust mixture that will give good growth and is found locally is preferred.

Action Steps:

1. Discover rock dust. Visit your local gravel quarry, ask for the chemist, get several bags of rock dust (they should be free), and throw and sprinkle the dust directly into the soil around your trees and garden.

If local rock dust is not available, contact Don Weaver at: Earth Health Regeneration, P.O. Box 620478, Woodside, CA 94062-0478, USA. He can provide you with the best and most economical sources of rock dust available world-wide.

2. Read John Hamaker and Don Weaver's book **The Survival Of Civilization**.

Lesson 20:
Teeth

One of the ways anthropologists date human fossils is by looking at skull teeth. The more modern the fossil, the more tooth decay. Analyses of striations on fossilized teeth show no decay or premature wear when hominids ate a raw-vegan diet. Most paleontologists agree that tooth decay coincided with the discovery of fire and accelerated with the advent of agriculture.

An unbalanced cooked diet lacking in alkaline minerals (calcium, magnesium, silicon) and high in sugar and acid-forming minerals (phosphorus, chlorine) damages teeth formation. Because teeth begin to be formed in the pre-natal stage, the diet of the mother has a lifelong influence. Due to improper nutrition, the body does not have the energy or minerals with which to properly control the eruption of teeth into the mouth. Poor nutrition results in crowded and malformed teeth, along with an altered bite. These structural dental challenges begin essentially as birth defects and are exacerbated by continuous improper nutrition. T.C. Fry reported in an article entitled, "The Myth Of Health In America" which appeared in Dr. Shelton's **Hygienic Review** (37:7, p. 150-152) that 98.5% of the US population suffers from dental problems of one type or another. These may often be reversed and corrected in one or more generations of eating significantly more mineral-rich organic green-leafed vegetables.

The average adult human has 32 teeth: 4 canines (the dullest of any primate), 8 incisors, 20 molars: 12.5% dull canines, 25% incisor teeth, 62.5% grinding teeth. This indicate that the majority of what we should eat is food which must be chewed (ground up), such as fibrous plant matter.

Calcium combines with phosphorus to form calcium phosphate crystals which build the structure of bones and teeth. These crystals are incredibly light and are formed into a pattern similar to that found in a diamond. They have a weight-bearing capacity which is four times greater than an equal amount of reinforced concrete.

Teeth and bones are dynamic living tissues that are constantly being replaced and rebuilt. To support this process, both calcium and phosphorus are required in a 1:1 ratio. Most people follow a diet high in phosphorus (foods such as: cooked rice or grains, nuts, potato and corn chips, and meat), but they do not balance their diet with easy to assimilate calcium-rich foods (green-leafed vegetables). This creates an acid-condition which leaches calcium from the bones, and especially the teeth, to neutralize the acid, thus leading to tooth weakening and decay.

Meats, nuts, and seeds (grains) are the heaviest foods in acid-forming minerals. Undoubtedly, the introduction of milk products (high in calcium) into the human diet coincided with the explosion in meat and grain consumption when humans domesticated grazing animals and wild grains. Because pasteurized (cooked) milk products are not suitable for human consumption (and for other reasons mentioned in earlier lessons), calcium should come primarily from green-leafed vegetables and/or their juices.

Contrary to the belief that fruits are alkaline, many fruits are slightly acidic in their end-mineral breakdown, meaning they contain slightly more phosphorus than calcium (reference **Lesson 14: Sapoty Brook's CaPNaK Chart**). Even alkaline fruits, such as oranges, have such a strong citric acid content that, if eaten excessively, may damage tooth enamel, unless the teeth are cleaned with a brush or green leaves after a meal. Fruitarians can develop dental challenges if green leaves are not included in the diet in adequate proportions to provide alkalinity and an excellent calcium-phosphorus balance.

Green-leafed vegetables help clean sugar from the teeth. The harmful effects of refined and processed sugars on the teeth have been well established, but even excessive fruit sugar can damage the teeth, although not to the degree as these other types.

The body best assimilates calcium, when both magnesium and manganese are present together. Green-leafed vegetables are high in magnesium, manganese, and silicon. Spinach is the best source of all three of these minerals together. When eating, one should daily consume 1,000 mg of calcium, 300 mg of magnesium, and 5 mg of manganese (2 pounds of whole or juiced green-leafed vegetables will be adequate).

Silicon-residue foods play a major role in bone and teeth formation in the body. A high-intake of silicon-residue foods has been shown to heal broken bones at an accelerated rate (see Louis Kervran's book **Biological Transmutations**). Silicon-residue foods include: cucumbers, horsetail (an herb), lettuce, nopales (prickly-pear cactus leaves), okra, ripe bell peppers, radishes, and tomatoes.

Chewing green leaves helps clean and repair the teeth. I like to say in my seminars, "A few days of 'leafarianism' (eating leaves) naturally brushes the teeth and heals mineral deficiencies."

Wadging like the primates is an excellent way to heal the mouth of pyorrhea, gum disease, and cavities. Wadging means to load your mouth with greens and chew and compress the pulpy matter into the teeth and gums like a ball-player who chews tobacco. Continue to chew and compress the pulpy matter in the mouth for 30 to 45 minutes without swallowing. I have done this every day for weeks at a time for lunch by chewing on mouthfuls of wild malva for 20-30 minutes — wadging with wild food heightens the healing potential.

To radically remineralize the body, and rebuild the teeth, do the following daily for at least two weeks consistently: get plenty of Sunshine, exercise outdoors, eat at least 1.5 pounds (1.5 kg) of spinach and other deep greens with avocado or stone-crushed olive oil daily, drink 0.5 quart (0.5 liters) of fresh green-vegetable juice (kale, celery, cucumber), drink one 12 ounce (0.35 liters) glass of fresh orange juice as your only sugar food (but keep the juice away from the teeth), eat no hybrid vegetables (beets, carrots, corn, potatoes, rice), and eat no nuts or seeds.

Be sure to maintain excellent dental hygiene by doing the following:

1. Be sure to daily floss between all of the teeth. Unlike a natural animal's teeth, the average person's teeth are crowded together.

2. Brush your teeth daily. The apes are often seen cleaning their teeth with small chewed up branches rich with resin, much as we use a toothbrush. Consider using sea salt and/or baking soda instead of toothpaste. Brush your teeth, rinse, and gargle with fresh ocean water if at all possible. Although I brush with water, I do not use toothpaste and have not since 1992 — occasionally I will brush my teeth with sea salt and/or baking soda. Be sure to also brush the gums and tongue.

3. Eat green-leafy vegetables. Green leaves are the best source of calcium and mineral salts. Chlorophyll is a medicine. Our teeth are living bones whose primary mineral is calcium.

4. In my experience working with people, I have found that fasting is a good way to heal a minor toothache. A minor toothache may be the body's signal that it needs a rest from the constant food bombardment, so that it may heal. After fasting on water for a few days, brush your teeth clean, and then consider giving your gums a chance at a complete physiological rest from food and brushing for several more days. If you have severe pain in a tooth, have lost a tooth, have an infection, have a chipped tooth, have bleeding gums, or if teeth problems persist, please see a holistic dentist.

Action Steps:

1. As you begin The Sunfood Diet, set up an appointment to have your teeth cleaned by a dental hygienist. Have all the excess residue removed from your teeth. This will help give you a fresh start.

2. Have mercury amalgam fillings removed from your mouth as soon as you are capable. Mercury is one of the most toxic substances known and should not be in our mouths! I have clients and friends who were close to death from mercury poisoning from amalgam fillings which were leaching into their bodies. They had the mercury removed, discovered eating raw plant foods, and healed. Consult a holistic dentist for proper removal and replacement. Be sure you are protected from mercury amalgam dust by a "rubber dam" when you have your fillings removed.

The presence of metals in the mouth causes an 'electrical short circuit' of the vital nerve energies. This is true not only for the specific area where the metal is located, but will also be reflected in other parts of the organism that correspond to that area in the brain's circuitry. Thus an amalgam filling in the lower, left molar(s) may affect the sigmoid colon, or an amalgam filling in the "eye tooth" may affect the eye, etc.

3. Read **It's All In Your Head** by Dr. Hal Huggins.

Lesson 21:
Sun

"We choose the god-like splendor
Of the best-loved Sun
To inspire us;
May the shining Sun
Brighten your Life!"
— **Ramayana**

"If gorillas had a religion, they would surely be Sun worshippers."
— Dr. George Schaller, **Year Of The Gorilla**

Have you discovered absorbing nutrition directly from the elements —
the air, the water, the Sun?

All life on this planet derives from the Sun. The Sun beats like a great
heart through every living organism. They say the molecules that make
up our bodies were born in the great infernos of our superabundant star.

The air we breathe is transformed Sun energy. During photosynthesis,
as plants absorb Sun energy, they transform carbon dioxide (CO_2) into
vital oxygen (O_2) for animals to breathe. Here, at the first step, Nature
dictates the necessity of animal life upon the underlying matrix of Sun-
imbued plant life — animal respiration depends specifically on solar
energy.

The foods we eat are energy reservoirs of transformed Sun energy. Through photosynthesis, plants capture energy from the Sun and lock that power into their stems, leaves, seeds, roots, and fruits. All animals are transformed plants. The body of the zebra is nothing more than grass. The body of the lion is also grass, as it preys on the grass-eaters.

To a great extent we are heliovores — beings nourished directly by Sun energy. Sunlight can transform your health. The human body, with many capillaries in the skin surface, draws in Sunlight which is converted directly into nourishment by hemoglobin in the blood, just as chlorophyll converts Sunlight into nourishment in the plant. Remember, hemoglobin and chlorophyll are identical except for one mineral. Hemoglobin contains iron, chlorophyll contains magnesium.

Sunlight makes us bright and cheery. It cultivates a healthy positive attitude. A lack of Sunlight has the opposite effect. We see that people in colder climates are often afflicted by a seasonal depression which has been attributed to a lack of Sunshine during the winter months.

The same elements in green-leafed vegetables which protect the leaves from ultra-violet radiation also protect you when you ingest those leaves. One of these substances is beta-carotene, which literally shields the nucleus of each cell.

The benefits of Sunshine are improved by eating correctly as the Sun and fresh air act like magnets in drawing toxic matter to the skin. When the body is clean and internally protected with beta-carotene you will be amazed at how long you can be in the Sun and how well you tan. When people eat correctly and are detoxified, exposure to the Sun cannot lead to skin cancer.

A diet high in cooked fat (free radicals), chemicals, and low in green leaves has been positively linked to skin cancer. This is because free radicals and toxins in the unprotected skin are baked and mutated by the Sun's rays. Recently, researchers at Baylor College of Medicine found that people on a low-cooked-fat diet had a greatly reduced risk of developing pre-malignant growths and non-melanoma skin cancers.

Sunlight improves our health in many different ways:

A good Sun bath is an incredible waste eliminator, as it draws toxins out of the skin. The skin is the body's largest eliminative organ.

Dr. Kime tells us in his wonderful book **Sunlight** (which I highly recommend):

> "Cholesterol [formed by the body, not foreign cholesterol] turns to vitamin D — a vitamin needed for proper bone formation — when Sunlight or ultraviolet light strikes the skin. Without this vitamin the bones do not become calcified and will bend easily. This condition is called rickets."

Dr. Kime describes that Sunlight builds the immune system and increases the oxygenation of the skin.

Dr. Kime writes:

> "A study of the results of combined Sunlight and exercise, showed that group that was getting the Sunlight treatments with exercise, had improved almost twice as much as shown by their electrocardiograms, as had those who only exercised, even though both groups were on a general health resort treatment program."

Sunlight lowers blood sugar. It is a natural insulin. A diet high in sweet fruit must also be accompanied by Sunshine on the skin to help metabolize the sugar. Sunlight helps to store the sugar as glycogen in the liver, muscles, and cells for later use.

Exposing the skin to the Sun stimulates the capillaries and brings more blood to the skin surface. This helps to heal cuts, bruises, and rashes. In

World War II it was discovered that exposing abrasions, open wounds, and broken bones to direct Sunlight led to quicker healing.

Fungus is destroyed by direct Sunlight. Candida cannot survive in direct Sunlight. I have worked with numerous people with candida. The first step to overcoming candida is Sunlight on the naked body (reference **Lesson 13: How To Use The Sunfood Triangle**, **Eating To Overcome Candida**).

Sunlight increases the strength of digestion. Sunlight increases the body's internal "fire." In Chinese oriental medicine we find the concept of yin-yang balance and we see that "cold" raw foods may be balanced with hot Sun energy.

Sunlight improves the eyesight and regulates the hormones. Occasionally bringing direct Sunlight into the eyes just for a brief moment, unmitigated by glasses, windows, or filters, will help balance the body's hormones. *It is important that if you look directly at the Sun, it only be for a split second, or else you can burn your retina.*

Sunlight directly on the skin, especially on the breasts and reproductive organs heals impotence and dysfunction in those areas. A contributing cause of challenges in those areas is restrictive clothing and a lack of Sunshine.

Action Steps:

1. Try fresh aloe vera juice as a Sun lotion. By following The Sunfood Diet your resistance to ultraviolet (UV) radiation and Sunburns will increase dramatically. I have found that it is literally impossible for me to get burned under the Sun; even if I have not been in the Sun for several weeks. *The best UV protection is inner protection.*

Commercial sunscreens disable the body's natural sunburn alarm mechanism. Most suntan lotions, creams, and butters are made of chemicals mixed with cooked fats which produce free radicals in the skin just like dietary cooked fats. For these reasons I do not recommend commercial sunscreens.

2. Seek out at least 30 minutes of direct Sunlight each day on as much of your body as possible. No matter where one lives, the practice of simply allowing the Sunlight to reach one's exposed face will provide benefits.

There is no mistake in Nature. We are designed for a life of "Fun in the Sun!" Enjoy the abundance Nature has to offer — soak in the golden rays of life. Sunlight is good mood food.

Consider the the following: "Everyone, ill or well, looks better, feels better, gets healthier and functions more gracefully after exposing every part of their naked bodies to the beautiful Sunshine. Sunbathe each moment you can. It enlivens you in every possible way!"

Lesson 22:
Breathing (Pranayama)

"And the Lord God formed man of the dust of the ground
and breathed into his nostrils the breath of life;
and man became a living soul."
— Genesis 2:7

"For the rhythm of thy breath is the key of knowledge
which doth reveal the Holy Law."
— The Essene Gospel of Peace, Book I

I have provided you thus far with a detailed treatise on how to lighten the diet to liberate more energy for achievement, but before I go further, let me tell you: Do not be deceived — little energy comes from food — stimulation comes from food! The digestion of food takes energy away from the body. Energy comes first from the spirit, and then primarily from the air — from oxygen — and from a lack of obstructions in the body. A lack of oxygen makes people weak, and food is what they turn to for strength (stimulation). For more energy, start breathing!

All scientific considerations aside, air contains some life principle (prana) which keeps the human body functioning. This life principle (prana) is passed from the air to our bodies by breathing. Isn't that fascinating?

When you sleep you automatically breathe, but you do not automati-

cally eat! One can live for weeks without eating, for days without drinking, but only fleeting minutes without breathing. Yet breathing is the most
neglected science in the health field. All other organs operate to keep the
lungs functioning. The lungs, in turn, keep the internal organs healthy by
pushing and squeezing them, allowing the fluids to move around, within,
and through them.

Every breath contains more air by weight than would be eaten at a typical meal, and we are taking thousands of breaths a day! One is just as
poisoned by toxic air as by toxic food.

The power of breath is four-fold:

First and foremost, the breath controls the energy level in the body. We
know that everything is energy — matter is just a form of frozen energy.
The more oxygen available to your cells, the more energy you have to
accomplish your goals and the less food you desire. Many people overeat
because they are not breathing deeply.

If you feel hungry, sick, tired, or worn out, a good way for you to quickly rejuvenate yourself is to go outside and take 30 deep diaphragmatic
breaths.

Second is the fact that the lungs play a major role in the human immune
system. The lungs are the pump for the lymph system. There is four times
as much lymph in the body as blood; lymph bathes every cell of the body.
*As long as the lymph is kept clean and pumping through the body in an
orderly fashion by daily deep breathing, the immune system will become
incredibly strong.*

Deep breathing alkalizes the body by removing carbonic acid (dis-
solved carbon dioxide) from the blood and lymph.

Third, controlling the breath allows you to begin to also control the so-
called autonomic (automatic) functions of the body (i.e. heart rate, blood

flow, body temperature, etc.). The yogis of India have long-known that every state of the mind and body is associated with a corresponding respiration pattern. Long slow breaths slow the heart (that is why Ehret called the heart a valve, not a pump). Deep breathing warms you up. If you feel cold by eating raw foods, then take deep breaths to warm your body! Take deep breaths to increase your inner "fire" energy.

Fourth, oxygen eliminates pain. Pain in the body is always associated with a lack of oxygen in that area. Athletes who strain a muscle often continue to play, in fact prefer to play, because by staying active the strained muscle remains oxygenated and will be less painful. One can find relief from back aches and sore muscles by deep breathing.

It is the control we exert over our own breath that most distinguishes humans from the other primates. The only other mammals that can control their breath are those with aquatic characteristics, such as the dolphin, the hippo, the seal, the whale, and even the elephant.

Longevity is associated with slowing the breath. Those species which breathe very slowly live the longest. The giant tortoise breathes only four times a minute. Humans in comparison, breath 18 times a minute, and a restless monkey 32 times a minute.

While breathing in through your nose, hold your mouth lightly closed, and leave your tongue comfortably pressed to the roof of your mouth. Ideas and inspiration come to us by breathing through the nose. Experiment with making your breathing so slow that it would not disturb a feather on your nose.

Exhaling is more important than inhaling. To fully help detoxify the body, blow out all the air from the bottom of the lungs, then hold your breath. The vacuum produced in the lungs will exert a drawing force which will pull more poisons from the blood into the lungs for elimination.

A rarely discussed reason why people become addicted to smoking cigarettes derives from the breath control that smoking entails. When someone smokes a cigarette they fall into a habitual breathing pattern that fun-
damentally alters their state and energy level until they feel "relaxed."
Practicing deep breathing helps overcome addictions to smoking.

By breathing deeper and more rhythmically, you become calmer and
can concentrate and work better. Slow, deep diaphragmatic breathing was
the first health discipline I mastered. I credit late-night deep breathing
exercises with improving my performance in college when I was studying engineering and political science. I often would need an additional
two extra hours every night to do work, so at midnight I would go outside
and do at least ten deep diaphragmatic breaths in the 1:4:2 ratio. From
this practice my mind would clear and my energy would soar.

We are breathing all night as we sleep and the exhaled carbon dioxide
accumulates in stuffy homes. Keep your home windows open as much as
possible, especially at night to allow fresh oxygen to continuously revi-
talize you. Consider, bringing a plethora of house plants into your bed-
room and home to provide you with fresh oxygen.

Breathing is our most vital experience. Be silent, breathe deep. Silence
is power. Silence is an art. Long life is a matter of deep rhythmic breathing and keeping extremely quiet. Be silent and you allow your conscious,
doubting, warring mind to listen. The best performers have the calmest
breathing and quietest minds during the moment of truth.

Action Steps:

1. In my opinion, the best pattern for deep diaphragmatic breathing,
which I have used daily since age 19, is the following 1:4:2 ratio:

Breathe in (through the nose), for a multiple of 1 count. The nose
simultaneously filters and humidifies the air we breathe. The cribriform

plate above the septum in the nose also regulates the temperature of the air entering the lungs.

Hold that breath, for a multiple of 4 counts. This fully oxygenates and stimulates the body.

Breathe out (through the mouth), for a multiple of 2 counts. The out breath releases toxins.

An example of this breathing ratio:
Breathe in for 6 seconds.
Hold that breath for 24 seconds.
Breathe out for 12 seconds.

2. I have also had much success with the following 1:1:1:1 yogic breath ratio:
Breathe in (through the nose), for a multiple of 1 count.
Hold that breath, for a multiple of 1 count.
Breathe out (through the mouth), for a multiple of 1 count.
Hold the lungs empty, for a multiple of 1 count. This creates a vacuum suction which draws toxins out of the tissues on the following inhalation.

An example of this breathing ratio:
Breathe in for 6 seconds.
Hold that breath for 6 seconds.
Breathe out for 6 seconds.
Hold the lungs empty for 6 seconds.

3. Practice 30 deep diaphragmatic breaths each day following either of these patterns or both. Tune your lungs to these patterns. Initially, some dizziness and light-headedness may be experienced by breathing in this fashion as the brain becomes fully oxygenated; but this phenomena will pass as the body grows accustomed to deep breathing practices.

Lesson 23:
The Physiology of Excellence

"The higher your energy level, the more efficient your body.
The more efficient your body, the better you feel and the more
you will use your talent to produce outstanding results."
— Anthony Robbins

Excellence is a habit. Good health is an achievement — there are certain things you have to do. When your health improves, every other aspect of your life improves simultaneously. The ways you view your potential and the world improve too.

Physiological things, such as muscle tension, what we eat, how we breathe, and our posture all have a huge impact on our mental imagery, emotional state, and spiritual strength. A physiology of vibrant health produces a mindset, emotional attitude, and spiritual power of vibrant health. A physiology of vibrant health has an uncanny knack of attracting the right people, foods, and exercises that we need, right when we need them. That is the law: things produce after their own kind.

The As If Principle

We are physical, mental, emotional, and spiritual beings — it is a four-body system and each dramatically influences the other. The As If Principle demonstrates that we can use physiology (the way we are holding and moving our physical body) to influence our mental, emotional, and spiritual states. The As If Principle is invoked by taking on the physiology of the state we wish to reach.

Stand up tall and proud. Smile like you have never smiled before, from ear to ear. Breathe in deep. Now, try to get depressed. But do not stop smiling and do not change your physiology. Go ahead, try and feel sad. You cannot do it without changing your physiology. Every mental, emotional, and spiritual state is associated with a certain physiology.

Excellence is a state of physiology. Excellence is created by the way you carry yourself. Robust deep breathing, a knowing smile, a confident stride, and good posture, all create excellence.

Act as if you felt more energized, powerful, and resourceful than you ever have before and pretty soon you begin to become that way. When you act like a winner, you become a winner. Act as if you already are one of the healthiest individuals on the planet and pretty soon you begin to become that way.

If you ever feel mental, emotional, or spiritual trauma, change the way you are moving your physical body. You can change the way you are using the muscles in your face, the way you are moving your eyes, the way you are carrying your entire muscular system. Anthony Robbins tells us: "Emotion is created by motion." You are in control of your mental, emotional, and spiritual state. Tell yourself: "I am the master of my state. Nothing or no one can change how I feel except me. Through motion, breathing, and posture, I alter my state in a moment."

Eating food at the physical level accesses different mental, emotional, and spiritual states. Beautiful food accesses beautiful states of consciousness. The great thing about The Sunfood Diet is that it is something you can physically do! You just take action and the mental, emotional, and spiritual benefits automatically arise.

Empower Your Physiology

In addition to diet, the more exercise and stretching you do, the greater will be your health, and the more you will empower your physiology. Those who are in excellent physical shape are more in tune with their bodies. They have more control over their bodies and, as a result, are better able to control their mental, emotional, and spiritual states.

Fitness and health are not the same. Fitness is the ability to perform athletic feats. Health is a state of overall well-being, excellent digestion, and vibrant aliveness. Many professional athletes have excellent fitness, but poor health. This is why we often see some former athletes end up as physical wrecks after illustrious careers.

Daily exercise and stretching are as essential to excellent health as diet. Exercise and stretching move the lymph fluid and elevate the immune system. Low-impact lymphatic exercises, such as jumping on a trampoline or rebounder, are particularly powerful because they softly exercise each cell against the pull of gravity.

Exercise consists of two elements: endurance and strength. Endurance has to do with inner cleanliness. The less obstructions you carry around inside of you, the greater is your endurance. Strength has to do with overall muscular power. Muscular power is built by consistent yet varied training. I learned years ago to consistently "surprise my muscles" to overcome plateaus.

Stretching consists of two elements: flexibility and alignment. Both are developed and enhanced by yoga.

When you combine raw foods with yoga, you tune into a phenomenal state of being. The Sunfood Diet radically improves your metabolism and the biochemistry of your body. Yoga reforms physiology by the consistent practice of different stretching poses. Yoga helps squeeze toxins out of the tissues, open up tensions, and improve the mechanical functioning of the body. Yoga is about "letting go" to increase flexibility. Yoga will get the spine straight beginning with opening up the hips and sacrum. Practice yoga stretching after sleeping, sitting, or walking. If you have chronic back pain, start looking into yoga and eating more green-leafy vegetables to get your body alkaline (also consider sleeping without a pillow to allow the spine to rest in its natural position).

To achieve your true potential, you must cleanse your body of tension, free your mind of stagnant knowledge, and open your spirit to the physiology of pure excellence.

Action Steps:

1. Begin exercising daily. Engage in the type of exercise you enjoy, whether it be: walking, swimming, cycling, weight lifting, jumping on a rebounder, etc. Exercise outside in Nature whenever possible.

2. Enroll in a yoga class today. Read books on the subject; rent yoga videos, find an experienced teacher. Attend one of Nature's First Law's raw-food yoga retreats.

Lesson 24:
The Power Of Association

"No success is possible without a change in your peer group."
— Peter Lowe, success philosopher

"Burn bridges, not your food."
— Nature's First Law

Your mind is like a garden. The visiting birds and bees and bugs and winds are like television, radio, computers, friends, and relatives. If you fail to control and carefully plant the seeds of positive thought in your garden-mind with positive media, friends, or relatives, then negative seeds will grow by default.

Computer programmers know GIGO: Garbage In, Garbage Out. It is just as dangerous to feed junk information to your mind as it is to feed junk food to your body.

If we do not provide our minds with the programming we desire, others will provide that programming for us. Unless you control your suggestive environment carefully, you will be deluged with civilization's current frequency of negativity.

You are greatly influenced by your immediate suggestive environment. Anything which gets through to your conscious mind is influencing you. Are these influences helping or hindering the unfolding of the flowering potential within you? If they are hindering, you must decide to remove those influences, or remove yourself from such influences.

Unhealthy people are like sponges. They will try to gain energy from whomever they can. They draw the energy out of others. Since their energy is low, and they do not know how to create it on their own, they will try to take it from those around them. These are the people who steal your most valuable asset: your vital life energy! You know who they are. They are always ready to criticize rather than compliment. They are full of subtle verbal abuse and softly negative comments. They constantly try to keep you indebted to them. When they go into their routine, turn away. Disassociate from these people. The power to walk away from negative people is the best gift you can give to yourself.

Napoleon Hill has pointed out that the most common weakness of all human beings is the habit of leaving their minds open to the negative influence of other people. You must remove yourself from the range of influence of every person and every circumstance which has even the slightest tendency to cause you to feel inferior or incapable of obtaining the object of your purpose.

It takes a lot of energy to achieve your goals. You cannot afford to have negative people around you who drain your energy. Even if you make tremendous efforts in improving the quality of the information reaching you, if you still allow the same negative people in close, you will stumble. Select the people you associate with carefully — whether they be in person, on the phone, or on the Internet.

Join an inspiring crowd. The people around you are a reflection of yourself.

In **Unlimited Power** Anthony Robbins writes: "If you can surround yourself with people who will never let you settle for less than you can be, you have the greatest gift that anyone can hope for. Association is a powerful tool. Make sure the people you surround yourself with make you a better person by your association with them."

Only through the harmonious relationships with other living things may an individual have full, unhindered, complete use of all mental faculties.

Weed your life of negative influences. Protect your garden. Develop a garden so rich, so abundant, that after many years you won't need to weed it at all; it will be perpetually growing so many positive beautiful plants and offering forth such incredibly vibrant fruits that a weed will not be capable of growing in it.

Action Steps:

1. Surround yourself with plants, animals, people, books, pictures, motivational mottoes, and other suggestive reminders of your beauty and greatness. Build around yourself an impenetrable atmosphere of prosperity and achievement. Saturate your life in every way and by all means available, with those people, places and things which promote your visions and goals. Make each day one continuous positive affirmation. The only things we have in life are our moment to moment experiences. Make each moment a sensational joy.

2. Take a page in your journal and draw a line down the middle of it. On the left side, list 6 people with whom you are willing to spend less time with due to their negative influence on you. On the right side, list 6 people with whom you would like to spend more time with due to their positive influence on you. Make this page a goal; act on it immediately.

Lesson 25:
Saturation Point

"Information is the commodity of kings."
— Anthony Robbins

We live in an era where all knowledge is available to all those who seek it out.

There is an abundance of useful information out there in the world. We are at the source. We can choose. We may tune into any frequency we like. We can learn anything we desire.

Learning is never what one expects. Every step of learning is a new task. Learning is an unending quest. There is something for you to learn from every experience, every individual you encounter, every book you read, every audio/vidcotape you listen to or watch.

A commitment to life-long learning is an essential part of health. Positive information is to the mind what Sunfood is to the body. A malnourished body cannot thrive. Neither can a malnourished mind. A body fed by the negative energy of fired foods becomes ill. A mind fed by negative energy and wrong thoughts becomes ill. A diet of raw food is necessary to health, but if the mind is not also given pure food, the body will suffer. A mind fed evil, unkind thoughts of destructive criticism, condemnation, hate, jealousy, fear, and doubt will reproduce such emotions in the physical body, leading to illness.

You are made or unmade by your own education. You are at the source; you can control what information you are allowing to enter your awareness. You may study anything you desire. You can recapture a child's ability to learn by becoming inspired by new information. Studies presented in progressive educational books, such as **The Learning Brain** by Gorden Dryden and Jeannette Vos, prove that learning causes the brain to physically grow and rewire itself in a whole new way.

We learn in many ways: by repetition, by emotional impact, but the absolutely most powerful way to learn and master any subject is by saturation.

In my experience, the entire secret of success is saturation. Start bombarding yourself with words and pictures consistent with your goals. Just have fun. Read books which forward you in the direction you are headed. Listen to success tapes in your car. Listen to success tapes while you eat. Watch educational videotapes at the end of the day. Attend seminars which provide additional inspiration to accelerate your goal achievement. I guarantee that, when you start this program of massive saturation, you will dramatically improve your entire life and begin to manifest your dreams rapidly.

The most successful individuals in any field remain so by continuously adding to their own stock of knowledge by appropriating the thoughts, phrases, and ideas of geniuses through a program of information saturation. A mind nourished continuously by the ideas of genius minds will remain alert, brilliant, flexible, and receptive. If this renewal is neglected, the mind will stagnate — we see this in musicians who seem to have lost their "edge." "If you don't use it, you lose it," is a common phrase of simple yet profound truth — it is in strict accordance with the cosmic laws.

The way to make a radical change in your life is to consistently bombard your brain with a new stream of personal-development information, presented by different people, and presented in different formats. Since your number one goal is to be totally healthy, all the information entering your mind should be furthering that goal and none of the information should be detracting from it.

To achieve vibrant health, educate yourself on the subject of gardening, herbs, natural living, raw foods, and related subjects. through reading. This has been a major factor in my own health, as my organization Nature's First Law offers the largest selection of raw-food and natural-health information in the world — the content of which I have fully accessed.

Saturation means attending every health seminar possible. Attend every success seminar possible. Attend every seminar given in your specialty area. Each speaker can provide you with wonderful distinctions which can transform your life. Any one speaker might say something you have heard before, but in a slightly different way, a way which immediately applies to you. The energy of a live performance cannot be matched. Go to success seminars for fun.

When you are healthy, and your suggestive environment is cleared, you can accelerate your success by converting all information entering your mind into one focused field — the field in which you desire to excel. Make all information input positive, uplifting, and focused on the items necessary in this field for your goal achievement. You can become an expert in any field in less than five years, and if you truly saturate yourself in the way I have advised, you can become an expert in any field in two or three years.

If you want health, you have to study health. If you want success, you have to study success. In my own life, I have made a study of superior health and incredible success. I am fascinated by vibrant health. I am fascinated when I see someone who is totally alive. I am intrigued by phenomenal success. I love hearing success stories. It is so interesting to hear the stories behind mega-music bands, such as The Beatles or The Bee Gees or ABBA. Saturating my mind with the secrets of health and the stories of super success has revolutionized my life. The mystery of incredible success is unlocked when one's fascination is met with saturation.

Reading

If you want to get good at something, read a book on it. Read many books on it. More is better.

The successful individual with a purpose in life makes it a business, a responsibility, and an exciting and fun use of time to read books relating to that purpose. In that way, important knowledge is acquired which comes from the experiences of others who have gone before.

An individual's reading program should be as carefully chosen as the daily diet, for that too is food, without which mental growth will stagnate.

Business philosopher Jim Rohn says, "Miss a meal, but don't you miss your reading." What excellent advice! Reading a book written by a person you admire puts you in a mental and emotional state similar to theirs. Those with a purpose devour books like paradisical fruits.

We intuitively know that readers are achievers. Leaders read. Feed your mind with good reading.

Success philosopher Brian Tracy describes that one hour of reading in your chosen field each day will make you an authority in that field in 3 years, a national authority in that field in 5 years, and an international authority in that field in 7 years. Just reading alone!

Read

Do you want to lead?
Read.
Do you have a mind to feed?
Read.

Read every chance,
During each snippet of time.
Choose a variety of
Prose and Rhyme.

"The Secrets of the Ages
Are found on written pages."

Five years hence,
You'll be the same as now,
Except for the people you meet,
And the books you browse.

Learn from those
Who've gone before.
Find out how
They opened the door.

Discover wild stories,
Get a new feel.
Don't spend your time,
Reinventing the wheel.

Take notes on your books
And write them all down.
The results you reap
Will amaze and astound.

The answers to your questions
Have already been found,
They exist somewhere —
Written down.

Read every page on your bookshelf,
You'll laugh out loud
And attract brilliant wealth.
You'll cry without sound,
And breathe in new health!

Words through your eyes,
Deeply impress;
Transformed they become
The thoughts you express.

Read an hour a' day,
In the field you choose.
With persistent action,
You can't lose!

Everything you read
Is a marvelous seed!
Which explodes into fortunes
And inspires great deeds.

I once had read, "Success leaves clues."
So I asked a genius, "What do you do?"
After much probing, the genius did say:
"Well, I read three books a day."

There is a vast world
To explore,
If you'll just read—
A little bit more!

How To Begin Saturating Your Mind

Ideally, your entire day should be one continuous bombardment of positive, uplifting information.

The first waking hour sets the pace of the day. Whatever you do, listen to, or read in that first hour stays with you all day long. Have you ever woke to a song, and that song was in your head throughout the day? This is the principle in action. What if you awoke each morning to the most uplifting music, or the most powerful success literature possible? It is great to feel those inspirations coursing through the body all day long.

The alpha-wave state of the brain is the state of highest mental activity. It is the state you are in when you awaken in the morning and right before you sleep at night. You may achieve the alpha-wave state by taking 10 long deep breaths. You may achieve higher performance on tests or in physical competitions by saturating the mind through positive affirmations, goal writing, goal reviewing, reading, success audio listening, etc. when the brain is in the alpha state.

Begin each morning with empowering messages and then continue the bombardment throughout the day. Raw foods action supplemented by daily self-improvement information saturation is a success formula which cannot be topped.

Chaos theory teaches us that even tiny differences of input could quickly become overwhelming differences in output — a phenomenon mathematicians have termed "sensitive dependent on initial conditions." In weather this translates into what is known as the "Butterfly Effect" — the notion that a butterfly stirring the air today in Peking can transform storm systems next month in New York. Since this is true, imagine how a *massive* difference in mind input through focused information saturation will equate into an extraordinary difference in output. The Butterfly Effect would become a Phoenix Effect.

Action Steps:

1. Everyone has their own way of learning things. Find out what works best for you. My preference is for reading and audio tapes. What is the best learning modality for you? If this is not clear, ask yourself: "How can I figure out what learning modality works best for me?" Try different approaches. Try alternative learning strategies.

2. Invest in good books. Invest your money in you and your family's education. Find the best health books and read them!

3. Make plans this week to attend a health or success seminar in your area.

4. Record all good ideas in your journal. Become a collector of good ideas you have gathered from live seminars, books, audio tapes, videos, and personal experiences.

5. Become a success-tape addict. Listen to success tapes while driving, eating, or exercising. Dispose of cooked-food addiction and replace it with success-tape addiction.

6. During your first waking moments each morning, listen to a song that inspires you and will keep you charged throughout the day. During the first 30-60 minutes each day, read success books or listen to empowering audio tapes.

7. Tape a new motivational quote to your nightstand or bathroom mirror every week.

Lesson 26:
The Inverse Paranoid

"Verily the most necessary thing is contentment under all
circumstances; by this, one is preserved from morbid conditions
and from lassitude. Yield not to grief and sorrow: they cause the
greatest misery. Jealousy consumeth the body and anger doth
burn the liver: avoid these two as you would a lion."
— Baha'u'llah

"Nothing has any power over me other than that
which I give it through my conscious thoughts."
— Anthony Robbins

"All bad things must come to an end."
— Nature's First Law

In order for you to remain in "flow" all the time, in order for you to
achieve the health levels you desire daily, you must be able to convert
negative thoughts into positive thoughts.

You can create an aura of positive energy around you by a positive
mental attitude. A positive outlook means confidently expecting to learn
and benefit from every situation. When you are in the right frame of
mind, any obstacle may be transformed in a moment into greater effort
which will bring you closer to the massive success of which you are capable.

Attitude is everything. A bad attitude does not come by chance — it is constructed by negative thoughts and emotions.

Negative emotions are always harmful. They serve no useful purpose. They poison and acidify the body. Negative emotions are the primary reason why people fail to achieve the highest levels of material and spiritual success. Feelings of doubt and fear always lead to failure.

If you experience negative emotions in your life, let them flow through you rather than bottle them within you. You can dispel negative emotions physically by: hitting, kicking, yelling, and/or biting. Dispel anger by driving a golfball, kicking a football, screaming aloud, and/or chewing dark green-leafy vegetables. Let the anger pass through you into the physical object. Transmute anger into positive action.

You can dispel negative emotions through normal exercise (although not as quickly as through the methods mentioned above). Dancing, lifting weights, surfing, or walking are all effective ways to manage negativity.

You can also dispel negative emotions mentally by reframing the experience, by changing what the experience means to you. When you look for the good in any situation, then the good looks for you and you dispel negativity.

All experiences may be transmuted into useful service. No experience need be a negative mental liability. Through the power of thought, one may transform sadness to happiness in a nano-second. Your ability to reframe any situation, to find the positive benefit, is unlimited.

It is not what happens to you, but your reaction to what happens to you that counts. No mental challenge is stressful in itself, only your response to a mental challenge can cause stress.

Nothing is entirely good or bad for you until you say so. If you believe that everything which happens to you in life contains some good within it, then everything will come forth to strengthen you and help you to rise to a higher level of consciousness.

Problems are challenges; challenges are good; challenges are inevitable. Every challenge in your life is heaven-sent to teach you a valuable physical and spiritual lesson. Every challenge contains its gift.

Use your willpower to keep any disappointment from dampening your spirit. Every disappointment builds character, knowledge, strength, and stamina. Use each setback as a stepping stone for advancement.

Accept defeat as an inspiration to greater effort and carry on with the belief that you will succeed. Convert defeat into a challenge to greater effort.

Most people sense intuitively that there is another side to life — a better way. But when they advance towards it, they are struck by a bombardment of contradictory information and negativity which stumbles them. This is the test you must pass to achieve success. Napoleon Hill discovered in researching his **Laws Of Success** that the greatest achievers he interviewed found their greatest successes just beyond their greatest failures. So, even following an enormous perceived failure, keep yourself in a state of total resourcefulness and you will eventually succeed. Success lies on the far side of failure.

There is one unbeatable rule for mastering frustrations and disappointments, and that is to accept the lesson learned and continue to work diligently and intently towards one's goals. Use strong emotions, whether positive or negative, to inspire the creation of ideas through your imagination, then take action upon those ideas.

You are in control. You either make yourself miserable, or you make yourself strong. The amount of work is the same. In fact, it takes even more energy to be miserable than to be strong. It takes more energy to be a "paranoid" than to be an "inverse paranoid." Consider this: it takes 13 muscles to smile and 112 muscles to frown.

An inverse paranoid is someone who believes the universe is conspiring to do her/him good. The personality of the inverse paranoid is characterized by a positive mental attitude. A positive mental attitude is one of the best indicators of how healthy a person really is. Due to a positive mental attitude, the inverse paranoid is always more likely to succeed.

The inverse paranoid expects to win and is always swift to make decisions based on intuitive feeling without fear or regret. My experience as an inverse paranoid has taught me this is true as I feel I am a good decision maker. I have always trusted my gut feeling. The inverse paranoid trusts her/his instincts! Instinct is a direct download of information from infinite intelligence.

The inverse paranoid continues to smile and expect the best results, in even the worst situations. The mind of the inverse paranoid is a transformer which takes all challenges and transmutes them into creative opportunities. Every discordant word and thought becomes transformed into greater things.

The inverse paranoid calls upon spiritual powers through which obstacles may be removed at will. That spiritual power changes the biochemistry of the mind and body to access greater resources to overcome any challenge.

In my journal I have written the following: "Nature is conspiring to do me good, to keep me young, and to place me at the top of the world." That is the attitude of the inverse paranoid.

Indian philosophy explains that once we state something ten thousand times it becomes a mantra, a thought form which shapes the future. The word "mantra" in its sanskrit derivation is a combination of two words

"man" (thought) and "tra" (liberation). A mantra should be a thought of
liberation. The slogan, mantra, or motto of the inverse paranoid is: "Don't
worry about it, embrace it." Try saying that aloud or to yourself ten thousand times! I have — and the results are revolutionary.

Action Steps:

1. Understand the messages of failure and pain. Failure and pain speak
one language — they directly communicate to us what kind of change
must take place. They tell you where you have gone wrong and where
you have gone right! They chart your course and tell you when and where
you are off target.

2. The next time you are faced with a stressful situation, say to yourself: "Don't worry about it, embrace it." Repeat this over and over in your
mind.

Don't Worry About It, Embrace It

From:
Frustration to
Fascination.
Bust to
Boom.

Misery to
Magic,
Thrilled,
And Ecstatic.

Disgust to
Delight.
Heavy to
Light.

Weakness to
Might.

Shadow to
Sun.
Fear to
Fun.

By power of mind
You'll discover and find
You can go from:
Vanquished to
Victorious.
Drab to
Glorious.
Tense to
Joyous.

Don't worry about it,
Embrace it.
Every adversity carries,
A seed of great benefit.

Substitute good thoughts
For bad.
Happy thoughts
For sad.
Rule your brain,
Join the few.
You can only think:
One thought, not two!

Go from:
Devastation to
Procreation.

Labor to
Recreation.
Irritation to
Innovation.
Desperation to
Inspiration.

Turn it around,
You're in control.
Why not happily attain
Your every goal?

Worse is better.

From anger
To laughter,
And sorrow
To smiles.
Go from rags to riches
In the shortest of
Whiles.

Don't hate,
Feel great.
Lift yourself up to
The highest state.
You are the master, of
Your fate.

Failure to
Success.
Insult to
Jest.
Worst to
Best!

Don't grieve,
But perceive:
What happens,
Happened.
Its already the past.
Only in your mind,
Can an event last.
Stress won't ever change it.
Don't worry about it —
Embrace it.

Lesson 27:
Tapping Infinite Intelligence

Spiders have always constructed their webs as they do now, and each type weaves its own style of web. They were never taught nor needed any experience. From where does this knowledge arise?

Birds have always built their nests as they do now, and each type constructs its own style of nest. They were never taught nor needed any experience. From where does this knowledge arise?

Science has no reasonable answers to these questions. Science says these creatures are guided by "instinct." But science fails to explain what "instinct" is, how it arises, and where it is stored. It is more intuitive to look at a spider and understand it is a perfectly tuned being accessing infinite intelligence through an unobstructed nervous system when it spins a perfect web during its first try. An unobstructed nervous system is connected with the ability to tap infinite intelligence. The cleaner the body, the purer the instinct; instinct is infinite intelligence working through the living being.

Based on studies of the neocortex region of the brain, researchers at Stanford University concluded the average person uses only about 2 percent of her or his mental powers! Why are so few people tapping their mental abilities? Because they are constantly poisoning themselves with improper foods, associations, thought patterns, and ideas. When you clean away the poison, you open up dormant areas of your brain capacity. Your true potential is vast!

Within you is a vast genetic library containing all the wisdom you need to accomplish everything you desire. The essence of your spirit has the capability to tap infinite intelligence.

Infinite intelligence is the ether, the storehouse of eternal knowledge, the sum of all thoughts past, present, and future. It is likened to a "cosmic circuit board" we may tap into through specific questions, silence, and pure living. It is the spiritual energy which turns seeds into plants and plants into flowers. It arcs flowers into the lovely face of the Sun. Though it may be quiet and extremely subtle, it is there and it stays there, never to be underestimated.

When you purify your body after several months on The Sunfood Diet you get in touch with infinite intelligence. This is, in my opinion, the greatest value of eating raw plant foods. The proper diet can literally unlock dormant genius as it allows one to increase the intensity of thought to the point where one can freely communicate with sources of knowledge not accessible to the average person. By the process of fine-tuning the body into its natural state, The Sunfood Diet allows you tap into the resource of "cosmic vibrations."

How does this happen? Consider Dr. Norman Walker's words in **Colon Health: The Key To A Vibrant Life**:

> "The entire universe is composed of an infinite number of vibrations which, by their very condensed numbers, form matter, substance, or intangible things, much like the thousands of individual threads in a weaver's loom form a piece of cloth by the warp and woof — or crossing and re-crossing — of the threads. Cosmic energy vibrations are vibrations (or wave lengths) in the universe of inconceivably astronomical numbers per millimeter in length or per second in time."

Dr. Walker also describes the cosmic energy receiver or antenna, the hypothalamus.

"The human organism is, a mysterious, miraculous electronic computer administered by a tiny gland, the hypothalamus, located in the mid-brain. Nothing goes on in the human organism that is not watched over, controlled, and administered by the hypothalamus."

"Considering the fact that nerves spread out to every part of the brain from the hypothalamus, and that the cleaner the body is, the higher the cosmic energy vibrations available to the brain, it certainly pays to cleanse the body and keep the colon in a constantly clean and healthy condition....The hypothalamus is a transformer which lowers the cosmic energy vibrations of the universe from untold millions of volts down to the degree of energy-voltage which the individual needs from moment to moment."

It is now understood that the pineal gland governs the hypothalamus, making the pineal gland the master gland of the entire body. On a diet of cooked food, the pineal gland calcifies and hardens. The brain becomes dense and obstructed with waste matter which would have distorted the cosmic receiver and blocked out the cosmic life energies. A diet of alkaline-plant food dissolves these obstructions and calcite deposits, freeing the flow of energy. Thus we see that the cleaner your body, the greater your latent powers of mind.

After you go on a raw diet, and especially when you fast, moments of inspiration from infinite intelligence will drop into your mind, sometimes at random. As you tune your physical body, inspirational moments will occur more and more often. The mind becomes tuned to the broadcasting signals of infinite intelligence. Through purification you can tap a mighty power you never knew you possessed.

Consider what Henry David Thoreau wrote in **Walden**, "...Every man who has ever been earnest to preserve his higher poetic faculties in the best condition, has been particularly inclined to abstain from animal food, or from much food of any kind."

Let your body become a receiver through which the energy of the cosmos can flow. When you feel pure intelligence flowing into you, rays of genius will strike you — follow these intuitions. From infinite intelligence comes the solutions to all challenges. Each ray of its divine radiance is an idea which may illuminate the world. When we align ourselves through diet, through belief, through focus, through optimal physiology, we are in contact with infinite intelligence. The goal is to live in contact with infinite intelligence at all times while flowing from grace to grace.

Embrace the infinite intelligence which bathes all of the Earth's life. Every individual is a receiver and a broadcaster within this realm of intelligence. As such, the individual has no limitations on what information s/he can tap into, except those which are accepted and set up by the individual in her/his own subconscious mind.

The subconscious mind is the connecting link between the conscious mind and infinite intelligence. It is a pump through which thought power may flow. The pump is activated by thoughts which are inspired by emotional and spiritual feelings.

Self-discipline means using your will-power to focus on only those emotional thoughts which fulfill your desires so as to begin the flow of infinite intelligence into the conscious mind, and to eliminate those emotional thoughts which lead to self-doubt and ruin.

Professor Arnold Ehret described that the lungs are a pump (they actually move the blood and lymph) and the heart is the valve which is stimulated by the flow. In the same way, the subconscious mind is a pump, which (by its control through self-discipline) moves infinite intelligence. The conscious mind is the valve that receives and is stimulated by the flow. If the body is obstructed physically, the lungs will be hindered and the blood and lymph will not flow cleanly into the heart; in the same way, if the subconscious mind is troubled, infinite intelligence will not flow clearly into the conscious mind.

After you emotionally drive an idea into the subconscious mind for a long enough period of time, the tables will turn and the idea will begin to drive you effortlessly!

Tapping infinite intelligence allows you to tap into the frequencies of other minds. Napoleon Hill described in his book, **The Master Key To Riches**, that our brains contain a vibration center, which is comparable to a sensitive radio broadcasting and receiving center. It is tuned into the life-force energy surrounding us. This powerful center projects thoughts and feelings, and receives unending swarms of vital messages. It is a tireless two-way communication system of infinite capacity. One mind can broadcast, and the thunder of that communication echoes through the cosmos, whereby it is picked up by those tuned to the same frequency and they share in the vibrations of that thought.

Synchronous living —
An antenna in your mind.
Broadcast to the world
And everything you'll find.

The flow of infinite intelligence is accelerated by what Napoleon Hill originally called *The Mastermind Principle*. He defined it as "an alliance of two or more minds blended in a spirit of perfect harmony and co-operating for the attainment of a definite purpose." This principle is invoked when another mind, operating at the same frequency as the first — with identical hopes, aims, and purposes as the first — is brought into communication with the first. When this synchronicity occurs, a third intangible cooperative mind is formed within the sphere of infinite intelligence. He discovered this to be one of the greatest secrets of success for the super-prosperous.

Action Steps:

1. Be sure to have your journal ready, near your bed or on your person, so that you may record your insights! As you purify your diet by eating more high-quality raw plant foods, you will tap into a higher power.

2. The flow of infinite intelligence is accelerated even further when a Mastermind Alliance is formed between two or more minds purified by eating raw plant foods. Attract others on the path of eating raw plant foods and join with them in activities, business ventures, family gatherings, etc.

Lesson 28:
Questions Are Answers

It is amazing what one can receive simply by asking for it.

"Ask and it shall be given you; seek and ye shall find; knock and it shall be opened unto you. For everyone that asketh receiveth; and he that seeketh findeth; and to him that knocketh it shall be opened" (Matthew 7:7-8).

How do you get whatever you want?...Ask! Ask yourself or others. Ask your superconscious mind. Ask specifically. Ask with emotion! Asking creates possibilities. Asking questions is how you change your own focus or the focus of others. If you ask for a dollar, you will receive a dollar. If you ask for the highest joy possible, you will get that too!

The challenge is not to find the right answers, but to find the right questions! Depending on how you ask the question, you get a more empowering answer.

Richard Bach wrote in **Illusions**: "Isn't it strange how much we know if only we ask ourselves instead of somebody else?"

Between your ears lies the most incredible computer on Earth. When you ask your own brain specific empowering questions, it will — every time — come up with precise answers. By asking your brain questions you are able to tap infinite intelligence which consists of all knowledge past, present, and future.

Years ago, I gave a health seminar to a corporate group. Afterwards, many people congregated around me and a young gentleman approached and asked a most potent, yet succinct question. To this man's question I gave a trite answer, although at the time, I didn't realize its profoundness. I still often think about the answer I gave. In reference to the world's challenges, he asked, "So what is the solution to all this craziness?" I stood there a moment and replied, "Grow your own food."

When a question is asked, the answer will make its appearance.

Stop for a moment and look around you. The world is filled with over-flowing abundance. All you have to do is have the courage to ask for your share of the infinite.

Do you remember the song?
"When you wish upon a star,
Makes no difference who you are,
Like a bird, out of the blue,
Your dream comes true."

Manifest your wonderful wishes by asking for them.

Why do people not ask for what they want? Because of the fear of rejection! Always remember: rejection is never final. Fear is conquered by acts of raw courage.

If you ask for anything in the world with enough commitment, courage, desire, and persistence, you will get it. Mark Victor Hansen and Jack Canfield call this principle *The Aladdin Factor* in their wonderful book of the same title. Everyone who asks receives — it is decreed by cosmic law.

Action Steps:

Ask yourself the following questions daily:

1. What specific actions can I make today to powerfully increase my energy levels?

2. How can I attain a state of health perfection and enjoy the process?

3. What can I enjoy doing that will greatly increase the beauty of the world and which is in harmony with my purpose for being on Earth?

4. How surprised would I be to discover incredible abundance in my life?

5. How can I improve the value of life for everyone I encounter each day?

When you feel moved, write down the answers to these questions in your journal.

Questions Are Answers

Ask yourself questions
That uplift and empower.
Ask your brain questions,
And answers will soon flower.

How do you tap into:
All that you've learned
All that you've seen
Every page you have turned.

It's all still recorded
In your subconscious mind.
It's all still there,
But difficult to find.

Ask yourself questions

Specific and distinct.
Draw out ideas from,
your deepest memory link.

No open-loop questions, like:
Why does this happen to me?
What kind of answers,
Would you expect to receive?

An answer comes at will,
If the question is asked right.
An answer written down,
Will let you sleep at night.

Answer with a question
No problem is unsolved,
Asking empowering questions
Is how your brain evolved.

Questions are the answer
To all life's maladies
The wisdom of the body
Is in your memories.

Lesson 29:
The Law Of Attraction

"To bring anything into your life,
imagine that it's already there."
— Richard Bach, **Illusions**

The Law of Attraction is:
1. Universal — it operates everywhere;
2. Eternal — it is ongoing;
3. Absolute — it operates whether you know it or not.

Your mind is a living magnet. You automatically draw people, things, and circumstances into your life in harmony with your dominant thoughts and desires. Every person, all the animals in your life, and every object you have are here because you have chosen to draw them here.

The Law of Attraction demonstrates that you will experience whatever you hold in your conscious mind long enough and deeply enough. Whatever your goals, whomever you want to meet, the law will magnetize them into your life. The more emotional and spiritual intensity you attach to your thoughts, the quicker that desire becomes reality.

Recall the following words from **Lesson 1: The Principle Of Life Transformation**: "Health is not something we can get; rather, it is something we attract, by the person we become. If we chase after health, it will elude us like a butterfly. However, if we calmly attract health by becoming the type of person who can be radiantly healthy, it will land upon us with a most radiant flutter."

Health attracts health. Happiness attracts happiness. Prosperity attracts prosperity. This is in absolute harmony with the foundational law that things produce more of their own kind. The happier you are, the happier are the people around you.

Things do not balance out. Success breeds more success. Failure breeds more failure. Like attracts like, it is the cosmic law again. Each produces more of its own kind.

We can only attract to ourselves a vibration which mirrors our own consciousness. Your present environment is a mirror reflection of yourself at this time. Your surrounding environment is constantly being recreated as your life progresses. Everything you have in your life right now is only a duplication of what you subconsciously believe you deserve.

You were created in the divine image and you possess within you the spark of that creative power with which, consciously or unconsciously, you create the conditions around you. You are always a creator of circumstance and never a creature of circumstance. You are at the cause, not at the effect.

Those people who feel they will be alone eating raw foods, might want to think things differently. Most people think at the "effect" side of things. They believe there are no other raw-foodists out there, so they can excuse themselves from going all the way. Or they excuse themselves by claiming high-quality organic fruit is not available. The truth is, they are always on the "cause" side of things and by the Law of Attraction they are in every moment attracting to them the reality they expect. If they went 100% raw, they would attract other 100% raw-foodists, and not before. If they committed to finding the highest quality organic food, they would attract it, and not before.

The change must first come within you and then you will attract what you need.

Highly advanced beings in all fields walk the planet Earth. How do you meet them? How do you learn from them? You must learn to match their frequency and attract them into your life.

I have worked with many people all over the world who I pushed to persist. They felt lonely, isolated by their diet and thus created that reality. However, as they persisted, and the Sunfood delivered its effect, their vibration changed, as did their consciousness. Even in the most remote locations other raw-foodists would show up in their lives. You will be absolutely astonished by how many people are into raw-foods, or are willing to go raw with you when you reach the right frame of mind!

You attract into your life those with a message for you. The message that "when one is ready for a thing, it presents itself" is proved by the indisputable fact that you have picked up this book and that you have found me at precisely the right time for you.

Embrace the Law Of Attraction. Accelerate your transition. Become more social, meet new dynamic people. Attract into your life beautiful people and relationships by becoming beautiful inside. Pair up with those (especially a lover) who are headed in the same direction as yourself. Employ The Mastermind Principle as discussed in **Lesson 27**.

The most attractive thing you can do is smile. Everyone knows that a beautifully happy being is a sight to behold. A smile profoundly affects all who see and feel it. Like the Sun, a smile brightens the entire day.

The most powerful vibration you can send out is love. Love is the very essence of the Law of Attraction. The most blessed, beautiful people are those who continually send out love vibrations towards all the living plants and creatures around them. By sending out love you always make the world a better place to live for all of the Earth's precious creatures.

Learn to love. Love helps heal every injury, every illness. Let love emanate from your being. Let your spirit sing with a new-found love for Life. Love is magical. It is the greatest gift and the most powerful force in the universe.

Love withheld, in the past or present, lies somewhere at the root of all psychosomatic illness. Attempting to compensate for the lack of love causes erratic, neurotic behavior. Love withheld cascades down from the emotional body into the mental body, causing neuroses and from there it slides into the physical body in the form of illness. In simple terms, love deprivation causes sickness.

Love is necessary to our being. It is our most vital Sunfood. It supports us, sustains us, gives us the power to overcome. You never can tell what a loving word can mean to someone. Speak loving, caring words to friends and family members, especially when they are ill, and they will become healthier. They will be physically, mentally, emotionally, and spiritually uplifted!

Send out waves of loving energy. We know by the Laws of Karma that what we put out comes back to us — multiplied! As much love as you put into your interactions, that is how much love comes directly back to you.

To be loved, we have to love ourselves. Loving yourself is very healthy. Only when we love ourselves do we have enough love to give away. By giving love we then receive love.

Action Steps:

1. Two key points to live by daily:
     Stop chasing, start attracting.
     Stop striving, start arriving.

2. Ask yourself: "What will it take for me to love myself?" When you love yourself, your journey through life will be so much more enjoyable and you can start to love others as well. Stop taking everything so seriously. "Seriousness addiction" plunders the joy of life.

The Law of Attraction

It is operating always
In greater or lesser forms.
It directs the roaring majesty
Of deep-blue tropical storms.

It masters mighty mountains
And rolls each grain of sand.
It alters the course of rivers
And pulls the tide to land.

It summons bee to flower
And drone to honey queen.
It is felt by primal wisdom
But rarely is ever seen.

It may shift its shape
And shape its shift
To bring two, eye to eye.
Try to grasp its power:
It eludes,
Like a butterfly.

It calls the bird to the tree;
It lays the eggs in the nest.
It turns the tides of fortune
And never does it rest.

It lingers in the mortal world
And filters through the dust.
To bond a fated pair
It takes the form of lust.

The Law is organic power
Captured by clean living;
Drawing forth Nature's favor,
When love is what you're giving.

Like and like beget,
'Birds of a feather' attract.
That purer bodies captivate
Is the ever-certain fact.

Success attracts success
Fortunes rising higher.
People, places, things
In harmony with your desire.

When you are ready,
For what you want.
When you truly believe
You deserve it.
All the resources will show up
With the people to support it.

Help is ever on the way,
Drawn by your conviction.
When you are absolutely certain,
You call the cosmic law to action.

The Law is eternal —
A mysterious, magical charm.
Multiplying Life:
It creates a jungle from a farm.

Nothing circumvents its pull.
Not one escapes its force.
Nothing is by chance.
It is part of every source.

It brings a hand to hand;
It touches a paw to paw.
Primal love vibrations —
The Mistress of Cosmic Law.

It magnetizes masterminds
And shapes the destiny of worlds.
It spins the cosmic froth about,
And giggles in little girls.

It is Nature's gravitation,
Method of motivation,
Modus of procreation,
Concept of creation.

The Law of Attraction —
The Logic of the Spheres.
Desire a thing deep enough,
And it suddenly appears.

Lesson 30:
The Mystery of Sex Transmutation
Revisited (Seeds Must Live)

"...The 'forbidden food' in the midst of fruits and herbs
(Garden of Eden) is their seed, which if eaten destroys
their own purpose of reproduction, and makes man and
woman 'go to seed'..."
— Dr. Johnny Lovewisdom,
Spiritualizing Dietetics: Vitarianism

The drive for sex is one of the most powerful of all desires. Success
philosopher Napoleon Hill found that when driven by this desire, people
develop keenness of imagination, courage, will power, persistence, and a
creative ability unknown to them at other times. He found that the desire
for sexual expression is so powerful that people will run the risk of life
and reputation to engage in it. He concluded that when harnessed and
transmuted into other channels, the driving force of sex energy maintains
all of its motivating attributes which may be used as powerful creative
forces in literature, art, or in any other profession or calling, including the
accumulation of wealth. What Napoleon Hill revealed was that those who
had achieved incredible accomplishments had a high degree of sexual
charisma. They had learned to channel their sex energy into success —
they had mastered the art of sexual transmutation.

Napoleon Hill also discovered that those who experienced great successes in their life did not achieve those lofty heights until the age of forty

or beyond. He attributed this to the ability, with age and experience, to transmute the sexual impulse into areas of creativity and achievement. Now this is possible to do without having to wait for age and experience to bring the sexual drive under control. The sex drive can be transmuted through the right use of diet.

Proper use of diet allows us to channel energies used for sex up the spine into the brain for superior mental performance. This is the secret of creative ability. Transmuted sex energy lifts the mind into a higher sphere, allowing communication with infinite intelligence.

A pure diet of fruits and green-leafed vegetables (no nuts or seeds) allows one to better control the sex drive. Foods that contain seeds (such as cucumbers) are okay to eat, however, the eating of individual nuts and seeds (e.g. almonds, pumpkin seeds, rice, etc.) is to be avoided. The teachings of Dr. Lovewisdom demonstrate that eating seeds causes us to "go to seed." The hormones in nuts and seeds drive the sexual organs.

To sublimate the sex impulse and use it to drive you forward and upward in great health, wealth (business and sales skills), and vitality, stop eating nuts and seeds of any type for a specific period of time. A pure seedless diet automatically sublimates the sex energies. Sexual sublimation cues up the mind so it works rapidly, efficiently, clearly, with real inspiration. The control of the physical side of sex expands the imagination. It lends mighty power to the creative faculties.

Male sexual fluids have extraordinarily high levels of trace minerals. For males, excessive ejaculation — "spilling the seed" — without nutritionally replacing what is lost, drains minerals and life-force energy from the body, which causes premature aging, leads to an accelerated loss of hair in men, and contributes to impotence. Men can replace sexual fluids by specifically eating nuts, seeds, seaweeds, avocados, olives, garlic, onions, and hot peppers. Breathing pure air and Sunbathing nude will also help restore sexual fluids and energy.

Due to the mineral deficit and toxicity caused by the standard diet, men often experience a "crash" or a mood swing after ejaculation, which is typically not pleasing to the sexual partner. This will reverse and may be totally eliminated once the diet is purified by eating a healthy balance of raw plant foods.

The books and articles I have read on diet, spirituality, and sex generally agree that between 25% and 40% of the life-force energy men accumulate from breathing, eating, Sunlight, spiritual power, etc. is transmuted into sexual energy, which is stored physically in male sperm. A single ejaculation contains 200 to 500 million sperm cells. If we consider each sperm cell as a potential human being, there are sufficient sperm cells for a man in a few days to generate the current population of the Earth. That is the power of the semen.

Complementary to dietary considerations, there is a Taoist technique for redirection of the sexual energy called the "big draw." This technique involves drawing back the discharge of sexual energy and redirecting it up the spine to the brain. Through practice one can develop this retention ability. The increase in sexual potency that follows is quite remarkable, it creates great libido, more subtle sexual enjoyment, remarkable capacity, and progressively increasing sensitivity.

For men, the point is to have sex, but not to ejaculate every time. Sex is essential to excellent health as it restores imbalances in the body chemistry, excites the sex hormones, and balances the other major glands (the adrenal, thymus, thyroid, pituitary, hypothalamus, and pineal). Sex clears the mind, frees the spirit, and helps build a wonderful relationship with one's partner.

A healthy body is a sexual body. Sexual people have a bountiful supply of attractive magnetism.

Two tuned beings consciously uniting their physical bodies invokes a powerful spiritual energy. There is no substitute for spiritual sex. Sharing pleasure and love unconditionally with another adds a new meaning to existence. Sex as a raw-foodist with a raw-foodist is one of the most amazing experiences in the world and a unique goal to achieve.

How To Increase The Sex Drive

"Having sex with another is usually more pleasurable
if the person smells appetizing, tastes,
and looks good (just like food)."
— Joshua Rainbow, **Biotrophic Protocol**

To increase the sex drive, eat nuts and seeds. Eating nuts and seeds creates the desire "to go to seed!" From personal experience I have found watermelon seeds to be quite an aphrodisiac. I am also convinced that the stamen-center of the cherimoya fruit has aphrodisiac qualities. Other raw plant foods that drive the sex impulse are: avocados, olives, raw organic olive oil, raw dulse (seaweed), pollen (pollen from the male date palm tree is an aphrodisiac for women), onions, garlic, and hot peppers (the yogis of India have long-known that spicy foods excite the sexual passions). By eating significantly more of all these foods, males will see a major increase in sperm count and females will experience a greater sex drive. (Eat organic food only! Pesticides, when absorbed into the body, end up in the sexual fluids; they decrease sexual vitality and cause sterility.)

Action Steps:

1. Set a period of one month aside to use the power of sexual transmutation. For that one month eat no nuts or seeds of any type. This will automatically sublimate the sexual energies and provide you with more creative abilities in other areas. Use that time to complete a project at home, with the family, or in business.

2. For men: experiment with having sex without ejaculation.

Lesson 31:
Avocados (Persea Americana)

Aboriginal to Mexico and Central America, the avocado tree has migrated its way into North America and has since spread throughout the world.

In English, avocados have been known by over forty different names, including: Alligator Pear, Butter Fruit, Butter Pear, Custard Apple, Laurel Peach, Midshipman's Butter, Shell Pear, Spanish Pear, Subaltern's Butter, Testicle Fruit, and Vegetable Marrow.

In her excellent reference book, **Whole Foods Companion**, my friend Diane Onstad has written: "The English word avocado is a corruption of the Nahuatlan Mexican ahuacatl, itself an Aztec shortening of ahuacacuahatl, which means testicle tree. The Aztecs explained that their ahuacatl was given the name not only because the fruit resembled a testicle and grew in pairs, but because it greatly excited sexual passion."

The avocado is the new world olive. It is the fatty fruit which dominates the Americas as the olive dominates the Mediterranean world.

The avocado has a huge variety of tastes and flavors — over 500 different types have been identified. Avocados very rarely ripen on the tree. They ripen on the ground as most fatty fruits do. Each variety in and upon itself is very sensitive to environmental conditions and picks up a superior taste when grown in mineral-rich soil and is left to ripen naturally.

Some of the heavier varieties, such as Reed, Cannonball, Pinkerton, etc. should be left on the tree for at least 1.5 years to allow their true oil content to set in.

Avocados are a rich, emerald cream. The gentle flavor, high-fat content, smooth texture, and natural oils within them make avocados an ideal beauty food and baby food.

There is no doubt about it, avocados are the best transition food from a cooked-food diet to a raw-food diet. Fatty foods in general (nuts, seeds, coconuts, avocados, olives, durians, etc.) transition you from cooked foods to raw foods — they are the bridge.

The avocado is in ascendancy right now worldwide; more and more people are discovering its secrets. You want to know how powerful the avocado is? The avocado can help save the human race because avocado fat replaces meat and dairy fat. The avocado replaces resource-depleting animal products in the diet. Keep in mind: 260 million acres (1.05 million square kilometers) of United States' forests have been cleared for cropland to fuel the meat-centered diet; the percentage of U.S. topsoil loss directly attributable to livestock raising is 85%; more than half the water used in the U.S. is used for livestock production; 2,500 gallons of water is required to produce one pound (0.45 kg) of meat.

Most raw foodists I have met have eaten 2-5 avocados nearly every day since they started on a program of natural nutrition. Most seem to never get tired of them! I know raw-foodists who have been eating 2-5 avocados nearly every day for 5, 10, even 20 years. Fatty raw plant foods are like that, you only need one or two and they seem to be totally satisfying. A good healthy body loves them. They are soft on the body, especially when eaten with green leaves.

One day I was at the beach looking for a place to surf while eating an avocado. A gentleman walked by, looked at me, and commented, "soul food." He was right. Avocados are soul food. They feed our essence.

Almost every raw foodist I have ever met is an avid fan of the avocado. But, some wonder whether or not they are addicted to the fruit. What they are feeling is not an addiction per se, but a manifestation of the body's desire for fat. To get off avocados, simply replace them with another fatty plant food. Soft, young coconuts make an excellent replacement. Nuts and seeds work great; Sun-ripened olives are also an ideal fatty food. Optimally, I think it is excellent to move around the fat category eating macadamia nuts for several weeks, then olives for several months, eating some avocados, bringing in some durian, then pecans. This is how I have come to eat raw plant fats. This gives your body some variety and makes your diet easy on the liver.

Avocado

A New World treasure —
Never found?
Which ripens amongst
Leaves on the ground?

The smooth, rich taste
The Mayan fruit.
The raw-wild flavor
Behind Pan's flute.

Sexual passion
An instantaneous connection.
Smooth, clear skin
A perfect complexion.

The emerald idol
An erotic oil
The polished leaves
From exotic soil.

Indulge your lips
In fertile cream.
Awaken to a
Wonderful dream.

The misty forest
The secret delight.
Urban fruit foragers
In avo-groves at night.

They gaze upon
The twilight sky
As silver jewels
Sway nearby.

The bass, the beat,
The tribal drum,
The Sunfooder singing:
"I've got to have one."

The dictated cry, that:
"Thin is in"
Can never bring forth
The beauty within.
"Fat's where it's at!"
Says the tribal man.
A filled luscious body
Is Nature's plan.

Sensual compassion
The Avocado transition;
The jungle fruit
Has come to fruition.

The searching masses

With food to burn
Perhaps one day
Will listen then learn
That the golden secret
Of El Dorado
May be found within
The Avocado.

Lesson 32:
Olives (Olea Europea)

"Olives — Their lubricating, cleansing, beautifying, and
rejuvenative power is the greatest among all fruits."
— Vera Richter, **The Cook-Less Book**

Olives are quite possibly the world's most perfect food. Olives are a
biblical fruit associated in the scriptures with symbols of goodness, happiness, purity, and prosperity. In ancient Greece, during the height of their
culture, Solon, the great law-giver, enacted laws protecting all olive trees.
He made it a capital offense to kill a tree or to cut one down. The Romans
were the first to perfect the stone-press with which they extracted the
olive's oil. The Romans believed the olive to be an incredibly sexual fruit,
an aphrodisiac, especially when eaten in large quantities.

If I had to pick one fruit to live on for the rest of my life, it would be
the olive. Once you delve into the olive, you will become privy to the
great Mediterranean secret of health, happiness, and longevity. The olive
is a magical fruit. But the olive remains a mystery to almost everyone I
know, including other raw-foodists! Few people know how to eat an olive
naturally!

It took me several years to unravel the olive's mystery. The first clue I
discovered about olives is that they are a type of fruit which ripens on the
ground. Avocados, dates, cherimoya, and even citrus fruits fall into this
category (I have noticed citrus fruits reach their peak maturity after

weeks, or even months, on the ground in the Sun; if you buy citrus fruits in the store, leave them outside under the Sun if possible or in the windowsill to allow them to reach their full ripeness).

Olives must be picked fresh and Sun-ripened. As the olive ripens in the Sun, the bitter component (oleuropein) is converted and the fruit suddenly becomes edible! The black olives commonly grown in United States and the Mediterranean reach their ripe maturity when the fruit softens and the internal flesh of the fruit changes from white or red to brown or black. The olive skin may begin wrinkling at this stage as well. Though there are these markers to watch for, olives are a food you acquire a "feel" for. I can look at an olive or pick one up and know if it is ripe or not, even if it has undergone no obvious external changes.

The second clue I unraveled was that olives taste best and are most digestible in their juicy ripened state before they become too dry. Olives are an ancient biblical fruit, yet very few people have ever eaten them in their juicy ripened natural state! Juicy Sun-ripened olives are beyond description. The olive has such a marvelous variety of flavors. I might eat 10 in a row, all from the same tree, while noticing a different flavor in each olive. I usually do not stop with 10, I might eat 50 olives with a salad for dinner. On some days as many as 150 have passed my lips!

The third clue was that olives are an extremely sensitive fruit. Olives are very perishable. They are especially perishable when taken out of the Sun. That is why we do not see naturally juicy olives in stores. Olives contain no sugar, thus they are not protected by sugar's antimicrobial properties. Olives must either be soaked in olive oil, salt-cured, or altered in some other way to remain stable over time.

I do not recommend pickled olives as they are extremely acid forming in digestion, though technically not cooked. Canned black olives have been pasteurized and soaked in ferrous gluconate (an iron compound which darkens them), and should be avoided. The only cured olives I recommend eating are "water-cured" or "raw sea-salt and olive-oil cured" olives (these should be eaten moderately because of their high-salt content, e g not more than 15 with a salad). Aside from the natural way, the best choice to eat olives is to find Sun-ripened olives which have been soaked in olive oil and a light sea salt. Nature's First Law is presently distributing the best Sun-ripened olives soaked in olive oil and sea salt available throughout North America. Nature's First Law is also currently distributing stone-crushed, cold-pressed extra virgin olive oil (pressed in the original way the Romans and Greeks did it). Regularly check our web-site (http://www.rawfood.com) for more details.

Olive trees are ubiquitous in the southwestern United States (California, Arizona, and Nevada) as well as throughout the Mediterranean world, the Middle East, and India. Olives grow abundantly in California, especially in Southern California; they have been naturalized here, and even grow wildly, having been spread by the birds. I have also seen olives growing abundantly in southern Nevada, especially in the Las Vegas area. They grow throughout Arizona as well. They love the desert.

Consider the power and benefits of the olive. The raw olive is:

(1) The highest fruit in minerals!

(2) The highest fruit in calcium. Olives contain twice as much calcium as oranges by weight.

(3) High in magnesium.

(4) High in amino acids, including: leucine, aspartic acid, and glutaminic acid

(5) An alkaline fruit.

(6) A fatty fruit (mostly monounsaturated fat).

(7) An alkaline fat source.

(8) Loaded with beneficial omega 3 and omega 6 fatty acids.

(9) High in vitamins A and E.

(10) In possession of many antioxidant properties. Antioxidants deactivate free radicals allowing us to live longer, overcome illness, and maintain more acute mental and muscular faculties.

(11) Available in different varieties, which fruit all year around.

(12) Pressable into a powerful oil, usable in a limitless number of ways all year around.

(13) Able to soothe the mucous membranes with its oil.

Olives have the greatest propensity of any fruit to dissolve toxic mucus in the system (in fact, they are three times more powerful than oranges in that respect). In Arnold Ehret's classic book, **Mucusless Diet Healing System**, he reprints Ragnar Berg's Table which organizes different foods by their acid-binding or acid-forming potential. The higher the food's acid-binding potential, the greater its ability to dissolve mucus and cooked-food residues in the body. The olive, it turns out, is the highest mucus dissolver of any fruit. It rates with a value of 30.56 with figs following behind at 27.81, no other fruit in the chart ranks above 20.00. To give you an idea of how high these values are, the orange, an excellent mucus-dissolver, ranks at 9.61.

Olive oil is a soothing fat for damaged and dry skin, hair, and nails. It can be used to soothe the skin after shaving. Olive oil may be used on baby skin instead of the harsh "baby oil" brands available in stores. Some olive oils are devoid of lipase (the fat-splitting enzyme), probably because they are made from unripe olives. This is why I recommend only stone-crushed, cold-pressed extra virgin organic American or European brands in dark bottles (oils are light sensitive). The Greek and Italian oils I find to be slightly better in taste and quality.

The Olive

The mysterious little fruit
Few can understand
Was there overseeing
Achilles last stand.

It rode the tides of war
Traveled the odyssey,
Even to be crowned as:
Athena's sacred tree.

A tree so rich with jewels
To cause an army to invade.
The bravery of Lycurgus
Can ever it...fade?

The prize, the wise
Would realize.
Is the food of the divine.
Ripened from soil
Made to oil.
Valued more than wine.

Grown erratic,
Rough between stones.
Dropping fruit which:
Builds strong bones.

Clearing the complexion
Building affection
Creating a fertile,
Instantaneous connection.

The symbol fruit of
Massive abundance.
The startling
Charisma of the ancients.

Across the seas,
For the royals,
Thales' secret,
To carry the oils.

The sea-farer's bed,
The sacred union,
It is time for a:
Mediterranean reunion.

The gnarled tree,
Grown by the seas,
Reveals the wisdom
This world needs.

Lesson 33:
Time Management Through Fasting

"Fasting is at once a journey near and yet so far.
By undergoing one, more will be learnt from it than
all the lands you visited or books you have read."
— Morris Krok

Fasting (resting the body from food) is part of life. People fast every night when they go to sleep; this abstainment from food and liquid may last eight to ten hours or longer. Now if humans lived in a normal and natural way, each night's repose would be adequate, but because humans live so far away from the natural state, the nightly nocturnal fast is not sufficient to completely rest or purify the body.

Isn't it interesting that the major religions of the world teach the benefits of fasting? I find that fascinating!

The journey into fasting is about becoming a finely-tuned spiritual instrument. Fasting is mentioned as part of nearly every religion on Earth. Fasting on water is a spiritual practice. Undertaking a fast measures self-discipline and self-control. Fasting tests the will.

Fasting is Nature's foundational law of all healing and revitalization. Nature's healing command is: "Don't eat, lie down, hide, be quiet." Fasting seems to be a part of every answer. Are you confused? Fast. Feeling ill? Fast. Sick to your stomach? Fast. Those who fast regularly know that not eating has a cleaning effect on all areas of the mind and body.

Fasting enables the body to start healing itself. The amazing thing about fasting is that it is Nature's supreme medicine. When one begins to fast, the elimination process is set in motion and the entire body commences a cleansing program. During a fast, the body can focus its enzyme power to autolyze (dissolve) tumorous formations and toxic residues.

While fasting, the blood thins (recall **Lesson 10: Detoxification** where we learned how the quality of the blood is formed at the intestinal villi). This allows the thick mucus trapped in the lymph to diffuse out into the blood for elimination. This is the process of diffusion, elements move from areas of greater concentration to areas of lesser concentration.

Roe Gallo, a fruitarian and natural healer, fasts the chronically ill on citrus juice until they are ready to transition onto a raw-food or fruit diet. She describes her experiences in her book **Perfect Body**. Roe has helped heal people of many types of illnesses, including cancer, by following this simple fasting procedure.

Orange, grapefruit, lime, and lemon juices dissolve toxicity, mucus, and excess calcite deposits so they may be washed out and eliminated. I recommend including the pith (the white inside of the rind) with your citrus juices, especially when fasting. The pith contains bioflavonoids, fiber, and calcium.

Case studies conducted by Natural Hygiene practitioners over this last century prove that the longer you fast, the more centered you become, the better you heal, the higher your intellectual activity, and the younger you appear. Digestive juices and enzymes are secreted by the pancreas when the stomach and duodenum are empty. These fluids travel into the intestinal tract, are absorbed by the intestinal villi, and then enter into the blood and lymph to digest undigested fats, carbohydrates, and proteins.

When your body is clean and tuned up through fasting, you will experience a continuous flow of vibrant health, electric energy, and mental strength. This will enable you to perform at levels you never thought possible. Time will slow down, but your brain will speed up. You will feel amazingly calm. Your consciousness will glow as ideas flow through you exactly when you need them.

Fasting is an art. One masters fasting by developing the ability to raise the functions of the body while the blood sugar is low.

If we are living with passion and with a purpose, then fasting is exciting, never boring.

Let us not lose sight of the truth: food is a means to an end, not an end in itself. The paradox of The Sunfood Diet is that food is not an issue! As long as the food is raw plant food, eat what you need for fuel and get on with accomplishing your goals! Be so busy accomplishing your goals that you don't spend any time even thinking about food. Use the secrets of diet and fasting to help you advance in life and business. Get more done in less time.

The best time to get tedious, organizational work done is during a fast. Time management is best accomplished through fasting. Eating food is a tremendous consumer of time.

How To Fast

One must be careful with fasting. There are health conditions which do not react well to fasting. For instance, a fast is not recommended for diabetics who have taken insulin for more than two years. Those taking medication or recreational drugs should also not fast, until they have detoxified their body and stopped the intake of all chemicals. Otherwise, fasting may cause too much poison to flow out of the lymph fluid into the blood too quickly.

One should build up stores of natural amino acids (greens), sugars (fruit), and raw plant fats in the system for at least 6 months before undertaking a fast of two days or longer.

To begin fasting, try the no breakfast plan initially — no break-fasting. Then go one day and continue farther.

Preferably choose to fast when the seasons change or on the full moon; that is when the body cleanses the strongest. During each change of seasons, Nature does its house-cleaning by expelling poisons; this is why people experience the flu (detoxification) during the seasonal changes. When the moon is full, the tidal energies are pulled, and this lunar position also triggers the body to detoxify.

I recommend fasting on distilled water mixed with fresh lemon juice (snow or snow water is better than distilled water if you have access to it). The lemon juice acts as an internal soap by dissolving mucus and cooked-food residues. The fasting I recommend for accelerated healing is designed to keep the blood sugar low — as a low-sugar fruit, lemon works perfectly.

The fasting I recommend for time management can include coconut water, fruit juice, and/or green-vegetable juices, but may also be done just on water with lemon juice. When you are fasting for time management, small fasts of two or three days may serve your purpose. I typically will fast on water all day, while working at my business, then accomplish an incredible amount of work in the evening and at night (reading or writing), wake up after 5 hours of sleep at 5:00 am and work 3 or 4 more hours before eating something the following morning.

If you are new to Sunfoods, fasts should be undertaken with care, ease into them. For those who are inexperienced, fast for small intervals (one or two days). Go on an adventure with a trustworthy friend or family member. Spend a day fasting out in Nature in a forest, at a pond, or near a waterfall, consuming only pure water.

As you begin to undertake longer fasts, you will recognize that the body first uses up the sugar in your system for fuel, then, after three days, clicks over to glycogen stored in the cells and liver. The body will eventually tap into the body fat and begin converting that to fuel until it is depleted. Protein breakdown is the last thing the body turns to for fuel.

During a fast, an individual should not be too concerned about bowel movements anymore than one should not be too concerned about regulating the flow of the bloodstream or the beating of the heart. The bowels will move when they need to. If you feel a bowel movement is necessary while you are fasting, administer an enema to yourself or visit a colon hydrotherapist. Colon hydrotherapy while fasting is very cleansing and tremendously healing.

The amount of water you drink during a fast should be dictated by thirst. Two quarts (liters) of water or juice each day should be adequate. The less fluids you take in, the more aggressive will be the fast. Do not push yourself beyond the bounds of reason, if you feel dizzy, weary, extremely thirsty, and/or experience pain in the kidneys (outer lower back) drink more water, or add fresh juice.

As you are fasting, read books on the subject to keep you focused and motivated. My organization Nature's First Law has gathered together and now distributes the highest-quality books on fasting to help all people learn more about this fascinating subject.

This brings up a crucial point: how you break a fast determines to a large extent the value of the fast and the degree of rejuvenation. Remember the rule that however many days you fast, it takes the same amount of additional days to fully recover. Break a fast with a juicy alkaline fruit, such as an orange or a papaya; fresh figs, grapes, or cherries also work quite well. This introduction of alkaline fruit will cause a peristaltic wave and a flush of all the dislodged toxins throughout the body. Keep in mind the stomach will shrink from days of fasting. Wait at least 2 hours before eating something else to allow the full cleansing peristaltic wave to sweep through the body (peristalsis is a muscular contraction which flows wave-like through the colon helping to expel waste). The next meal may consist of heavier foods, preferably blended, such as fruits and avocados mixed together. After one or more days, whole green leaves may be reintroduced into the body. Cooked food should be avoided following a fast.

Generally, the more toxic a person is, the more weight they will lose during a fast. Weight and size lost during a fast can be regained with no detrimental effects if desired; the body retains a "memory" as to its normal proportions. I have found that at this point I can fast 4 to 5 days on water with almost no weight loss.

What I Learned From The Yaqui Medicine Man

I once met a Yaqui Indian medicine man of the same race and ethnicity as Don Juan from the Carlos Castaneda books. He was a robust man who radiated an extraordinary vitality, grace, and simple gusto for life. I believe he was 82 years young when I met him. But his age was unguessable to anyone who did not know. He looked in some ways as if he were 10 years old; he had many of the features of a young boy. I looked at his hands closely and noticed no wrinkles and no liver spots.

He has followed a vegan diet since birth, as taught to him by his mother (overturning the false idea that indigenous peoples are not vegetarians or vegans). Only 3 times in his life has he eaten animal foods (raw rattlesnake twice as a ceremonial experience and turtle soup once). He can identify thousands of herbs.

He told me the story of how he crossed the Desert of Silence in the State of Sonora Mexico. He crossed without food or water for 8 days all the while sucking on a small pebble.

He described that fasting was the key to spiritual awakening. He fasts 2 days a week, taking in very little water. He also fasts 3 days every full moon.

Breatharianism

Recall **Lesson 2: The Foundational Law** — things produce after their kind. When you overeat one day, you are hungrier the next. The more you eat, the more you want to eat; the less you eat, the less you want to eat. The more you fast, the easier it is, and the less you desire food. Fasting becomes easier the more you do it.

I am of the opinion that when the body is finely tuned and totally purified on all levels (physically, mentally, emotionally, and spiritually), one can fast for an extremely long time.

In his fascinating book **Spiritualizing Dietetics: Vitarianism**, Dr. Johnny Lovewisdom describes exactly how he fasted for 7 months and 7 days on 99% distilled water (the other 1% consisting of citrus, tomato, or green juice), and then, 4 months later, again fasted for 6 months and 17 days on 99% distilled water. Pictures taken following these two amazing fasts are included in **Maitreya: The Lovewisdom Autobiography, Volume II**.

Jasmuheen of Australia, founder of The Self Empowerment Academy, describes in her book **Living On Light** how she has lived on herbal teas and very little food since June 1993. She writes: "It is not about fasting, it is about allowing, trusting, clicking into an energy pattern of knowing that our true sustenance is provided by Cosmic Light, which sustains many beings from many Universes, and is a possibility offered to us here and now. Nor is it a process of denial..."

I know Jasmuheen personally. She has stayed at my home here in San Diego while conducting a weekend seminar for Nature's First Law. She really does walk her talk. Every day we spent together, her energy levels were high and balanced. She is a lot of fun! She spent 2-4 hours meditating each morning and evening. I got the impression that her lifestyle is easy for her.

In my estimation, the end goal of natural nutrition and mind-mastery is "breatharianism" — a lifestyle involving regular long fasts and a pure, frugal diet.

Action Steps:

1. After eating plenty of raw foods for at least 6 months, prepare and undertake your first water fast. While fasting, read books on fasting. This will help strengthen your resolve. I recommend **Rational Fasting** by Professor Arnold Ehret, **Fasting Can Save Your Life** by Dr. Herbert Shelton, and **The Miracle Of Fasting** by Paul Bragg.

2. As a healthy life discipline, make routine fasting part of your life. Fast 3-7 days on water, fruit juice, and or vegetable juice during the change of seasons. Fast when you attend seminars. Fast for time management. Fast for fun!

Lesson 34:
Do What You Love To Do

"Indeed, there is no such thing as Truth in itself: there can
only exist the Process of Living Truly — in so living as to
constantly manifest the fullness of one's Being — in so living
that the actual process of one's life reflects fully the
Wholeness of the greater Cosmic Process."
— Michael Tobin

"If it makes your heart sing, do it!"
— Jasmuheen

You are here on Earth to become exceptional, to make a majestic contribution, and to achieve something wonderful which uplifts all living
things. You are part of a great plan which has been set in motion. Every
obstacle you face is filled with indispensible experience points which
lead you to higher and higher skill levels. Every adversity you face is
exactly what you need to face in order to allow you to rise further up.

You were put on this Earth for a reason. Everything has its place and
purpose, and so do you. Each individual has their own assignment. Your
existence is not random. You are endowed with a gift that only you have.
Within you is a Strong Exciting Essence Desire (SEED). Nourish it,
make your contribution.

You exist to fulfill the destiny conceived at your inception. Your destiny is not something you can get; it is something you already know.

Find your area of excellence and channel all your abilities, your entire focus into becoming the best there is in that field. Choose your garden and start planting. Get bent on a specific purpose in life and do only that which furthers the accomplishment of that purpose.

When you find your purpose in life — the job you were designed for — then you will be able to do it without even thinking of money or food. You will be able to do it with great joy and effervescence even while fasting — that is how you *know*.

The greatest successes in the world have found their area of excellence and focused all their resources into that area. There are no exceptions to this rule.

Those who are doing what they were meant to do have the wisdom to keep their own counsel and do not waste their time trying to discourage others. Healthy individuals seek only to lift their fellows to a new level of progress. They are so busily engaged in promoting their purpose on Earth that they have no time to waste with anyone or anything which does not contribute in one way or another to that purpose. This is not a self-centered mode of living, because those who do what they love to do are so good at what they do, they give others exactly what they want!

We are here to serve others. How is it that we may best serve others? By fulfilling our assignment on Earth. That is why this book is in your hands now — I am fulfilling my assignment. We always contribute to the betterment of all by focusing on what is best for our own state of mind and the Earth's integrity.

Your contribution is a spiritual force which has more power than your own brain. It has the power to live on, grow, and expand, even after you are long gone.

You will always feel happiest and most spiritually fulfilled by doing what you love to do no matter what the financial rewards. And you are in control of determining your financial rewards by answering the question: How can I do what I love to do and create financial abundance while doing it?

Just as you deserve an abundance of physical, mental, emotional, and spiritual health, you deserve an abundance of financial health. Money in itself is neither good nor bad, it is neutral. Financial abundance can be used to support tremendous projects to help save tortured animals, grow trees, protect the land, and heal the planet.

One common attribute of self-made millionaires is that they are doing what they love to do. They love what they do so much that they challenged themselves continuously to achieve the highest levels of success in that field, and the financial abundance followed.

The best, most fun, and most exciting way to attract financial abundance is to find out what you really enjoy doing in life, the thing you have always loved doing, the thing you always wanted to spend all your time on, and then leverage your mind to figure out how to attract money while doing it. Make your favorite hobby your livelihood. When you are greatly enjoying what you are doing, people will be glad to invest their money with you! Turn what you have in your heart into something thousands, even millions, of people can enjoy, and you may use your rewards to live an abundant life spiritually, emotionally, mentally, physically, and financially. Remember: wherever your heart is, there you will find your treasures.

What you do for a living each day should be enjoyable for you. If it is not, you are on the wrong track. If you are stuck doing something each day you do not like to do, you must figure out a plan of how to stop doing it, and how to start doing what you like to do.

All of Nature is part of a single giant organism in which every living creature has her or his own place and purpose. When you undertake a raw-Sunfood diet you will become more attached to the great workings of Nature and your true place and purpose will become more obvious to you. You will be "compelled" to let it unfold. Eating raw "compels" you to get into your own true pattern of life.

Zero-based thinking states: If the situation is wrong for you, if it is emotionally draining you, get out. Anything which emotionally drains you may cause you to do unhealthy things. This is why a pure diet and lifestyle compels you to get into situations that are right for you.

Would you be surprised to discover that one of the keys to health is to do what you love to do? Doing what you love to do is actually the easiest way to become, not only wealthy, but healthy as well!

Destiny

No two lives are alike, each attempts to unfold a divine pattern, a great and holy destiny, a unique form of abundance. As you live true to your own deeply-known destiny, you will radiate as perfectly and as beautifully as the most divine wild fruit tree. No one can stop you from reaching your highest potential, if you will but follow your own true pattern of life.

Wasted is every thought, feeling, or vibration which is out of harmony with your true pattern of life. Learn to live by the pattern of life which is contained within you. You already know what it is. Now it is time for you to remember.

I have found my own true pattern of life is not that of an ascetic peace-lover wandering in bliss. I am animated by strong Sun-fired passions. I am driven by an overpowering internal fire. I will draw the line and take a stand. I feel that this is true to who I am and to try and be otherwise, based on some model of cooked spirituality, is not true for me. I live my life with a great intensity to bring this beautiful raw-vegetarian lifestyle to the world.

There is a force which wants you to realize your destiny; it wets your appetite with a taste of success. For it is not only possible that you have your dream — it is necessary.

The closer you get to realizing your destiny, the more your destiny becomes your true reason for being. When your desire is highest in intensity, then you are closest to the true spirit of the world. When you want something so powerfully that literally nothing can stop you, then you have found your mission on Earth and all the universe will conspire to help you achieve it.

Life is generous to those who pursue their destiny. Those who live out their destiny know everything they need to know. Pursue your aspirations and goals in every moment and one day your destiny will be realized!

To attract health, wealth, peace of mind, emotional beauty, and spiritual fulfillment, do — all the time — what you do best. That is the path to incredible success in life, and is always the path of least resistance. You are more apt to succeed when you do what comes naturally. Develop your life's dreams along the line of least resistance. Is this not how the potent seedling sunders the cement?

Tilt your head and listen, now is the time to finally hear the unmistakable invitation ringing down the years — the call of your destiny. For the sake of a future for us all here on Earth...DO ONLY WHAT YOU WERE PUT HERE TO DO!

Action Steps:

To uncover your true path in life, there are many things you can do; begin by answering the following questions on paper and recording them in your journal:

1. Begin by thinking about your childhood. Tap into your subconscious mind. What did you really love to do between the ages of seven and fourteen? What captivated your attention? What still captivates your attention?

2. Make a list of the twenty things you enjoy doing most in life. What gives you the greatest excitement? This will stimulate the creative action mechanism within your subconscious mind into revealing your purpose.

3. The subconscious mind may also be activated by reading. Start reading everything you can, this will help you uncover your purpose more quickly. Which books will you read this month to help you discover your life's passion?

4. Ask yourself: Where will I be and what will I be doing ten years from today if I keep doing what I am doing now?

5. Ask yourself: In what area do I express an extraordinary passion? When you know the answer to that question, then you know what you need to be doing.

6. Ask yourself: How can I do what I love to do and create financial abundance while doing it?

Heightened Prosperity

Each one
Teach one.
Each one
Reach one.
Each one
Grasp more
Each one
Reach for

The most
Of what you can be.
The best
Of what you can see.

Each one
Teach fun.
Each one
Love Sun.

What excites you
You should do.

Each one
Reach back.
Each one.
Heal lack.

Each one
Release strife,
Each one
Live more life!

Be alive,
Happily achieve.
It's all yours
If you believe.

Each day
Plan a way.

Each night,
Plan a site.
That you will see
When your dreams become —
Reality.

Each dawn
Listen long
To an uplifting book
An enchanting song.

Set the pace,
Win the race,
Give to all,
A smiling face.

Each life
Touch deep.
Bigger dreams
Less sleep.

Break bounds,
Become the best.
Leverage your mind
Surpass the rest.

Lesson 35:
Persistence

Begin Again
(Author Unknown)

Begin again — you can, you know.
Seek out a better way to go.
Forget the past — the past is dead,
And all tomorrow lies ahead!
There's never a time too late to start
To bring to fruition that dream in your heart.
Begin again now, this minute, this day!
A new life is waiting — don't wish it away!

"Do the thing and you shall have the power."
— Emerson

"By being persistent you are demonstrating faith."
— Earl Nightingale

"All great success in life is preceded by long, sustained
periods of focused effort on a single goal, the most
important goal, with the determination to stay with it
until it is complete. Throughout history, we find that
every man or woman who achieved anything lasting
and worthwhile, had engaged in long often unappreciated

> hours, weeks, months and even years of concentrated,
> disciplined work, in a particular direction. Fortunately,
> the quality of self-discipline is something that you can
> learn by continuous practice, over and over, until you
> master it. Once you have mastered the ability to delay
> gratification, the ability to discipline yourself to keep
> your attention focused on the most important task in
> front of you, there is virtually no goal that you cannot
> accomplish and no task that you cannot complete."
> — Anonymous

There is a rite of passage all must pass before they enter the hallowed halls of immortality. To pass those gates, one must possess the one key which opens all doors. A key which eludes all those who have not aligned their lives with their divine blueprint. A key which only opens the gates of fate when one has committed oneself entirely. That key is persistence — relentless persistence.

Before persistence, no army can stand, no wall can hold, no limit can remain. Absolutely nothing can take the place of persistence. There is a magical place awaiting those who will persevere. Persistence pays off.

Don't quit, no matter what. Decide to hold on in advance.

When Buster Douglas knocked out Mike Tyson it was the biggest upset in boxing history. When Buster Douglas was knocked down in that fight, it was time for his test. Before that fight ever started, he had decided he was getting up no matter what — he had committed himself to go all the way. He had just gotten out of an alcohol recovery center, his mother had just died, his wife was going down with disease. He was considered a nothing, a bum. When he got knocked down, Buster Douglas had a reason to get back up. He got back up and knocked out Mike Tyson. Reasons come first, answers come second.

The same holds true for you. Why will you persist when you get knocked down? You already have powerful reasons to get back up; what are they? *It is going to take everything you have got to become all you can be.* From some final reservoir of courage and determination, you will summon all of your strength and triumph. You will persist and make it to the top.

The lessons in this book have provided you with the diet and success information, now it is time for action.

Persistence is the science of continuous movement. Action is the key to abundance. Action is what it takes. As long as we keep making efforts, even if we stumble, we are still moving, making progress, and learning. Isaac Newton told us a body at rest tends to stay at rest, but a body in motion tends to stay in motion! Keep moving!

It is never too late to be who you "might" have been. Keep acting until you become who you want to become. It is never too late to get what you "might" have gotten. Keep looking until you have found what you are looking for.

The more you try, the more likely it is that you will find the right approach. You have to overcome the fear of failure by understanding that the more you fail, the more likely it is you will succeed at an exceptional level. Babe Ruth struck out almost twice as much as he hit home runs. Thomas Watson Sr., the founder of IBM (International Business Machines) said, "Do you want to succeed? Then, double your failure rate. Success lies on the far side of failure." Thomas Edison tried ten thousand types of filaments for the electric light bulb before he found the one which worked. Did he look at himself as a failure? No, he remained persistent. The only guaranteed way to fail is to not make the effort. I heard a success seminar speaker once say, "Successful people fail their way to the top." Taking action is always better than doing nothing, because if you fail, at least you know what doesn't work!

Courage Versus Conformity

People do not lack courage, they simply are overburdened by an abundance of conformity. Persistence requires courage, while quitting requires conformity.

It is better by far to live a vital life of commitment, rather than a shallow existence of compromise. After you commit to your goals, then you begin to move down a new trail, paths will open up to you that you never would have seen before. You will discover how you will become something more.

Keep in mind that the higher you rise, the greater and more clever is your opposition, and the greater will be the pressure to compromise. Always return to the basics when doubts arise. As I mentioned earlier, the greatest sports coaches the world has ever seen taught the basics over and over and over again. Practice the fundamentals daily. Conquer the critics by mastering fundamentals.

Have the raw courage to stand out. The great vice of the ages is conformity. Be strong and fear not, for all obstruction melts away before real strength of deed and sincerity of character. When you triumph, thrice blessed are you. Glory and honor be unto those who have the courage to win.

The time has come when every individual must rise from the slumber of indifference, from the orthodox complacency of the standard rules and regulations of society, and reach out, pioneering new fields of beautiful, ethical, and spiritual progress. It is now time to experience the incredible majesty of living.

Instantaneous Change

At a certain point in our lives, after assiduously applying the principles of mind-mastery and circumstance creation, our lives are taken into the nourishing arms of destiny and we are catapulted forward to places beyond our wildest dreams. We enter hallowed halls of instantaneous change. Everything can change suddenly, without a single warning. In the Bible it says, "Behold, I show you a mystery; we shall not all sleep, but we shall all be changed, in a moment, in the twinkling of an eye..." (I Corinthians 15:51-52).

When real change happens in our lives, it happens instantaneously. The secret of instant change is to continue to *persistently* practice fundamentals until you hit what in non-linear mathematics is called a point of instability. In science and mathematics, it is known that a chain of events can have a point of crisis which can instantly magnify small changes. But chaos theory teaches us that such points are pervasive — they are everywhere. This means that no matter where your station in life, it can be changed instantly; you can arise out of obscurity to the very highest level of intensity in any field. But, to do so, you must practice fundamentals daily!

Go forth and win! Gather all you can of the Earth's good things. As you persist, remember: "That which you are seeking is also seeking you." Employ the trial and success method: learn from your mistakes and adjust your behavior accordingly.

It is for you to travel the path, no outside power can do it for you. It is as detrimental to have some outside force travel the path for you as it would be to tear open a cocoon before the butterfly has emerged. You have to free yourself through persistence, and in the struggle to obtain your freedom, you will have acquired the strength to fly.

Behold and understand that you are now standing upon the threshold of a splendid dawning Sun. With persistence, you hold the key to the future.

Action Steps:

1. Open your journal and review the top 5 yearly goals established in

the **Action Steps** at the end of **Lesson 5: Goals**. Rewrite exactly why you will faithfully persist until you achieve your top 5 yearly goals.

2. Consider the following aphorisms: "Do the thing you fear and the death of fear is certain," "Feel the fear and do it anyway," "Act in spite of your fear." Ask yourself: "How can I make conquering my fears fun?" Record the answer in your journal.

Don't Quit
(Author Unknown)

When things go wrong, as they sometimes will,
When the road you're trudging seems all uphill,
When the funds are low and the debts are high,
And you want to smile, but instead you sigh,
When care is pressing you down a bit,
Rest if you must, but don't you quit.

For life is strange with its twists and turns,
As everyone of us sometimes learns,
And many failures turn about,
When they might have won, had they stuck it out.

So don't give up though the pace seems slow,
You may succeed with another blow;
Success is failure turned inside out,
It's the silver tint of the clouds of doubt.

And you never can tell how close you are,
It may be near when it seems so far.
So stick to the fight when you're hardest hit,
It's when things seem worst that you must not quit.

The Far Side Of Failure

On the far side of failure,
Beyond the path of rejection
Far past the ghosts
Of doubt and dejection.

Just a bit farther
Than life's toughest question.
Over the stream running,
After each lost election.

Farther along
Than the extra mile.
Floating further
Than the lonely isle.

Beyond the sign:
"The buck stops here."
Over pools reflecting —
The faces of fear.

Over chasms deep
Where things seem worst,
Through hardened deserts,
Overcome by thirst.

Even surpassing
The road traveled less
Lies the hidden valley
Of massive success.

Lesson 36:
My Personal Challenge To You

"In the last analysis, great human achievement
rests on perfect physical health."
— Emerson

"It's a funny thing about life; if you refuse to accept
anything but the best, you very often get it."
— W. Somerset Maugham

"What the caterpillar calls the end of the world,
the master calls a butterfly."
— Richard Bach, **Illusions**

"I challenge you to make your life a masterpiece.
I challenge you to join the ranks of those people
who live what they teach, who walk their talk.
Live with passion!"
— Anthony Robbins

"Outlive and outdo everybody."
— The Raw Courage Challenge

My challenge to you is to become the divine being you are capable of becoming. We are creators of circumstance, never creatures of circumstance. We can become anything we desire. We can fulfill every goal. We can achieve a state of total prosperity, perpetual health, and youthfulness.

The cosmic laws are always in operation. The Laws of Nature are here, and they remain here. "As you think, so shall it be" is part of the code — it is written into everything. From the seeds of your thought spring all the events and material objects around you. From great thinking arises a great life.

You get out of life what you expect to get. If you expect massive abundance, you shall receive massive abundance. Your state of mind controls your state of results. You create your own reality. Cultivate within your garden-mind an abundant success consciousness.

Life is a self-fulfilling prophecy. *Whatever you truly want will happen.*

Dare to take possession of your own mind! Your thought habits are created by the mental food that your mind consistently dwells upon, just as your eating habits are created by the food you consistently eat. When you plant the seeds of prosperity in your garden-mind, they will always grow.

What you think dramatically affects the way you eat. What you eat dramatically affects the way you think. Food has a consciousness. One cannot remain positive long by ingesting a consciousness of fire, poison, pain, and death. When one takes in positive, living food and positive, living thoughts, one also becomes positive and living! What an amazing truth this is! Dead food and negative thoughts lead to ruin.

Eat the divine food offered to us by the Sun-God Ra (Raw)! The Raw Law is unlimited. It does not end today or tomorrow. It persists for all time.

Increase your energy. Digestion is the number one energy sapper. To increase your energy, eat less and breathe more!

Make your body a supreme physical support system, so that it will carry you to distant goals and your most treasured dreams. Purify! Get there I say! From purity arises divinity.

Eden is here on Earth. It is right where you are at this moment. You are standing right now on your own "Acres of Diamonds." *Paradise is a state of health. All you have to do is purify yourself and you automatically arrive.*

The Sunfood Diet Success System works — every time. Simplicity is the key. Use the 36 lessons in this book to help you lead a simple and beautiful life. As the philosopher Friedrich Nietzsche wrote: "To live simply and naturally is the highest and final goal."

The Sunfood Diet Success System places you in a magical world of continual renewal. When you stay this path long enough, many of the profound mysteries of the world will be revealed to you. You will come to discover that for the complete reconstruction and rejuvenation of this planet and its inhabitants, there are tremendous projects afoot.

Life is an incredible adventure. You should spend every moment of your life fully alive, never bored. You should be growing, becoming better in every single way.

Surround yourself with those who can push you to your limits, who can challenge you to be everything you can be and more.

Transform all your trials and tribulations, your battles of mind and diet, your thirsting in the desert of knowledge, into flowing grace. Allow grace to embrace you.

Transform an ephemeral life into one of dynamic longevity. Allow age to ennoble you.

When your time is passed, let others say: "Now there was one who really lived life! There was one who chose the uncommon path, and achieved an uncommon destiny of health, happiness, and success." The choice is yours: a long life of glory, or a short, uneventful life in obscurity. What will it be?

You are the heir to all the ages, in the foremost ranks of time. You are a genius, a masterpiece of Nature. Embrace the abundance life has to offer. Trust your judgment. Take action! (Nothing is more fulfilling than taking action). By your fruits you shall be known! *Your actions speak so loudly that no one can ever hear a word you are saying!*

What counts is action — acting instead of talking. When you decide to do something you must go all the way. You must know exactly why you are doing it. Then you must proceed with massive action without having doubts or remorse. Keep moving forward, until it is done.

Success is not a goal, but a process, a way of living, a series of habits. Successful people practice fundamentals every day. Successful people take daily consistent action towards their life's purpose.

Everything in life is cumulative. Everything counts. Stack the odds in your favor whenever possible. When you use any one of the lessons in this book today, you have made a positive choice for your future, your children's future, and the planet's future.

It is time to awaken, to think, to believe, to desire, to act in faith, and fulfill. Within you are the seeds of greatness. Revel in the joy of your true Nature. Step into your mastery and climb the ladder of your destiny.

Fulfill your purpose! Walk your talk! Become more than you ever thought possible. Reach the highest state of perfection imaginable. Attract to yourself an abundance of spiritual, mental, emotional, physical, and financial wealth! Cultivate a philosophy of perfect health consciousness. Enjoy every moment of life's adventure. Laugh your way to the top!

A great transformation in a single individual can alter the destiny of the human race.

What would your life be like if you were to do the impossible?

Take on heroic, sacred attributes. There is a mysterious, almost magical charm about the personality of true greatness. A magical being is a sight to behold.

Dare to be bold. Spiritual forces will come to your aid. The bolder you are, the more magnetic is your presence. Boldness has a mystical quality to it, it creates an invisible force-field around you which deflects all attacks and attracts everything you need.

Go after what you really want, that state which humankind has always aspired to, the manifestation of the divinity within, here and now. The spiritual power lies within you. It is the unlimited power which provides superhuman strength of body, mind, and spirit. It is yours to use. Use it.

We sense there are two sides to our nature. You exist in this form as part animal, part deity; we are a spirit animated in a physical body. The glorious journey is to become as much of a deity as possible and ascend to our highest potential. To that end we desire a health which allows the full expression of our spirit through our physical body. You are a divine being who walks the Earth — start living like one.

Decide to *be*, and command forth, the youthful spirit. Become powerful, passionate, outstanding in all fields. Accelerate the energy within you at any moment. Live your dreams. Succeeding is so much fun!

Best wishes on your journey. May the force be with you.

Keep facing the Sun and the shadows will fall behind.

The Master

A friend of the brave,
Gives strength to the weak.
Who loves the Beautiful,
And builds up the meek.

Who breathes in:
To win.
Who breathes out
All-doubt.

Who calls up high-daring,
And casts down despair.
To rule the Earth,
To run with the Fair.

The Solar Vibration
And wild charm,
Impeccable to live
Without causing harm.

The choice of word,
And dramatic timing.
Passion, deep meaning.
Eyes: clear and shining.

Light of foot,
Intuition,
Heavy wit, Grace,
Decision.

Glory,
Great Fortune,
The Effortless,
In action.

The Grand Logic,
Magnetic.
Abundant
Symmetric.

The Cosmic Forge
A dance of the stars.
The Destiny,
The smooth sea —
Perfection.

A Message To All Sunfoodists

"And when much of the people were gathered together,
and were come to him out of every city Jesus spake by a
parable: 'A sower went out to sow his seed: and as he
sowed, some fell by the way side; and it was trodden
down, and the fowls of the air devoured it. And some
fell upon a rock; and as soon as it was sprung up, it
withered away, because it lacked moisture. And some
fell among thorns; and the thorns sprang up with it, and
choked it. And others fell on good ground and sprang up,
and bare fruit an hundredfold.' And when he had said these
things, he cried, 'He that hath ears to hear, let him hear.'
And his disciples asked him, saying, 'What might this
parable be?' And he said, 'Unto you it is given to know
the mysteries of the Kingdom of God: but to others in
parables; that seeing they might not see, and hearing they
might not understand. Now the parable is this:
The seed is the word of God.'"
— Luke 8:4-11

"There is nothing more powerful than
an idea whose time has come."
— Victor Hugo

This book is the flower, you are the fruit. Go out and spread the seeds
of good fortune. Let others devour your knowledge.

It is imperative for us as Sunfoodists to become attractive artists, wonderful parents, friendly farmers, great inventors, glorious statesmen, spiritual giants, magical millionaires, famous actresses and actors, and mystical musicians. By our achievements we will attract attention to this diet. We will spread this information by our inspiring example to the farthest corners of the world.

You are an incredible human being. I have tremendous respect for you being the type of person who took the time to read this book.

My message to you is to walk your talk; example is not the main thing influencing others, it is the only thing. Especially if you are teaching **The Sunfood Diet Success System**, first go to work on yourself, then set about the business of attracting new interest.

The eye's an amazing student,
And more telling than the ear,
Fine words are important,
But the example's always clear.

Unfortunately, in the past there have been many promoters of raw plant-food diets who did not walk their talk. Therefore, their information was not accurate, and even though they carried the message forward transforming many lives, it did lead many people astray.

The Sunfood Diet is about massive abundance. The Sunfood Diet cannot be about restriction and denial. When you are teaching the raw plant-food diet, let people know that their choices are abundant. If they want to eat a lot or a little, it does not matter. If the food falls within the "raw plant food" category, and the guidelines of The Sunfood Triangle are followed, the result of vibrant health and living in harmony with the Earth will be achieved.

After many years of promoting a raw-food lifestyle, I have found that the best way to introduce The Sunfood Diet to other people is to be a shining example of health and vitality myself. This is always the best way to attract people to the Sunfood lifestyle.

Become the example. You are in a much better position to communicate with people when they approach you, rather than when you approach them. Have them ask you about your amazing state of health. I have had women approach me from out of the blue and ask to touch my skin or ask me what is my secret. When this occurs you are in a powerful position to forward this vital Sunfood information. When someone approaches you like this, when they see your vitality, your transformation, don't give away the farm. Make them work for the information. When they ask, "What's your secret?" Just smile and say, "It's a secret." That will arouse their curiosity and make it much more likely they will take action on the information when you do eventually tell them about this success system! It will also make the situation much more fun!

Aside from the charismatic power of your own example, I have found the top two approaches to help people discover the raw-food truth for themselves are as follows:

Approach #1. "Life is designed raw." Out of trillions of organisms that were alive at the beginning of time, are alive now, and will be alive at the end of time, only one tampers with its food. You do not want to bet against those kinds of odds!

Approach #2. "You can't convince a child." Children naturally gravitate towards brightly-colored fruits! My friend Lenny Watson, a long-time raw-foodist and natural healer from Maui, tells us, "You don't start a child on macrobiotic food." Children intuitively know that their natural foods are raw fruits and vegetables.

As you communicate this information, people will say "no" to you. The best salespeople know how to do deal with doubters, pessimists, the dis-interested, and the apathetic. The best salespeople have overcome their fear of rejection. They just say, "Next." Move on to someone else. There are billions of people who need this information and millions who will listen and take action. Go forth, find them, leverage your mind to present this diet to them in the most attractive way possible.

Some Do. Some Don't.

Some do.
Some don't.
Some will,
Some won't.
Some do now,
Some do later.
Some never do
And say : "See you later."
Some get it,
Some don't.
Some grasp it,
Some won't.
Some live,
Some die.
Some ask:
"Why?"
Why it is? Who knows.
It's just how it goes.

Some laugh,
Some cry.
Some are honest,
Some lie.
Some win,
And some tie.
Some say: "Just try."
Be curious.
Move on.
Some pro,
Some con.

Some fake it.
Some make it.
Work with it,

Not against it.
Some slip,
Some rise.
Some see
With clear eyes.

You can't
Change it,
Rearrange it.
It's the set up,
Just face it.
But you can
Change yourself.
To attract some —
Living wealth.

Your goal
You control.

Some believe,
Some achieve.
Some reach,
Some hold.
Some are shy,
Some are bold.
Some grow,
Some won't.
Some do.
Some don't.

Dynamic Communication

Start talking to people about raw foods. Become a dynamic communicator. The more precise our communication with ourselves and others, the more effective we are; because we humans are gregarious, social beings.

Communication is more than it seems. Discover how to communicate! First, tell your voice it is in harmony with the sounds of Nature. Then, tell your skin it glows with smooth perfection. Next, begin to talk health into every organ of your own or another's body. Tell yourself or another that their muscles are limber, shapely, and beautiful. Tell your mind, or another's mind, that it is functioning at peak efficiency. Master personal communication skills. Choose your body language, tone of voice, and words carefully.

Be aware of the 55:38:7 communication equation. 55% of your communication (as it is perceived by others) is non-verbal. This includes: physiology, body language, eye contact, and gestures. 38% comes from the sound and tone of your voice. 7% of your communication is the based on the actual content of what you are saying.

Be there in the present moment with anyone you find before you throughout the day. Really listen to what they are telling you. Ask questions. Some of the most incredible stories I have ever heard came from seemingly boring people. I find something fascinating in every person I meet. When you are a good listener, you not only know what you know, but you also know what the other person knows!

Teaching is not about preaching, it is about asking questions. How can I know how I can help someone nutritionally if I do not know anything about them? By asking questions, I can discover everything I need to help!

Questions are answers. Just as you can focus your own brain's energy by asking yourself specific questions, you can also direct the focus of someone else's brain by asking her/him specific questions.

As individuals who live the Sunfood lifestyle, we should understand cooked food causes more than raw food alone can cure. Other healing modalities: massage, yoga, meditation, walking, playing, laughing...all have their place. But the raw-food information is the key to the whole thing — it makes everything else work amazingly well. This information is absolutely vital to the future health and happiness of the planet. People can always use a boost, they need **The Sunfood Diet Success System** in their hands and hearts. Challenge yourself to push this message into the world. Speak up when you would have held your tongue.

My organization Nature's First Law is dedicated to capturing the attention of all media with this message. Help us spread the word! How can you help us, help yourself, and enjoy the whole process?

Pass It On

If there is a blessing known,
If a better way is shown,
Pass it on.
Send it out on waves of thought.
Let it find one who has sought.
Pass it on.
Inspire it in each holy mind,
Let it produce after its kind.
Pass it on.
Let it travel down the years,
Let it dry another's tears,
Until in heaven the deed appears,
Please pass it on.

I want you to know that I feel tremendously fortunate to be the individual to bring this blessing to you. It seems almost uncanny that such an opportunity would befall me. I would like to thank you for your interest in becoming all that you can possibly be.

Together we must carry the Sunfood Diet message forward. Together we can turn this world into a paradise. You, who have glimpsed your true potential, will be among the leaders of a new dispensation on Earth.

"We, the new, the nameless, the hard-to-understand, we firstlings of a yet untried future — we require for a new end also a new means, namely, a new healthiness, stronger, sharper, tougher, bolder, and merrier than any healthiness hitherto. He whose soul longs to experience the whole range of hitherto recognized values and desirabilities, and to circumnavigate all the coasts of this ideal "Mediterranean Sea," who, from the adventures of his most personal experience, wants to know how it feels to be a conqueror and discoverer of the ideal — as likewise how it is with the artist, the saint, the legislator, the sage, the scholar, the devotee, the prophet, and the godly Nonconformist of the old style: — requires one thing above all for that purpose, great healthiness — such healthiness as one not only possesses, but also constantly acquires and must acquire, because one continually sacrifices it again, and must sacrifice it! — And now, after having been long on the way in this fashion, we Argonauts of the ideal, who are more courageous perhaps than prudent, and often enough shipwrecked and brought to grief, nevertheless, as said above, healthier than people would like to admit, dangerously healthy, always healthy again, — it would seem, as if in recompense for it all, that we have a still undiscovered country before us, the boundaries of which no one has yet seen, a beyond to all countries and corners of the ideal known hitherto, a world so over-rich in the beautiful, the strange, the questionable, the frightful, and the divine, that our curiosity as well as our thirst for the possession thereof, have got out of hand — alas! that nothing will any longer satisfy us!"

— Friedrich Nietzsche, **Joyful Wisdom**

"Don't worry about it, embrace it."

Selected Poetry

The Logic Of Today

It was thought that ruled,
When Augustus fueled,
The ships of ancient Rome.
It was thought that led Columbus,
Over the Atlantic's foam.

It was thought that guided the astro-nauts,
To the Moon's Tranquillity Bay.
Thought is the power which rules the world:
This is the logic of today.

Thought alone is the building stone,
The total of which you're the sum,
The strangest secret of success in life is:
What you think about you become.

Behind the world's greatest minds,
Lies the primordial law,
Brilliant thoughts, radiant ideas,
To hold the world in awe.

The thinking mind creates the future,
All "luck" is a fraud.
Each mind is a creative force,
With the potential of a god.

Actualize your thoughts
Through deeds of splendor and renown.
Face your inner fears,
And they retreat without a sound.

Creative minds may free the Earth,
When action is taken thereon,
And Liberty to those who know:
What you think about — you become.

For thoughts command when people reach,
Outward towards the stars,
And it was thought which dropped the probe,
Onto the surface of Mars.

It was thought that ruled,
When the druids built
Astronomic Temples of stone and clay.
This is the testimony of the ancients:
And the logic of today.

And thoughts direct when empires sink,
In storms of steel and flame.
And it is by thought alone
That seeds are sown —
And it will always be the same.

The powerful thoughts
Of those who act,

Rush forth to fill the mass,
Of thoughtless minds
Who should invest their lives,
Growing gardens instead of grass.

Harmonize with the Earth and trees,
People and plant are one,
The greatest truth of all the world is:
What you think about you become.

Thought governs all organic life,
Inspires all right and wrong.
It's Nature's plan to give a helping hand,
To those whose thoughts are strong.

By thought you may ride to glory —
Let nothing bar your way,
And if you decide to rule your thoughts:
You've grasped the logic of today.

Ye Are Gods

"...Is it not written in your law, I said, **Ye Are Gods**?"

A fascinating abstraction.
The pranic interaction.

The Empyreal Living Sea.
Pantamorphic energy.

Galama. Air. Radiation.
You are a —
Perfect Creation.

Bubbling springs of sweet, clear blue.
Ye are Gods! I tell you!

Humans need little here.
The simple needs are few!
Some fruits to smell and herbs to feel,
Good thoughts for an evening meal,
The truths the immortals knew.

The secret trite
and simple rite:
"Air for dinner,
Makes a winner."

Bathed within
Oceans of gas
Billions of sparks unseen.
The purest fuel of immortal Life,
Burns so pure and clean.

No residue remaining.
No ash to remove.
Air alone sustaining.
Float instead of move.

The secret now revealed:
Grow in the open air,
Breathe and sleep with the earth,
Dream deeply of the fair.

To see the good in everybody,
Think what is only true,
Breathe in life above the strife,
And show what you can do.

Emanate the impeccably true,
Ye are Gods! I tell you!

Obey your own conviction,
Love. Wisdom. Perfection.

Touch what can't be touched,
See what can't be seen.
Let the drama unfold,
No need to intervene.

Float on intuition,
Go with what you feel,
Only what you sense is true,
Can ever become so real.

An energetic forcefield,
An energetic seeing,
Not eating for a living,
Is a new way of being.

Stop tho world, right on cuc.
Ye are Gods! I tell you!

Paradox is reality,
Life is Destiny.

"As above you so below".
See the living planet glow.

Rhythm and antiquity.
Deep unsolved history.

Stillness, solitude, open space.
The beauty of being in this place.

The Earth is bliss
Between the worlds.
At the dawn,
A mystery unfurls.

Clear view of Sun,
Sky, stars, clouds,
Moon, cliffrock, canyon.
Dance among the sounds.

Time enough to allow
Thought and feeling to range far.
From here to the end of the world and back.
Travel from star to star.

The more harmonious you become
To the beat of the vital heart,
The more you will attract to your being
The whole, instead of the part.

Surrender all your ideas,
Things are not what they seem.
Here, within all worlds,
We can only live our dream.

Action. Life. Manifestation.
You are a —
Perfect Creation.

Trust the spirit, desire it too.
Ye are Gods! I tell you!

Transmit the signal,
Harmonize the storm
The Ascended Masters
Are here in form.

Abundant love
You attract.
Abundant health,
No turning back;
Abundant life
It's a game, you see,
Abundant world
Fulfill your Destiny.

The Ascended Ones shower you;
Their vibration soon to strengthen you!
They seed your creative fire,
It's reality as you desire.

Be extremely quiet
Have no diet
And create,
Gather your spirit

Emanate:
The master work,
The philosopher's stone,
The elixir of life,
Few have known.

Materialized before you,
The mysterious, secret chain,
The Cosmic Circuit Board
Connecting every plane.

The white powder of gold
What Enoch left untold.

Ascended Master
Impeccable Faster
You are Creators upon this plane.

The NeFiLim
Are upon the Earth.
This is the moment
Of your rebirth.

As you ask you shall receive.
What you see is what you believe.
What you think in life you are.
Your breath alone will take you far.

With focus you surpass
All the expectations.
Manifestation is instant,
In this time of transmutations.

Float so high you find yourself
In constant states of joy and health!

Then you'll know with ease and grace.
The mystery of the secret face.

The divineforce
In physical form.
Magic presence.
Beyond the norm.
Perfect potential.
Life abounds.
Slow the breath,
Hear cosmic sounds.

You're obsidian, volcanic
A pulsing ember, organic.
You're a limitless being, creating anew,
Ye are Gods! I tell you!

All is perfection,
All is divine.
Don't eat...listen
And soon you shall find.

Majesty

Nature's test is:
The trial by fire.
To fall with the ash
Or rise ever higher.

You may become:
An elegant being.
A genetic titan
With entirely new meaning.

A spiritual giant
Baroque, classic,
Masterful, effective,
Totally dynamic.
A great, bold spirit
With impeccable logic.
Embodied pure form
Majestic, high-gothic.

But a challenge awaits.
One truth you must face:

It stumbles the beggar,
It fells the queen,
A gift of the gods?
Or a curse cast unclean?

The eternal lie,
The primitive flame
It's sapping potential
The most dangerous game.

It's flaming wings:
Dispel the magic,
Bring paradise lost,
Give birth to the tragic.

Confusing the mind,
Emotions entwined,
Forging a path where
Life's not designed.

The flames are about
And nearing they seize:
Life, love, and laughter,
Even the trees.

The peril is high
The passion arising
The flames upon you
The urgency rising.

Choosing now
What to believe.
To trust in You.
Is not to deceive.

Summon the symbol,
A Courage long past.
The Sun-Fired crest,
Revive it at last.

It's a trial by fire.
None excepted
Who will pass?
Each is tested.

The cosmic law.
Of paradox shifting,
That which destroys
Is also uplifting.

The flaming wings of divine tragedy,
Can uplift you to a soaring majesty.

Must all the gods die?
Have you found out why?

Age ennobles
The legends untold
Thrust through the ages
The karmas unfold.

The Fates deciding
The zodiak throw,
The pantheon crumbles
Impending overthrow.

Obscuring the Sun,
The ominous clash,
Mind-states in ruin,
Consumers of ash.

Descending now
The savage curtain,
And for the noble
The test is certain.
It's the twilight of the gods,
The wolf-god's unleashed,
Will you choose beauty...
Or the beast?

The destruction, ecliptic,
Ruins, apocalyptic.

The queen stares
The cities in fire
But the phoenix flames
Are rising higher.

It's a trial by fire.
None excepted
Who will pass?
Each is tested.

The cosmic law:
Of paradox shifting,
That which destroys
Is also uplifting.

The flaming wings of divine tragedy,
Can uplift you to a soaring majesty.

The killing words,
The elegant whisper:
"You will become more than you were."

It's the cosmic law:
That opposition breeds
A fertile ash for
Transforming seeds.

The solar beat,
A rhythm drumming,
You are pure life
Pure becoming.

Gather your strength,
Arise from the ashes!
Grasp now
What intuition flashes!

The biological aim,
The inner direction,
The fulfillment of what
Was ordained at conception.

A new royal
Dynastic crown,
You may be reborn
Of the sky and ground.

It's a trial by fire.
None excepted
Who will pass?
Each is tested.

The cosmic law:
Of paradox shifting,
That which destroys
Is also uplifting.

The flaming wings of divine tragedy.
Can uplift you to a soaring Majesty.

Faustian life striving
For infinite space.
A rhythm alive
From Rome to Thrace.

The love of wild Nature,
The mysterious compassion,

The ineffable forsakeness
An intangible fashion.

Will-to-power,
The passionate striving,
Uncompromised truth,
Forever is driving.

The electric thrill
In overthrowing
Regressing life
Never growing.

Aristocrat features:
Wild-animal eyes.
Staring deeply,
See through the lies.

True conviction belongs to the wise,
There is no strength in compromise.

Surpass, overcome,
Overwhelm all denial,
In Nature there is
Only one trial.

It's a trial by fire.
None excepted
Who will pass?
Each is tested.

The cosmic law:
Of paradox shifting,
That which destroys
Is also uplifting.

The flaming wings of divine tragedy.
Can uplift you to a soaring Majesty.

The heavenly bodies,
Both hemispheres,
A celestial symphony,
The conjunction nears

The maximum moment
The cosmic flowing
The zodiak spinning
Inspiration growing.

The destiny appears,
The mind-world showing
The tarot spinning.
Vision overflowing.

Insight deep from
A simple deduction:
"Wrong thinking leads on to destruction."

Insight clear from
A cosmic instruction:
"All death is caused by internal obstruction."

Opposition leads
to transformation.
You are complete:
A perfect creation.

Draw in the knowledge
A meteor shower,
Tune in the body,
Embrace its power!

A feeling of flowing,
Wondrous grace,
To always be found
In the right place.

"You are the reflection of transcendent perfection."

Unstoppable volition.
Philosophic insight.
Mystic premonition.
This is your right.

Purify the body,
The cosmic receiver
Dismiss away doubt
The greatest deceiver.

It's a trial by fire.
None excepted
Who will pass?
Each is tested.

The cosmic law:
Of paradox shifting
That which destroys
Is also uplifting.

The flaming wings of divine tragedy.
Can uplift you to a soaring Majesty.

The planets in glory
The ocean in pearls
Throughout the ether
The nebulae swirls.

The desire for life,
A cosmic imperium
Begins a thought seeking:
Mind-world dominion.

You are the sculptor,
You build the worlds.
From the font of a thought
Your destiny unfurls.

The gehenna fire
The cosmic joke.
Disintegrate now
Its plume of smoke.

Extinguish the fire
In which life burns;
Release pain's liar
From whom one learns.

How many times
Will you rise from the ashes?
With each death,
The Phoenix flashes:
The perception brighter,
The mind more alive,
Sensitive, elastic,
A new call to thrive.

Dragon Mistress,
The ancient quest,
Put down the flame,
For massive success.

Abundant life of
Archaic Earth
Now undergoes
A Gothic rebirth.

Architect of archetypes
In the mind-world array.
Actualize your form
Tomorrow is today.

It's Twilight in Olympus.
A mystic rage for order
Magic-moment chaos:
The You World Order.

It's a trial by fire.
None excepted
Who will pass?
Each is tested.

The cosmic law:
Of paradox shifting,
That which destroys
Is also uplifting.

The flaming wings of divine tragedy.
Can uplift you to a soaring Majesty.

It's the ineffable truth,
The eternal test,
That fire captures
All but the best.

Appendix A: Anatomy Chart

	CARNIVORE	**HERBIVORE**	**HUMAN**
Is a human being a carnivore, herbivore, or omnivore?			
1	Teeth are long, sharp, and pointed. No flat molar teeth. Sharp canine teeth.	Front and canine teeth may be sharp or pointed. Back teeth are flattened for grinding.	All teeth are flattened, especially the back molars. Dullest canine teeth of all primates.
2	To facilitate tearing and biting, jaw can move up and down (vertically).	To facilitate the grinding of vegetable foods, jaw can move both up and down (vertically) and side to side (horizontally).	To facilitate the grinding of vegetable foods, jaw can move both up and down (vertically) and side to side (horizontally).
3	No lip or pouchy cheek structure.	Adaptable lip and pouchy cheek structure.	Refined lip and pouchy cheek structure.
4	Shape of the face allows the carnivore to dig into a carcass and rip out the entrails.	Shape of the face allows the animal to pull vegetation off of plants.	Shape of the face clearly indicates that humans have no ability to rip out entrails with their mouth.
5	Forward facing eyes; binocular vision.	**Herbivores with predators:** radial eyeset allowing for wide field of vision. **Herbivores without predators:** forward facing eyes; binocular vision.	Forward facing eyes; binocular vision. Humans have no natural predators.
6	Drinks water by lifting it into the throat with the tongue.	Drinks water by suction.	Drinks water by suction.

	CARNIVORE	HERBIVORE	HUMAN
7	Tongue is rough and thin.	Tongue is smooth and thick to manipulate vegetable matter into the back molars for grinding.	Tongue is smooth and thick to manipulate vegetable matter into the back molars for grinding.
8	Zonary placenta.	Placenta non-deciduate.	Discoidal placenta.
9	Intestines are 3 times as long as the trunk of the body; their design facilitates rapid expulsion of fleshy matter.	Intestines are at least 8 to 12 times as long as the trunk of the body; they are designed for extracting all nutrients from plant fiber.	Intestines are at least 12 times as long as the trunk, and an integral part of the most sophisticated juice extractor in the world: the human digestive system.
10	Liver contains uricase, an enzyme used to break down uric acid; it can break down 10 to 15 times as much uric acid as a herbivore.	Liver has a low tolerance for uric acid.	Liver has a low tolerance for uric acid.
11	Bowels are smooth and short for quick expulsion of waste matter.	Bowels are sulcified and complex for the reconstitution of waste matter.	Bowel walls are puckered, convoluted, and full of deep pouches for the reconstitution of waste matter.
12	Digestive system has the capacity to expel large amounts of foreign cholesterol.	Digestive system has no capacity to expel foreign cholesterol.	Digestive system has no capacity to expel foreign cholesterol.
13	Saliva is acidic.	Saliva is alkaline; it contains enzymes specifically designed to break down starchy carbohydrates.	Saliva is alkaline; it contains ptyalin, an enzyme specifically designed to break down starchy carbohydrates.
14	Blood is acidic.	Blood is alkaline.	Blood is alkaline.

	CARNIVORE	**HERBIVORE**	**HUMAN**
15	Urine is acidic.	Urine is alkaline.	Urine is alkaline.
16	Cools itself primarily through action of the tongue and mouth (panting).	Cools itself primarily through perspiration.	Cools itself primarily through perspiration.
17	All four feet are clawed (to rip into flesh).	All four feet are hoofed (cloven) or hands and feet contain individual digits (fingers or toes) with nails.	Hands and feet contain individual digits with nails and opposable thumbs. Hands are perfectly designed to reach out, grab fruit, and peel it.

Appendix B: The Sunfood Diet Weekly Guideline and Menu Plan

Green-Leafy Vegetables, Fruits, and Fats:

A fruit is any natural food containing seeds (e.g. tomato is a fruit, cucumber is a fruit). Eat fruits with seeds (avoid seedless hybrid fruit).

All types of vegetables are great, however, preference should be given to green-leafed vegetables. Avoid hybrid vegetables (i.e. carrots, beets, potatoes).

All types of raw plant foods which contain fats help transition over from cooked foods to The Raw-Food Diet. They fill you up and satiate your hunger. These include avocados, olives, coconuts, nuts, seeds, etc.

If one is sensitive to sugar, it is a good idea to add oils (flax, olive, etc.) to smoothies or fruit salads. This will allow a slower time-release of sugar into the blood. If one is extremely sensitive to sweet fruits, replace sweet fruits in the morning with grapefruits, cucumber, tomatoes, or other low-sugar fruits. Some sweet fruit, however, is necessary in the diet.

Eat nuts and seeds moderately. Quantities should be kept to less than 2.0-2.5 pounds (0.9-1.2 kg) of nuts per week. Eat nuts together with green-leafed vegetables for ideal digestion. If one is sensitive to nuts, then replace all nuts listed in the menu below with avocados or olives.

All daily menus should contain a healthy balance of green-leafed vegetables (i.e. chard, collards, lettuces, kale, spinach, etc.), sugary fruits (oranges, melons, mangos, papayas, etc.), and fatty foods (i.e. avocados, olives, nuts, seeds, etc.). Chlorophyll foods build the structure of the body. Sweet fruits fuel the system with glucose. Fats lubricate and oil the body.

Salad Dressings:

For salad dressings, combine a raw plant fat with a sugar. For example, we can blend half an avocado with an orange in the blender and pour that on our salad as dressing. If we look at most commercial salad dressings on the market, we can see they consist of two basic ingredients — a fat (oil, pasteurized dairy milk) and a sugar (high fructose corn syrup). People love fats and sugars with greens because they complete The Sunfood Triangle!

Water:

The amount of water one drinks should be dictated by thirst. Raw fruits and vegetables contain so much high-quality water one may find that thirst disappears. If you do drink water, drink distilled water with a squeeze of lemon at least 30 minutes *before* you eat a meal — drinking water after a meal dilutes the digestive juices and interferes with digestion. If distilled water is not available, look for Evian water in glass or, when not available, in plastic.

Alcohol:

One should preferentially choose wine over all other alcohols. Most wines have not been heat-processed. Seek out organic varieties with no sulfites added.

All beers are brewed (cooked). If one does choose to drink beer, one should preferentially choose dark beers with more minerals over refined commercial beers. Dark beers have a less dramatic effect on blood sugar levels.

Gradually letting go of alcohol will strengthen one's immune system and decrease the risk of an early death in an accident.

Dairy Products:

Any pasteurized dairy products have long-range destructive effects on health and the digestive system. The only reason pasteurized dairy products are found in stores is because they have a longer shelf life than raw dairy products and thus they bring more money to the dairy industry.

If dairy products are included in the diet, they should be raw. Children who simply refuse to eat healthy portions of green-leafed vegetables may have raw dairy products in their diet for calcium.

Soy milk is also a better option than cooked milk. It has a high-fat content, and may be used to "cut" tea or coffee.

Chewing:
Be sure to fully chew every mouthful of food. The famous Dr. Fletcher recommended 50 chews per mouthful.

Try eating with chopsticks instead of kitchen utensils as they will help to slow the rate of your eating.

Sea Vegetables:
On the raw-food diet, sea vegetables have a balancing effect because they contain a dense amount of trace minerals and alkaline-mineral salts. Sea vegetables, however, grow in the sea, and are subject to intake the pollution found there. Reputable sources for these products are important. Nature's First Law distributes several varieties of sea vegetables (dulse, nori) which are tested for contaminants. Please call for more information: 888-RAW-FOOD.

Variety:
Among wild primates, approximately 25 different raw plant foods are eaten each week. In a year, wild primates eat up to 115 different varieties of raw plant foods. This provides us with some great guidelines and goals for our own diet. Enjoy a wide variety of fruits, vegetables, nuts, and seeds. Rotation is the natural way of eating. Always err on the side of eating more variety.

Transitional Strategy:
Eat as high a percentage of raw-plant foods in your diet as possible. Feel free to eat large quantities of raw plant foods if you feel so inclined. Discover sources for raw organic foods either locally or through mail order (reference the **Resources** section at the end of this book). Items

which may be unfamiliar, such as flax seed oil or spirulina, may be found at the natural-food store or through mail order.

Any cooked foods should preferentially be eaten in the evening and then only one type at a time. Always combine any cooked food with the evening's large salad and freshly-made vegetable juice.

Cooked starches should be those which are lower on the **Glycemic Index Chart** shown in **Lesson 11: The Secret Revealed**, **Sugar** such as yams or sweet potatoes.

Transitioning off of red meat initially, then pork, chicken, and finally fish is an excellent way to let go of animal foods. For all the reasons I have outlined in this book, it is very important for our own health and success to let go of these foods quickly.

Remember the simple rule: Simplicity is bliss.

Be flexible. Be easy on yourself. Transition at your own pace.

Three complete menu plans, corresponding to three stages of transition, are provided in the following pages: **The Basic Sunfood Diet**, **The 80/20 Sunfood Diet**, and **The All-Raw Diet**.

Unless otherwise stated, all menu items should be raw, plant-based, and organic.

The Basic Sunfood Diet

At this level, the focus is to include significantly more raw plant foods and their juices into the diet. At this level, one should make the commitment to seek out organic foods.

This diet is about abundance, not denial. Therefore, on **Day 5: Friday** and **Day 6: Saturday** one may still eat their favorite meals in the evening...but with a salad! Over time, as one eats more raw foods containing the 3 food classes, and less cooked foods, the taste buds will change and a dietary shift will happen automatically.

The Basic Sunfood Diet Weekly Menu (Spring/Summer)

Day 1: Monday
Morning:
> 3 pounds (1.4 kg) of watermelon (not seedless).

Afternoon:
> One small green-leafed vegetable salad. Squeeze lemon into the salad as dressing.
> One sandwich made with: toasted sprouted grain bread, avocado, clover sprouts, diced red bell pepper, and diced cucumber.

Snack:
> 2 mangos.

Evening:
> One large lettuce, cucumber, tomato, and green onion salad with two avocados, and a fresh-squeezed lemon.
> One meal of cooked starch (baked yams or sweet potatoes are preferred over potatoes or rice).
> 1/2 quart (1/2 liter) of freshly made vegetable juice containing at least 60% green vegetables, 40% other vegetables or fruits (i.e. apple, cucumber, etc.).

Notes:

Day 2: Tuesday
Morning:
> 14 ounce (0.4 liters) of a blended berry smoothie containing: blueberries, blackberries, raspberries, and strawberries. Add 3 tablespoons of stone-crushed, cold-pressed extra-virgin olive oil and/or 2 tablespoons of spirulina if desired.

Afternoon:
> One small green-leafed vegetable salad with one avocado. Squeeze an orange into the salad as dressing.
> One item of cooked starch (baked, no-salt corn chips would be preferred) eaten with one avocado.

Snack:
> 2 oranges.

Evening:
> Large salad containing 80% green-leafed vegetables, 2-3 avocados, and an orange squeezed as dressing.
> Steamed vegetables (cauliflower or broccoli).
> 2 apples.

Notes:

Day 3: Wednesday
Morning:
> 1 cantaloupe.

Afternoon:
> Cucumber, tomato, zucchini mixed salad. Squeeze an orange into the salad as dressing.
> One item of cooked starch (baked, no-salt corn chips would be preferred) eaten with avocado.
> One sandwich made with: toasted sprouted grain bread, avocado, sprouts, diced red bell pepper, and diced cucumber).

Snack:
> 1 bowl of figs.

Evening:
> Large salad containing 80% green-leafed vegetables including kale or spinach eaten with 20-30 raw macadamia nuts, and an orange squeezed as dressing.
> One meal of cooked starch (brown rice or baked squash).

Notes:

Day 4: Thursday
Morning:
> 1/2 quart (1/2 liter) of freshly-blended peach and nectarine juice. Add 4 teaspoons of flax seed oil and/or 2 tablespoons of spirulina if desired.

Afternoon:
> 2 bowls of berries (strawberries, blueberries, etc.).
> One small lettuce salad with cucumber. Add 2-3 tablespoons of olive oil if desired.
> One avocado.
> One serving of cooked starch (brown rice or wholegrain bread).

Snack:
> 2 oranges.

Evening:
> Large salad containing 80% green-leafed vegetables, and an orange squeezed as dressing. Add several servings of raw dulse seaweed to the salad.
> Dehydrated or sprouted crackers or bread eaten with one avocado.
> Steamed vegetables (cauliflower or broccoli).
> 1/2 quart (1/2 liter) of freshly made vegetable juice containing at least 60% green vegetables, 40% other vegetables or fruits (i.e. apple, cucumber, etc.).

Notes:

Day 5: Friday
Morning:
> 1 honeydew melon.

Afternoon:
> Cucumber, tomato, okra, zucchini mixed salad. Add high-quality extra virgin cold-pressed olive oil and a fresh-squeezed orange as dressing.
> One sandwich made with: toasted sprouted grain bread, avocado, lettuce, sunflower greens, sliced tomato, and diced cucumber.

Snack:
> 1 bowl of grapes (with seeds).

Evening:
> Large salad containing 80% green-leafed vegetables including parsley, 2 avocados, and blended mango juice as dressing.
> Include your favorite meal here!

Notes:

Day 6: Saturday
Morning:
> Drink the water of 2 coconuts.

Afternoon:
> 1 quart (1 liter) of freshly made vegetable juice containing apples and celery.
> One sandwich made with: toasted sprouted grain bread, avocado, clover sprouts, sliced tomato, diced zucchini, and cayenne or garlic powder.

Snack:
> 2 mangos.

Evening:
> Large salad containing 80% green-leafed vegetables including 3 ribs of celery, 2 avocados, and high-quality extra virgin cold-pressed olive oil as dressing. Add several servings of raw dulse seaweed and grated raw garlic to the salad.
> Include your favorite meal here!

Notes:

Day 7: Sunday
Morning:
      14 ounces (0.4 liters) of herbal tea. Squeeze in fresh lemon if desired. Use fresh maple syrup or raw honey to sweeten.

Afternoon:
      1 bowl of strawberries and/or blueberries.
      1 quart (1 liter) of freshly made vegetable juice containing cucumber, lettuce, and yellow bell pepper.

Snack:
      2-3 pears.
      2 ribs of celery.

Evening:
      Large salad containing 80% green-leafed vegetables, 30-40 pecans, dulse seaweed, and an orange squeezed as dressing.
      Include your favorite raw-food recipe here. Experiment!

Notes:

The Basic Sunfood Diet Weekly Menu (Fall/Winter)

Day 1: Monday
Morning:
      8 ounces (1/4 liter) of herbal tea. Squeeze in fresh lemon if desired. Use fresh maple syrup or raw honey to sweeten.
      One blended super smoothie containing: apple, pear, berries (all types), spirulina (2-3 tablespoons), and flax oil (2-3 tablespoons).

Afternoon:
      1 shot (1 ounce) of wheatgrass juice.
      One sandwich made with: toasted sprouted grain bread, avocado, clover sprouts, sliced tomato, diced zucchini, and red onion.

Snack: 3 oranges.

Evening:
      One large spinach salad containing cucumber, tomato, and green onion with 1 avocado and fresh-squeezed lemon.
      Dehydrated or toasted wholegrain bread with one cup of raw unhulled tahini.
      Popcorn eaten with stone-crushed, cold-pressed extra-virgin olive oil.

Notes:

Day 2: Tuesday
Morning:
      8 ounces (1/4 liter) of herbal tea.
      One blended smoothie containing: apple, pear, papaya, spirulina (2-3 tablespoons), and flax oil (2-3 tablespoons).

Afternoon:
      One small green-leafed vegetable salad (containing kale or spinach) with 10-20 water-soaked almonds. Add fresh-blended lemon, basil, and avocado as a dressing.
      One item of cooked starch (baked, no-salt corn chips would be preferred) eaten with avocado.

Snack: 2 oranges.

Evening:
      Large salad containing 80% green-leafed vegetables, 2 avocados, and an orange squeezed as dressing.
      Hummus (preferably raw) with fresh vegetables and fruits: celery, broccoli, cauliflower, cucumbers, and tomatoes.
      1 quart (1 liter) of freshly made vegetable juice containing at least 60% green vegetables, 40% other vegetables or fruits (i.e. squash, peppers, okra, etc.).

Notes:

Day 3: Wednesday
Morning:
　　8 ounces (1/4 liter) of herbal tea.
　　1 quart (1 liter) of freshly-made orange juice mixed with 1/2 avocado or 3 teaspoons of flax seed oil.

　Afternoon:
　　One shot (1 ounce) of fresh wheatgrass juice.
　　Warm vegetable soup.
　　One sandwich made with: toasted sprouted grain bread, avocado, lettuce, clover sprouts, diced tomatoes, diced cucumber, and cayenne powder .

　Snack: 2 persimmons.
　　Assorted green leaves (lettuce, spinach, endive).
　　Popcorn eaten with stone-crushed, cold-pressed extra-virgin olive oil.

　Evening:
　　Large salad containing 80% green-leafed vegetables eaten with 1 cup of unhulled tahini and a squeezed persimmon as dressing. Add several servings of raw dulse seaweed to the salad. Add 30-40 Sun-ripened olives (if available).
　　Dehydrated or toasted wholegrain bread.
　　Warm vegetable soup.
　Notes:

Day 4: Thursday
Morning:
　　8 ounces (1/4 liter) of herbal tea. Squeeze in fresh lemon if desired. Use fresh maple syrup or raw honey to sweeten.
　　One blended super smoothie containing: apple, pear, berries (all types), spirulina (2-3 tablespoons), and flax oil (2-3 tablespoons).

　Afternoon:
　　Greek salad containing: lettuce, tomato, cucumber, red onion, salt-cured black olives, 1-2 ounces (30-60 ml) of olive oil.
　　Blended pudding containing: dates, avocado, cinnamon powder, and distilled water.
　　One serving of cooked starch (wholemeal bread, wheat tortillas).

　Snack: 2 asian pears.
　　1 handful of raw pumpkin seeds.

　Evening:
　　Large salad containing 80% green-leafed vegetables, 30-40 almonds, and an orange squeezed as dressing. Add several servings of raw dulse seaweed to the salad.
　　One sandwich made with: toasted sprouted grain bread, avocado, lettuce, clover sprouts, diced tomatoes, diced cucumber, and cayenne powder.
　　1/2 quart (1/2 liter) of freshly made vegetable juice containing green-leafed vegetables (i.e. spinach, collards) and apples to sweeten.
　Notes:

Day 5: Friday
Morning:
>   1 whole blended papaya.

Afternoon:
>   1/2 quart (1/2 liter) of freshly made vegetable juice containing green-leafed vegetables (i.e. spinach, collards), apples, and pears.
>   10 almonds eaten with 6-8 dates (not medjool).

Snack:
>   2 tangerines.
>   1 grapefruit.
>   1 item of cooked starch (tortillas or baked, no-salt corn chips).

Evening:
>   Spinach salad using dulse as bacon bits. Add stone-crushed, cold-pressed olive oil mixed with one squeezed orange as dressing.
>   Include your favorite meal here!

Notes:

Day 6: Saturday
Morning:
>   1/2 quart (1/2 liter) of fresh-squeezed grapefruit juice.

Afternoon:
>   One shot (1 ounce) of fresh wheatgrass juice.
>   One small green vegetable salad.
>   One item of cooked starch (brown rice, wholegrain bread, etc.)
>   2 oranges.

Snack:
>   2 apples.
>   10 almonds.

Evening:
>   Large salad containing 80% green-leafed vegetables (including kale or spinach), 2 avocados, and high-quality extra virgin cold-pressed olive oil as dressing.
>   Include your favorite meal here!

Notes:

Day 7: Sunday
Morning:
> 14 ounces (1/2 liter) of herbal tea.

Afternoon:
> Seaweed salad containing: 2 cups dry dulse, 8-10 shittake mushrooms, 30 ground walnuts, 3 tablespoons of raw soy sauce (nama shoyu), 1 tablespoon of cayenne powder, and the juice of one whole lemon.
> One item of cooked starch (toasted rye or sourdough bread).

Snack:
> 2 pears.
> 1 zucchini.

Evening:
> Large salad containing 80% green-leafed vegetables, 2 avocados, and a lemon or lime squeezed as dressing.
> Include your favorite raw-food recipe meal here!

Notes:

The 80/20 Sunfood Diet

At this level, the goal is to consistently eat 80% raw plant foods containing a balance of green-leafy vegetables, sweet fruits, and raw plant fats.   Once one has stabilized at eating 80% raw-foods, major improvements will be seen at the physical, mental, emotional, and spiritual levels.

The 80/20 Sunfood Diet Weekly Menu (Spring/Summer)

Day 1: Monday
Morning:
>   3 pounds (1.4 kg) of watermelon (not seedless) eaten whole or juiced.

Afternoon:
>   1 shot (1 ounce) of wheatgrass juice.
>   One sandwich made with: toasted sprouted grain bread, avocado, clover sprouts, sliced tomato, diced zucchini, and red onion.

Snack: 3 mangos.

Evening:
>   One large spinach salad containing cucumber, tomato, and green onion salad with 2-3 avocados, and fresh-squeezed lemon.
>   Popcorn eaten with stone-crushed, cold-pressed extra-virgin olive oil.

Notes:

Day 2: Tuesday
Morning:
>   14 ounce (0.4 liters) of a blended berry smoothie containing: blueberries, blackberries, raspberries, and strawberries. Add 3 tablespoons of stone-crushed, cold-pressed extra-virgin olive oil and/or 2 tablespoons of spirulina if desired.

Afternoon:
>   One small green-leafed vegetable salad containing soaked sunflower seeds, 2 servings of dulse seaweed, fresh-squeezed lemon.
>   One item of cooked starch (baked, no-salt corn chips).
>   2 oranges.

Snack: 1 small melon.
>   Assorted greens (lettuce, endive, bok choy).

Evening:
>   Large salad containing 80% green-leafed vegetables, 2 avocados, and an orange squeezed as dressing.
>   Hummus (preferably raw) with fresh vegetables and fruits: celery, broccoli, cauliflower, cucumbers, and tomatoes.
>   1 quart (1 liter) of freshly made vegetable juice containing at least 60% green vegetables, 40% other vegetables or fruits (i.e. apple, cucumber, yam, etc.).

Notes:

Day 3: Wednesday
Morning:
> 2-3 apples.
> 10-20 pecans or macadamia nuts with lettuce.

Afternoon:
> Silicon salad (see **Appendix C: Sunfood Recipes**). Add stone-crushed, cold-pressed extra-virgin olive oil blended with orange juice as dressing.

Snack:
> 2 mangos.

Evening:
> Large salad containing 80% green-leafed vegetables including kale or spinach eaten with 1 avocado, and an orange squeezed as dressing.
> Live berry pie! (see **Appendix C: Sunfood Recipes**).

Notes:

Day 4: Thursday
Morning:
> 1/2 quart (1/2 liter) of freshly-blended peach and nectarine juice. Add 4 teaspoons of flax seed oil and/or 2 tablespoons of spirulina if desired.

Afternoon:
> 2 bowls of berries (strawberries, blueberries, etc.).
> One small lettuce salad with cucumber and tomatoes. Add a dressing containing blended avocado, lemon, and raw sunflower seeds.
> One avocado.
> One serving of cooked starch (brown rice or wholegrain bread).

Snack:
> 2 mangos.

Evening:
> Large salad containing 50% green-leafed vegetables along with tomatoes, cucumbers, parsley, cilantro, cayenne, and hemp oil as dressing. Add several servings of raw dulse seaweed to the salad.
> Dehydrated or sprouted crackers or bread eaten with one avocado.
> 1/2 quart (1/2 liter) of freshly made vegetable juice containing at least 60% green vegetables, 40% other vegetables or fruits (i.e. apple, cucumber, etc.).

Notes:

Day 5: Friday
Morning:
> 1 honeydew or sharlyn melon.

Afternoon:
> One smoothie containing: mango, orange, and peach. Add 2-3 tablespoons of olive oil if desired.
> One sandwich made with: toasted sprouted grain bread, avocado, lettuce, sunflower greens, sliced tomato, and diced cucumber.

Snack:
> 1 bowl of grapes (with seeds).

Evening:
> Large salad containing 80% green-leafed vegetables including parsley, 2 avocados, and blended mango juice as dressing.
> Include your favorite cooked meal here! (Notice how you feel in the morning!)

Notes:

Day 6: Saturday
Morning:
> 30-40 berries (strawberry, blueberry, etc.) blended with lemon. Add 1/2 avocado if desired.

Afternoon:
> 1 cantaloupe.
> 1 quart (1 liter) of freshly made vegetable juice containing apple, cucumber, and kale.

Snack:
> 2 mangos.

Evening:
> Sequoia's Calcium Soup (see **Appendix C: Sunfood Recipes**). (Make a thick, hearty raw soup, and enjoy until satiated!)

Notes:

Day 7: Sunday
Morning:
> No breakfast.

Afternoon:
> One smoothie containing: mango, orange, and peach.

Snack:
> 10-15 almonds.
> 2 apples.
> 2 ribs of celery.

Evening:
> Large salad containing 80% green-leafed vegetables, 1 avocado, dulse seaweed, and an orange squeezed as dressing.
> Include your favorite raw-food recipe meal here!

Notes:

The 80/20 Sunfood Diet Weekly Menu (Fall/Winter)

Day 1: Monday

Morning:

One blended super smoothie containing: apple, pear, berries (all types), spirulina (2-3 tablespoons), and flax oil (2-3 tablespoons).

Afternoon:

1 shot (1 ounce) of wheatgrass juice.

One sandwich made with: toasted sprouted grain bread, avocado, clover sprouts, sliced tomato, diced zucchini, and red onion.

Snack:

3 oranges.

Evening:

One large spinach salad containing cucumber, tomato, and green onion salad with 1 avocado and fresh-squeezed lemon.

Dehydrated or toasted wholegrain bread with one cup of raw unhulled tahini.

Popcorn eaten with stone-crushed, cold-pressed extra-virgin olive oil.

Notes:

Day 2: Tuesday

Morning:

One medium or large papaya eaten whole or blended with fresh orange or lime juice.

Afternoon:

1 large bowl of Sequoia's Calcium Soup (see **Appendix C: Sunfood Recipes**).

15 water-soaked almonds.

Snack:

2 cherimoyas.

Evening:

Large salad containing 80% green-leafed vegetables, 2 avocados, and an orange squeezed as dressing.

Cooked quinoa eaten with unpasteurized soy sauce (nama shoyu). Baked squash may be included with this meal.

1 quart (1 liter) of freshly made vegetable juice containing at least 60% green vegetables, 40% other vegetables or fruits (i.e. squash, peppers, okra, etc.).

Notes:

Day 3: Wednesday
Morning:
    1/2 quart (1/2 liter) of fruit juice containing: apples and pears. Mix with 3 teaspoons of flax or hemp seed oil if desired.

Afternoon:
    10 pitted dates, 1 avocado, and lettuce in a mixed salad. Squeeze an orange into the salad as dressing.
    1 bowl of hummus (preferably raw) eaten with celery, tomatoes, and cucumbers.

Snack:
    2 persimmons.
    Assorted green leaves (lettuce, spinach, endive).

Evening:
    Nori rolls! Be creative! (see **Appendix C: Sunfood Recipes**).

Notes:

Day 4: Thursday
Morning:
    Almond milk: blend 40 soaked almonds with 8 pitted dates.

Afternoon:
    Greek salad containing: lettuce, tomato, cucumber, red onion, salt-cured black olives, 1-2 ounces (30-60 ml) of olive oil.
    Blended pudding containing: dates, avocado, cinnamon powder, and distilled water.
    One serving of cooked starch (wholemeal bread, wheat tortillas).

Snack:
    2 asian pears.
    1 handful of raw pumpkin seeds.

Evening:
    Large salad containing 80% green-leafed vegetables, 30-40 almonds, and an orange squeezed as dressing. Add several servings of raw dulse seaweed to the salad.
    One sandwich made with: toasted sprouted grain bread, avocado, lettuce, clover sprouts, diced tomatoes, diced cucumber, and cayenne powder.
    1/2 quart (1/2 liter) of freshly made vegetable juice containing green-leafed vegetables (i.e. spinach, collards) and apples to sweeten.

Notes:

Day 5: Friday
Morning:
>2 young coconuts, with coconut meat and water blended together in a cream. If young coconuts cannot be found, blend 2 avocados with mature coconut water.

Afternoon:
>Cucumber, okra, zucchini, onion mixed salad. Add high-quality extra virgin cold-pressed olive oil as dressing
>>2 tangerines.
>>1 grapefruit.

Snack:
>2 cherimoyas or white sapotes.

Evening:
>Large salad containing 80% green-leafed vegetables, 2 avocados, and an orange squeezed as dressing.
>1 quart (1 liter) of freshly made vegetable juice containing at least 60% green vegetables (including 3 ribs of celery), 40% other vegetables or fruits (i.e. asparagus, apple, cucumber, etc.).
>Include your favorite cooked-food meal here. Notice how you feel in the morning!

Notes:

Day 6: Saturday
Morning:
>One fruit juice containing freshly-blended papaya and orange juice.

Afternoon:
>One small green-leafy salad containing kale or spinach. Add one squeezed orange as a dressing.
>>20-30 raw macadamia nuts.

Snack:
>1/2 quart (1/2 liter) juice containing apple and parsley.

Evening:
>Small salad containing 80% green-leafed vegetables (including kale or spinach), 2 avocados, and high-quality extra virgin cold-pressed olive oil as dressing.
>One large serving of spaghetti-sliced zucchini bathed in raw sauce (containing blended soaked nuts, basil, garlic, and lemon).

Notes:

Day 7: Sunday
Morning:
>No breakfast.

Afternoon:
>1/2 quart (1/2 liter) of freshly blended fruits containing apples, pears, and berries. If desired add one cup of raw sunflower seeds (soaked for 3 hours) with 1 tablespoon of cinnamon powder, and blend them in with the mixture.

Snack:
>Assorted greens (spinach, baby bok choy, endive).
>1 zucchini.

Evening:
>Large salad containing 80% green-leafed vegetables, 1 avocado, and one orange blended with two servings of raw, unhulled tahini as dressing.
>Include your favorite raw-food recipe meal here!

Notes:

The All-Raw Diet

The All-Raw Diet is where the real magic appears. One must take up The All-Raw Diet when ready — we want to avoid the "yo-yo" effect.

Calories

If we think of food as body fuel, then we can understand that the energy provided by food is measured in calories. According to the current standards, a male adult requires about 18 calories per day, per pound (40 calories per kg) of body weight. Women require about 16 calories per pound (35.5 calories per kg) of body weight, growing children and teenagers require about 20 calories per day, per pound (44.4 calories per kg) of body weight.. An increase in caloric needs follows from exercise. For example, a 165-pound (74.3 kg) male may need 2,970 calories for a normal day's routine. However, if the same man engages in vigorous exercise throughout the day, caloric needs may double, up to 5,940 calories.

As an example, I will analyze Day 1 of the Fall/Winter diet plan I have outlined below to demonstrate that enough calories are available on The Sunfood Diet:

Menu Item:	Calories:
2 young coconuts (spoon-meat & water)	=800
8 oranges	=1000
3 avocados	=1350
1 large bowl of spinach	=150
4 cucumbers	=100
4 tomatoes	=150
4 green onions	=25
1 lemon	=75
TOTAL	= 3,650 calories

Quantities On The All-Raw Diet

Feel free to eat large quantities of raw fruits and vegetables if you desire. Most of you will eat less than I recommend here, however, I want you to feel free to enjoy abundant natural foods. Over time you can refine your diet, increase your assimilation, and eat less and less. Follow the guidelines laid out in The Sunfood Triangle. Natural raw nutrition coupled with daily exercise is the foundation of perfect health. The All-Raw Menu is designed for an active 145-175 pound (66-80 kg) individual. Those of a lighter weight and/or who are less active can adjust the quantities down accordingly.

Women, suggested daily *maximum* intake:
6 pounds (2.7 kg) of fruit
2.5 pounds (1.1 kg) of vegetables (one-third in salad, two-thirds in juice)
0.25 pounds (0.11 kg) of nuts or seeds

Men, suggested daily *maximum* intake:
7.5 pounds (3.6 kg) of fruit
3 pounds (1.4 kg) of vegetables daily (one-third in salad, two-thirds in juice)
0.33 pounds (0.15 kg) of nuts or seeds

The All-Raw Diet Weekly Menu (Spring/Summer)

Day 1: Monday
Morning:
>   3 pounds (1.4 kg) of watermelon (not seedless).

Afternoon:
>   2 mangos.
>   1 avocado.
>   3 sticks of celery.

Snack:
>   2 mangos.

Evening:
>   One large lettuce, cucumber, tomato, and green onion salad with one handful of raw sunflower seeds, two avocados, and a fresh-squeezed lemon.

Notes:

Day 2: Tuesday

Morning:

One large honeydew melon.

The water of 2 coconuts.

Afternoon:

4 oranges.

One small green-leafed vegetable salad (containing at least 3 ribs of celery) with 10-20 walnuts and fresh-squeezed lemon.

Snack:

2 oranges.

Evening:

Large salad containing 80% green-leafed vegetables, 2 avocados, and an orange squeezed as dressing.

1 quart (1 liter) of freshly made vegetable juice containing at least 60% green vegetables, 40% other vegetables or fruits (i.e. apple, cucumber, yam, etc.).

Notes:

Day 3: Wednesday

Morning:

2-3 apples.

10-20 pecans or macadamia nuts with lettuce.

Afternoon:

Cucumber, tomato, zucchini mixed salad. Squeeze an orange into the salad as dressing.

Snack:

2 apples.

Assorted greens (green cabbage, lettuce, endive).

Evening:

Large salad containing 80% green-leafed vegetables including kale or spinach eaten with 20-30 macadamia nuts, and an orange squeezed as dressing.

Notes:

Day 4: Thursday
Morning:
> 1/2 quart (1/2 liter) of freshly-made grapefruit juice.

Afternoon:
> 2 bowls of berries (strawberries, blueberries, etc.).
> One small lettuce salad with cucumber.
> 1 avocado.

Snack:
> 2 mangos.

Evening:
> Large salad containing 80% green-leafed vegetables, 20-30 almonds, and an orange squeezed as dressing. Add several servings of raw dulse seaweed to the salad.

Notes:

Day 5: Friday
Morning:
> 3-4 oranges (eat the white pith too!).
> 10-20 macadamia nuts with lettuce.

Afternoon:
> Cucumber, tomato, okra, zucchini mixed salad. Add high-quality extra virgin cold-pressed olive oil as dressing.

Snack:
> 2 oranges.
> Assorted greens (spinach, baby bok choy, endive).

Evening:
> Large salad containing 80% green-leafed vegetables, 2 avocados, and an orange squeezed as dressing.
> 1 quart (1 liter) of freshly made vegetable juice containing at least 60% green vegetables, 40% other vegetables or fruits (i.e. pear, zucchini, asparagus, etc.).

Notes:

Day 6: Saturday
Morning:
      30-40 berries (strawberry, blueberry, etc.) mixed with lettuce or mixed with 1 avocado.

Afternoon:
      1 cantaloupe.
      1 quart (1 liter) of freshly made vegetable juice containing at least 50% green vegetables, 50% apples or pears.

Snack:
      1 handful of sunflower seeds.

Evening:
      Large salad containing 80% green-leafed vegetables including 3 ribs of celery, 2 avocados, and high-quality extra virgin cold-pressed olive oil as dressing. Add several servings of raw dulse seaweed and grated raw garlic to the salad.

Notes:

Day 7: Sunday
Morning:
      No breakfast.

Afternoon:
      The water of 2 coconuts.
      1 quart (1 liter) of freshly made vegetable juice containing at least 60% green vegetables, 40% other vegetables or fruits (i.e. asian pear, broccoli, cauliflower, etc.).

Snack:
      2 apples.
      2 ribs of celery.

Evening:
      Large salad containing 80% green-leafed vegetables, 1 avocado, dulse seaweed, and an orange blended with raw, unhulled tahini as dressing.

Notes:

The All-Raw Diet Weekly Menu (Fall/Winter)

Day 1: Monday
Morning:
> 2 young coconuts, with coconut meat and water blended together in a cream. If young coconuts cannot be found, blend 2 avocados with mature coconut water.

Afternoon:
> 5 oranges.
> 2 avocados.
> Spinach leaves.

Snack:
> 3 oranges.

Evening:
> One large spinach salad containing cucumber, tomato, and green onion salad with 1 avocado and fresh-squeezed lemon.

Notes:

Day 2: Tuesday
Morning:
> One large papaya eaten whole or blended with orange or lime juice.

Afternoon:
> 4 oranges.
> One small green-leafed vegetable salad (containing kale or spinach) with 10-20 almonds and fresh-squeezed lemon.

Snack:
> 2 oranges.

Evening:
> Large salad containing 80% green-leafed vegetables, 2 avocados, cayenne pepper, and an orange squeezed as dressing.
> 1 quart (1 liter) of freshly made vegetable juice containing at least 60% green vegetables, 40% other vegetables or fruits (i.e. squash, peppers, okra, etc.).

Notes:

Day 3: Wednesday
Morning:
>   1 quart (1 liter) of freshly-made orange juice mixed with 1/2 avocado or 3 teaspoons of flax seed oil. (Mixing a fat with a sugar for breakfast will time-release the sugar for more endurance energy).

Afternoon:
>   Cucumber, 10 pitted dates, lettuce mixed salad. Squeeze an orange into the salad as dressing.

Snack:
>   2 persimmons.
>   Assorted green leaves (lettuce, spinach, endive).

Evening:
>   Large salad containing 80% green-leafed vegetables eaten with 1/2 cup of raw nuts, and an orange squeezed as dressing. Add several servings of raw dulse seaweed to the salad. Add 30-40 Sun-ripened olives (if available).

Notes:

Day 4: Thursday
Morning:
>   2 large pomegranates and 3 oranges cut and juiced on a citrus juicer. Blend with 0.5 ounces (0.015 liters) flax oil if desired.

Afternoon:
>   8 dried prunes.
>   Silicon salad! (see **Appendix C: Sunfood Recipes**).

Snack:
>   2 asian pears.
>   Assorted greens (kale, spinach, baby bok choy).

Evening:
>   Nori rolls! Be creative! (see **Appendix C: Sunfood Recipes**).

Notes:

Day 5: Friday
Morning:
>   8 tangerines.
>   1 avocado.

Afternoon:
>   Cucumber, okra, zucchini, onion mixed salad. Add high-quality extra virgin cold-pressed olive oil as dressing.

Snack:
>   2 tangerines.
>   1 grapefruit.

Evening:
>   Large salad containing 80% green-leafed vegetables, 2 avocados, and an orange squeezed as dressing.
>   1 quart (1 liter) of freshly made vegetable juice containing at least 60% green vegetables (including 3 ribs of celery), 40% other vegetables or fruits (i.e. asparagus, apple, cucumber, etc.).

Notes:

Day 6: Saturday
Morning:
>   1 Papaya mixed with lettuce or mixed with 1 avocado.

Afternoon:
>   1 cup (0.25 liters) of wheatgrass juice blended or juiced with 3-4 apples or 1 quart (1 liter) of freshly-made vegetable juice containing at least 50% celery, 50% apples or pears.

Snack:
>   2 apples.
>   10 almonds.

Evening:
>   Large salad containing 80% green-leafed vegetables (including kale or spinach), 2 avocados, and high-quality extra virgin cold-pressed olive oil as dressing. Add 8 pitted dates to the salad for added zest.

Notes:

Day 7: Sunday
Morning:
> No breakfast.

Afternoon:
> 1 quart (1 liter) of freshly made vegetable juice containing at least 60% green vegetables (including 3 ribs of celery), 40% other vegetables or fruits (i.e. jicama, pumpkin, etc.).

Snack:
> 2 pears.
> 1 zucchini.

Evening:
> Large salad containing 80% green-leafed vegetables, 3 avocados, and a lemon or lime squeezed as dressing.

Notes:

Appendix C: Sunfood Recipes

There are so many options for designing beautiful meals with raw plant foods. Bring in two or more raw-food recipe books to enhance your kitchen. My organization Nature's First Law distributes every raw-food recipe book available in the world today. The forthcoming companion recipe book to this work is entitled: **The Sunfood Cusine** by the raw gourmet Fred Patenaude. **The Sunfood Cuisine** will contain a wide variety of recipe ideas and combinations, all of which are based on the recommendations in this book.

I do have a wonderful secret to share with all prospective live-food chefs. It would seem that the most ideal foods for human consumption would contain all three food classes simultaneously (review **Lesson 11: The Secret Revealed**). Since this does not occur, the secret to making totally satisfying live-food recipes is to combine all three categories of food: sugar, fat, and chlorophyll into one meal.

One of the most famous raw-food recipes is Doctor Ann Wigmore's "Energy Soup." Her soup contains avocado, apple, and wheatgrass juice among other items. The three main ingredients are a fat, a sugar, and a chlorophyll food. Doctor Ann would feed this balanced recipe to some of her patients as their sole nutrition for 3 months and they would be healed of disease! Doctor Ann's entire "Energy Soup" recipe may be found in her last book: **The Blending Book**.

I have developed some excellent healing combinations based on the Sunfood Triangle. Below I have included my favorite recipes, juices, and blends. All the ingredients in the following combinations should be 100% raw and organic. Many of these combinations require a juicer or blender; I highly recommend The Green Power Juicer, The Commercial Champion Juicer, The Miracle Wheatgrass Juicer, and The Vita-Mix Blender. I personally own and use them all. These are *essential* household appliances to create a healthy future for you and your family. To order any or all of these appliances, please contact Nature's First Law at 1-619-596-7979.

Recipes

Avocado Burritos
8 leaves of lettuce
2 avocados
2 jalapeno peppers
4 tomatoes
1 orange

Mix and mash the avocados, peppers, and tomatoes. Squeeze on the orange for sweetness. Place avocado mix into a lettuce leaf and roll up. Remove the jalapeno peppers if serving this dish to young children.

Ecuador
1 cherimoya
4 kale leaves
1 avocado

Pick the seeds out of the cherimoya. Dice the kale. Cut, dice, and mash avocado together with the other ingredients. The very center "stamen-like" growth in the heart of the cherimoya is excellent for replenishing male sexual fluids. This is a balanced meal.

Fats Avocado Salad
4-5 handfuls of wild greens
(dandelion, lamb's quarters, malva, mustard, etc.)
2 avocados
40 olives
4 teaspoons of high-quality extra-virgin stone-pressed olive oil

Mix in a salad. Combining olives with avocados is a powerful mixture. This is a trace mineralizer (wild greens are loaded with trace minerals) and a bone builder (as fats help with the assimilation of calcium). I feel I am on top of the world when I eat this!

Fats Guacamole
3 avocados
3 ripe jalapeno peppers
1 habanero pepper
3 tomatoes
1 bunch of cilantro
1 ripe yellow lime

Mix and mash. Squeeze lime into the mixture. The lime juice acts as an antioxidant allowing the mixture to keep longer and taste better. Keeping the avocado pits in the mix will also help the guacamole to last longer.

Live Berry Pie
Pie crust:
2 cups of soaked almonds
1 cup of shredded coconut
1/2 cup of monukka raisins
The juice of one lemon
1 teaspoon of cinnamon
1/2 teaspoon of nutmeg

Mix all crust ingredients together in a food processor and press into a pie shell.
Binder:
2 cups of berries (blueberry, blackberry, raspberry, and strawberry)
1 cup of peaches

Blend well in a food processor or blender. Stir the binder into the crust shell. Manicure the top of the pie with berries. Refrigerate for 2 hours before serving. This is a great recipe for children.

Nori Rolls
6-8 sheets of raw, sun-dried (not toasted) nori seaweed
2-3 avocados
1 bunch of clover sprouts
1 bunch of cilantro
1 cucumber

Dice all ingredients. Mix avocados, clover, cilantro, and cucumber into a flat spread on the nori sheets. Roll each sheet tightly with a sushi mat. Cut into bite size portions. Add raw soy sauce (nama shoyu) if desired. Nori is an excellent seaweed containing trace minerals.

Raw Candy
10 dates
10 almonds

Pit the dates. Insert an almond into the pit hole of each date. This can help any cooked chocolate lover to switch over to raw foods!

Raw Chocolate
8 dates
20 pitted black sun-ripened olives
1 tablespoon of raw carob powder.

Pit the dates. Blend these ingredients together. Use a little coconut water as a flowing agent. This recipe was originally created by the raw gourmet Fred Patenaude and fellow raw-foodist Andrew Durham. Experiment with the ratios of dates to olives. This is guaranteed to satisfy any chocoholic.

Sea Salad
10 strips of dulse seaweed
1 avocado
1 head of lettuce
4 tomatoes

Mix in a salad. Squeeze the lemon into the salad. Dulse is an excellent source of sodium and trace minerals and is a wild food.

Silicon Salad
1 head of romaine lettuce
4 cucumbers
4 tomatoes
6 okra
2 nopales
2 red bell peppers
3 tablespoons of horsetail herb
1 avocado or 1 ounce (30 ml) of organic
stone-pressed extra-virgin olive oil

Cut, dice, mix in a salad. Add avocado or olive oil for dressing. Excellent for silicon, which the liver can biologically transmutate into calcium. Silicon creates beautiful, elastic skin. Silicon remedies brittle fingernails and keeps the hair from turning prematurely grey. Silicon also relieves the pain of tendonitis and related tendon and ligament inflammation.

Winter Solstice
10 dates
10 dinosaur kale leaves (also known as black or lacinto kale).
1 avocado

Cut the avocado into 10 pieces. Pit the dates. Place a date with an avocado slice inside a kale leaf like a burrito. I lived on this food mixture for nearly the entire winter of 1997-1998.

Juices & Blends:

Almond Milk
40 soaked almonds
8 pitted dates
2 tablespoons of cinnamon powder
1 tablespoon of nutmeg

Mix and blend with distilled water. Almond milk is best when almonds and dates are mixed in an 8:1 ratio. An excellent warming drink for the winter. This drink replaces any egg nog!

Aloe & O.J.
2 aloe vera leaves
10 oranges

Juice the oranges on a citrus juicer. Fillet the aloe leaves until the green skin is removed. Blend aloe "gel" with orange juice. Aloe vera heals the skin and mucous membranes. Aloe vera juice is excellent for ulcers and hemorrhoids. Papaya makes a great addition to this drink.

Athlete
2 cucumbers
5 ribs of celery
10 kale leaves

Juice. I recommend this drink to all athletes. Fluid, sodium, and calcium...everything is there.

Captain's Powerhouse
Two handfuls of greens (preferably wild)
2 spoon meat coconuts with water
2 avocados

Blend. This is the raw-food bodybuilder Stephen Arlin's favorite drink which he describes in his book **Raw Power!**

Cherimoya Cream
1 avocado
2 cherimoyas

Remove pit, seeds, and skins from the avocado and the cherimoyas. Put the fruits in a blender. Blend. This is a splendid combination which one must taste to believe.

Estrogen Booster
2 yams

Juice. This drink is for young women looking for a boost, menopausal women, or anyone looking to taste something great.

Feijoa & O.J.
10 feijoas (pineapple guavas)
10 oranges

Cut all fruits in half. Juice on a citrus juicer. The smooth feijoa balances the acids in the oranges. This is my favorite winter juice.

Iron Boost
10 strawberries
10 raspberries
1 slice of watermelon
1 handful of parsley

Mix, blend, and serve! Red fruits, especially berries, contain high amounts of iron. Red watermelon has the highest iron content of any fruit. Parsley has the highest iron content of any green-leafy vegetable. This is an excellent drink for women just before and following menstruation.

Medicine
1 ripe red jalapeno or orange habanero pepper
5 ribs of bok choy
10 kale leaves

Juice. This drink helps detoxify the lymphatic system and boost the immune system. This drink relieves swollen glands in the throat. This is true medicine.

Molotov Cocktail
4 apples
1 clove of garlic
1 quarter slice of an onion root
1 red jalapeno pepper
1 slice fresh ginger root

Two cups of this drink a day: one in the morning, one in the evening. In conjunction with The Sunfood Diet plan I have outlined in this book, this drink is guaranteed to burn out all parasites in 30 days.

Performance
1 glass of coconut water
1 heaping tablespoon of spirulina

Spirulina is the highest protein food on planet Earth. Coconut water is the highest source of electrolytes found in nature. Both spirulina and coconut water are alkaline. Together, they can drive any athlete to superior performance in all areas. This is one of my secret drinks I advise to athletes.

Piece De Résistance
5 apples
1 lemon

Shave the outer skin of the lemon away, leaving the white pith. Juice. I was originally introduced to this recipe years ago by Jay Kordich's book

The Juiceman's Power Of Juicing. It is one of the all time best. I have been to Jay's beautiful home and we actually juiced this combination together — what a treat!

Potion Of Invincibility
2 heads of red-leafed lettuce
1 head green cabbage

Juice. A creamy drink. A powerful mineral boost. This is great to drink following a workout. My colleague Caleb "Kale" named this potion.

Raw Courage's Eyesight Enhancer
4 oranges
4 lemons
4 limes
2 grapefruits
2 tangerines
10 feijoas

Juice on a citrus juicer. Mix well and serve. These alkaline citrus fruits are internal cleansers and help to alleviate internal debris, even in the fine capillaries of the eye. This is an excellent drink to use on a juice fast.

Rejuvenator
1 bunch of kale
4-6 ribs of celery
1 cucumber
1 burdock root
1-2 apples (optional)

Burdock root is a blood purifier and an excellent base to help the body create hormones. Burdock contains one of the highest amounts of organic iron in any food. Kale provides a dense source of alkaline minerals. Cucumber and celery soften the taste. Apples may be added to sweeten (although better results occur without them). This is, all-around, perhaps the most effective juice combination I have found. This is a great juice to drink every day.

Remineralizer
8 ribs of celery
12 kale leaves

Juice. Loads the body with sodium and calcium. This is an important drink for those who have been taking mineral-depleting chemical medicines, antibiotics, or insulin as it restores heavy minerals to the body.

Sequoia's Calcium Soup
10 kale leaves (preferably dinosaur kale)
1 handful of parsley
2 cloves of garlic
1/3 of a red onion
2 lemons
1 avocado
1 tomato
2 yellow bell peppers
1 handful of dulse strips
1/2 teaspoon celtic sea salt
1 tablespoon of unpasteurized miso
3 tablespoons of flax oil
20 pumpkin seeds

Shave the outer skin of the lemons leaving the white pith intact. While blending all ingredients, add distilled water to reach a thick, soupy consistency. This is a great raw soup for kids! This is an excellent way to introduce important heavy minerals and calcium into a child's diet.

Super Smoothie
1 apple
1 pear
1 small bowl of blueberries, blackberries,
raspberries, and strawberries.

2 3 tablespoons spirulina
2-3 tablespoons of flax seed oil

Place all contents in a blender. Add distilled water and mix until the desire consistency is reached. This is an excellent morning drink in the winter. The pectin in the apples and pears stimulates a bowel movement. The berries are blood builders. The spirulina adds trace minerals. The flax oil allows a slower time-release of fructose into the blood.

Appendix D:
Remedies

My recommendation is to begin any disease or injury treatment program by first undergoing a series of colon irrigations. Unless the colon is clean and functioning properly, the body will not be able to heal or assimilate foods to optimal efficiency.

Burns

In my experience fresh, raw aloe vera juice heals burns faster than any other substance. Raw, fresh aloe vera juice should be topically applied 1-2 times a day (1st degree burns), 3-4 times a day (2nd degree burns), and 5-6 times a day (3rd degree burns). Accelerated healing will be noticed immediately.

stone-crushed, cold-pressed extra-virgin organic olive oil soothes the skin and may be rubbed directly onto burns *as long as* the wounds are closed, the skin is not raw, and the blisters are not oozing.

Eating plenty of avocados, olives, and olive oil with parsley will help accelerate the healing of burns.

Common Cold

Once your body is significantly detoxified by eating a balanced Sunfood Diet you will experience fewer and fewer flus and colds. An old saying goes: "You don't catch a cold; you eat a cold." Cooked foods and animal foods can depress the immune system making one susceptible to illnesses. Raw plant foods strengthen the immune system. Consider the ramifications of this startling fact in terms of saved time, energy, and expense!

Typically, cold symptoms make their appearance when the seasons change. When the seasons change, the body becomes more sensitive and detoxifies toxins more rapidly. Paul Bragg, the life-extension specialist, recommended in his books to fast four times a year (for seven days) during each change of seasons. As you purify your diet, take note of the seasonal appearance of colds, it will provide you with some interesting insights.

I know not everyone is ready right now to make a radical improvement in their diet, so I have provided my "Cantaloupe Cold Cure." I have prescribed this to many people over the years. I often hear their thanks days, weeks, even months later. If you or a loved one has a cold that just seems to hang on, try the following:

Cantaloupe Cold Cure

If sick with flu or cold symptoms, go to bed early. Upon awakening do not eat anything until 12 noon. After 12 noon eat an entire ripe cantaloupe. Do not eat anything else for the next 4 hours.

This will "break" a cold or the flu.

For the more disciplined individual, fasting (not eating) whenever sick works best. Energy is channeled away from digestion into strengthening the immune system.

Eating only juicy alkaline fruits or their juices (figs, papayas, oranges, tangerines, grapefruits, berries, etc.) while sick also accelerates the recovery. Try the "Alkaline-Fruit Blend" described in **Lesson 7: The Sunfood Diet, Recommendations For Rapid Results**.

If flu symptoms persist, daily drink 0.5 quart (0.5 liter) daily of the "Medicine" drink described in **Appendix C: Sunfood Recipes**.

Eczema

Eczema is a detoxification (often of drugs or medications) through the skin. Because it can be worsened by eating cooked eggs and cooked fat, especially pasteurized milk and cheese, these foods should be abandoned.

To heal this condition, after bathing, rub fresh aloe vera, avocado, and papaya into the eczema every other day.

If you have eczema (dry skin and eruptions) consider at least 6 colonics initially to allow the body to detoxify through the colon, rather than through the skin.

If colon hydrotherapy is not available, daily warm-water enemas while fasting on grapefruit juice will be helpful.

A raw herbal cleanse, such as the EJUVA program, can work wonders for those with eczema as I have seen first hand several times (for more on EJUVA, see **Resources** at the end of this book).

Eyesight

From years of observation and study, I am convinced that the primary cause of poor eyesight is the habit of reading in the dark or with dim lighting. To maintain excellent eyesight for a lifetime, please be sure to read under bright full-spectrum lighting whenever possible.

Eating 100% raw plant foods will definitely halt a continuous degeneration in eyesight. Eating 100% raw foods can gradually restore poor eyesight, but this can take years. My colleague Fred Patenaude gave up nearly a decade of wearing glasses after 10 months of eating 100% raw plant foods. His eyesight, though not perfect, is gradually improving.

To heal the eyes, stop eating cooked fats — especially animal fats. Large molecules of cooked fat, devoid of their lipase enzyme, can lodge in the fine capillaries of the eyes creating blockages and weakening the eye's fine-tuned motor muscles. John McCabe, in his excellent resource book **Surgery Electives**, cites a 1995 study of 2,000 people which linked the consumption of (cooked) saturated fat to blindness. He also concludes that a vegan diet can improve some vision imparities.

Also, to help improve poor vision, only drink distilled water or fresh juices for liquids. Inorganic minerals from tap and spring waters can enter the body, filter through the system, and damage the fine capillaries in the eyes.   For more information on this, read Dr. Norman Walker's book: **Water Can Undermine Your Health**.

Avoid all caffeine (coffee, tea, soft drinks) as it damages the fine nerve tissues in the eyes.

Table salt should be avoided as it tends to raise the blood pressure. This puts excessive pressure on the tiny capillaries in the eyes.

Several books describe specific programs including eye exercises you can do to restore eye strength and vision. **Relearning To See** by Thomas R. Quackenbush may be beneficial for you to study.

Hair Loss

Hair loss is a progressive decrease in hair growth typically resulting in baldness in men. It usually occurs due to poor oxygenation, acidification of the body due to a poor diet, and a lack of Sunlight. Genetic predispositions also play a factor.

Rubbing the oil of a slice of mashed up hot pepper directly into the hair loss area with your fingers will help dissolve waxy deposits which may have sealed off hair follicles. This oil will also cause blood flow to that area of the scalp oxygenating and enlivening the dormant follicles. Be cautious, pepper oil is very strong and can burn the skin — only 1/4 of a small pepper is required. Apply stone-crushed, cold-pressed extra virgin olive oil 2-5 minutes after the pepper oil as this will tone down the pepper heat and soothe the skin. Follow this procedure every day in the morning or evening for 3 weeks.

Dietary choices to restore hair loss should include significantly more organic alkaline fruits (papayas, figs, oranges), a wide variety of organic green-leafed vegetables to reverse any acid-condition in the body, and occasional dulse or nori seaweed for trace minerals.

For excellent scalp care, use only minimal amounts of organic, plant-based shampoos on the hair. Sometimes I simply use a dilute solution of lemon or orange juice as shampoo; I also occasionally use olive oil to maintain scalp and hair moisture and to avoid hair knots. Commercial shampoos and conditioners contain highly toxic chemicals and damage the scalp over time.

Mucous Congestion

Mucous congestion is a detoxification of the lungs and sinuses associated with sinusitis, discharges, headaches, earaches, eye pain, and fatigue. Mucus acts to both protect the system by acting as a buffer for the sensitive internal organs and it acts to transport toxins out of the body, typically through the lungs, mouth, and sinuses.

Anyone with a mucous problem should avoid raw or cooked dairy products of all types. Dairy products are notorious mucus-formers. Simply avoiding all dairy products is often found to eliminate sinusitis.

Direct Sunlight on the chest and face will accelerate healing this condition. Sunlight helps dry out mucus and recharge the sinus chambers.

Eating plenty of hot peppers (cayenne, jalapeno, habanero) will thin and flush sinus mucus.

Mucus and wax may have combined to form a hard ball in the inner ear. If you suffer persistent earaches, consider having your physician or naturopathic doctor flush your ears with warm water.

Muscle Soreness

Sore muscles are the result of too much lactic acid and uric acid having accumulated in the muscle tissue.

To counteract acids in the muscle tissue, drink at least 0.5 quart (0.5 liter) of green-vegetable juice. The "Potion Of Invincibility" described in **Appendix C: Sunfood Recipes** works extremely well. The alkaline minerals in green juices neutralize acids.

Long, hot epsom-salt baths may also help relieve muscle soreness.

Nail Biting

Nail biting is caused by an alkaline mineral deficiency and/or a parasitic infection. People typically bite their nails when nervous or stressed. This is an instinctive action to recycle the alkaline minerals (calcium) found in the nails into the body to neutralize the acids formed by stress.

Daily eating plenty of calcium-rich green-leafed vegetables, such as parsley or kale along with plenty of other alkaline plant foods, will help restore a mineral balance in the body. Plenty of garlic in the diet tends to flush parasites out.

Raw-foodist and health author R.C. Dini, a life-time chronic nail biter, completely reversed this condition by eating raw plant foods. He noticed a major shift after drinking a glass of parsley juice each day for two weeks. Results were also excellent after eating a bulb of elephant garlic every day with his salads for more than two months.

PMS (Pre-Menstrual Syndrome)

The body can use menstruation as a channel for detoxification. As toxicity is channeled out of the lymph for elimination during the monthly cycle, old substances will enter the blood. Because we crave what is in our bloodstream, cravings for toxic foods may surface during the cycle. These cravings appear just before or following a menstrual period — be aware and prepared for this. To get past cravings eat avocados. Avocados are excellent foods to help regulate the female cycle.

PMS is essentially a detoxification episode which always has physical, mental, and emotional components. PMS is the result of a toxic, cooked, animal-food diet (especially now with all the hormones fed to farm animals). The cleaner your body is by eating raw plant foods, the less PMS you will experience. After several months to a year of eating raw plant foods, PMS symptoms will disappear.

If candy, chocolates, or cooked carbohydrates are eaten this can lead to an overproduction of insulin and exacerbate PMS symptoms. Eat fruit to keep the blood sugar regulated throughout a PMS episode. On the day before and on the day after your menstrual cycle, drink at least 1 quart (1 liter) of the "Iron Boost" drink described in **Appendix C: Sunfood Recipes**.

When the body is totally purified, menstrual flow will be minimal. This is not a cause for alarm as it is the natural way of all mammals. When eating a diet of raw foods, avoiding nuts and seeds will greatly diminish menstrual losses.

Psoriasis

The quality of the skin (its glow, shine, radiance) reflects the state of the internal organs. The skin is specifically representative of the condition of the liver. Acne, rashes, spots, etc. are all indicative of challenges in the liver. The skin disease psoriasis is connected with liver dysfunction and enzyme deficiencies — especially a lipase deficiency.

To heal psoriasis, one needs to daily select an appropriate type of fat (one which digests well). Fats that are easier on digestion include: fresh young coconuts, coconut oil, and flax seed oil. One must ease into heavier dosages of fat in the diet as a weak liver (typical in those who have psoriasis) can be challenged by an excessive fat intake — even if raw.

To overcome psoriasis, all cooked fats, especially egg and milk products (cheese, milk) should be avoided.

For those with psoriasis, 6-10 colon irrigations should be undertaken. After two months of this treatment, one should fast on water for 3 days, then conduct a gall bladder flush (drink 8 ounces of stone-crushed, cold-pressed extra virgin olive oil followed by 8 ounces of freshly-squeezed lemon juice) (see **Lesson 10: Detoxification**). This will help flush the liver and gall bladder.

Rub avocado, extra-virgin cold-pressed olive oil, almond oil, or fresh aloe vera directly into the affected skin. Get the Sun shining directly on to the affected area. Sunlight will accelerate the healing process.

Regularly ingesting probiotic/soil-organism whole-food "supplements", such as **Nature's First Food** will be greatly beneficial to psoriasis sufferers. To find out more about probiotic/soil-organism products, please contact Nature's First Law at 888-RAW-FOOD.

Skin

For beautiful, healthy, glowing skin, eat plenty of foods rich in silicon (cucumbers, horsetail herb, lettuce, nopales, okra, radishes, etc.). Regu-

larly eat the Silicon Salad described in **Appendix C: Sunfood Recipes**.
Silicon-residue foods help to restore the elastic skin of youth.

For vibrant skin, sulfur-residue foods should also be eaten. Sulfur, "the
beauty mineral," provides smoothness and shine to the skin. Sulfur is
found in cruciferous vegetables (broccoli, cauliflower), ripe bell peppers,
ripe hot peppers, onions, and garlic.

For an excellent skin complexion, rub one or more of the following
items against the skin 2-4 times a week: papaya pulp, avocado, cucumber, and/or aloe vera.

For dry skin, rub stone-crushed, cold-pressed extra-virgin organic olive
oil directly into the skin as lotion. This will alleviate dryness immediately. Or use avocado on the skin directly. Avocado oil is almost identical to
our skin's oil.

To help dissipate scars, try applying the following formula directly to
the skin every other day for several weeks: 2 tablespoons raw aloe vera
juice, 2 tablespoons of parsley juice, 1 tablespoon of olive oil.

Thyroid Imbalance

The thyroid is a large endocrine gland situated at the base of the neck.
The thyroid controls the basal metabolic rate. An underactive thyroid
slows the metabolic rate and increases the possibility of obesity. An overactive thyroid speeds up the metabolism often leaving one excessively
thin.

For any type of thyroid imbalance I recommend removing all types of
inorganic salt (table salt) or sea salt from the diet and adding significantly more green-leafed vegetables (and green herbs) to the diet. Excess
inorganic sodium is positively charged and is attracted to the negatively-
charged thyroid gland and leads to dysfunctions. The calming effect of
the alkaline minerals, raw enzymes, and the restoring effect of the B-vit-
amins found in green-leafed vegetables (and green herbs) act to balance
the thyroid and other endocrine glands.

I have counseled people with hypothyroidism (a low functioning thyroid). Small amounts of iodine from dulse seaweed often corrects this situation (2 teaspoons of raw dulse seaweed flakes taken daily). Additionally, adding raw coconut butter as the major fat source in the diet will increase thyroid function. Also, Sunlight on the skin has been shown to stimulate the thyroid to increase hormone production.

Hyperthyroidism (overactivity of the thyroid) is a more difficult situation and has many causes which are all related to internal toxicity and an excessive amount of acid-forming minerals in the body. An individual with this condition should have their iodine levels checked by a naturopathic doctor or physician. If iodine is absent, 2 teaspoons of raw dulse seaweed should be daily added to the diet). If levels are excessive, no sea vegetables or iodized salt of any kind should be included in the diet. Additionally, adding raw polyunsaturated seed oils (flax, hemp, etc.) as the major fat source in the diet can slow thyroid function. Also, one with this condition should take 30 deep breaths daily in the ratio of 1:4:2 as described in **Lesson 22: Breathing (Pranayama)**, **Action Steps**. This will calm an overactive system.

Appendix E: Testimonials

Over the years, my partners in health and I at Nature's First Law headquarters in San Diego have received thousands of incredible phone calls, letters, and e-mails from inspired, rejuvenated raw-food eaters all over the world. Many have regained their youth by eating raw plant foods and/or attending our Eden retreats, others have found a new deep spiritual connection with their creator, still others have found a kinship with all life.

One day we received a telephone message from a gentleman exclaiming: "Your book is 20 to 50 times better than the Bible!" We laughed for days over that one. Another time we received a postcard with the words "Thank You" written 36 times on it, but with no other message.

We have encountered callers on radio and television shows who are delighted to discover others promoting the healing and rejuvenating powers of raw plant foods. I remember a woman who called into a show I appeared on to describe how her liver spots had disappeared within six weeks of eating raw foods.

I have included below clippings from some of the more interesting and inspiring letter testimonials we have retained in our files. Enjoy!

About The Sunfood Diet Success System:

Scott Brodie of San Diego, California writes:
"David, supreme job on the book. Thank you.
Somewhere around page 75-80 I really got inspired. Liked the beginning and also the format, action steps, quotes, poems, and references to people and their books. My favorite parts were: when you talked about Sergie's experience and the Russian family, your experience in the wild food chapter about the kids and the coyote, excellent chapter about hybrid food and the Sun. Lessons 27-29 are really, really good. Lesson 24 on the power of association is very important. Yes indeed olives!
Great statistics. I had no idea they were that good. The lesson on fasting very necessary. Perfect. The lesson on doing what you love to do was fantastic, especially the action steps. The Heightened Prosperity poem was great to see in writing. The paragraph on Buster Douglas in the lesson on persistence was very touching. Good stuff. The poem "Some Do, Some Don't" is absolutely amazing.
Over 500 pages in 10 days of fluid simple magic cover to cover. Now I am study-

ing, taking action, and gracefully healing. This book is the most complete work I have ever read. I never sailed through a book so easily. It is nice to know and respect the author. Thanks for everything."

Anita O'Neill of Corona del Mar, California writes:
"I must write you and tell you how much I love your new book, The Sunfood Diet Success System. It is truly the book I've always been looking for. After reading hundreds of books in my never-ending quest for truth, other than the Bible, yours is the most valuable book I've ever read. It just puts it all together.

You will certainly rank among the most important writers in the health and success fields. I put you write up there with Arnold Ehret."

Cheryl Stoycoff of Stockton, California, author of Raw Kids and Soul Speak, writes:
"I recently read The Sunfood Diet Success System and I must say it is the best book I've read on the subject of the living-foods lifestyle. You have encompassed the practical, physical, and spiritual and have related it in a way the "mainstream" can understand. It is obvious you have tapped into the infinite source that connects us all. What a wonderful thing, to have found your "calling" as such a young age and had the maturity to follow your inner intuition toward higher consciousness."

Shakti Maya of Lutz, Florida writes:
"David, Just a word of blessings. I want to honor you. Your book is wonderful, resourceful, well written, and beautiful. I have feelings of being proud of a divine brother. I am giving thanks for your time here on Mother Gaia. Shine on, grow bright, share and be fulfilled in all realms of life. May the Divine Light grace your walk. May the breath of life swirl a wind of Golden Love sweetly around you embracing the Beauty that your soul emanates. In Love and Light."

About David Wolfe's Inspiring Lectures:

Christina from New York State writes:
"Dear David, Thank you. I am sending you a profound, heart-felt thanks. You are a genuine leader. Authentic. The Real Deal. I sense this. I know this. A true inspiration and a pleasure to behold. You have a Great Mind and you are pure and generous with your message. Thank you."

Radha Williams of London, England writes:
"Dear David, enclosed is a picture of where my cooker used to be. It hadn't been used for a year, and it finally left my kitchen on the morning of June 15th, the day I said hello to you before your first lecture at Regents College, London. Very auspicious!

Sprouted seeds, nuts, and green leaves are in the fridge now, a second fridge has replaced the cooker. Now the room is transformed and it feels so good, being very light and clear, and uncluttered (by toaster, jug kettle, etc.) Just a Vita-mix, spiral slicer, and an abundance of fruit! Thanks again for inspiring me.

Gail Jackson of Encinitas, California writes:
"On February 12, 1997 I went to a local health food store to see a lecture on raw foods. I had known a little bit about this subject since I had read about it seven years prior. When I first learned about raw food, it was suggested to try to do it 75 or 80%. So I tried. Three quarters of each meal raw. Or two meals and a snack raw and one meal cooked per day. Or four or five days raw per week. Well, it was very difficult, so I gave it up. (I never thought of trying raw 100% because I thought it was too far out there, not a very sociable thing to do, and would be much too difficult to achieve given that I couldn't even accomplish 75-80%!

So, seven years later, here I was sitting at the health food store listening to a lecture about raw foods. The lecturer was David Wolfe, one of the authors of Nature's First Law: The Raw-Food Diet. He talked about raw food, of course, and suggested doing 100%. "Why wait until you're sick?" he asked everyone. And I thought: "that's what I am waiting for!" All I had previously read convinced me that 100% raw eating could reverse and prevent illnesses! But I was waiting for something serious! (At that point I didn't consider a major food addiction, memory loss, diabetes, and arthritis serious!)

So I'll give it a try, I thought. No! "Try" isn't going to make it happen. I will do it for a certain period of time (I hadn't yet decided how long). I will do this for my health. I absolutely will not let anything outside myself interfere with my 100% raw-food diet! No people, no food, no anything. I will go forward like an army tank!

That night I began. (I was actually eating raw sunflower seeds during the lecture!) That was February 12, 1997. Two days later — Valentine's Day — my daughter brought my two grandsons to my workplace and brought me my absolute favorite treat — dark chocolate covered almonds! (Uh! Oh! — Now what?) I decided to not eat them at that moment and to put them in my freezer. Today, fifteen months later, they are still in my freezer, along with other "irresistible" treats that came my way. But I guess they were not "irresistible" because I resisted them!

Even though David Wolfe had suggested keeping a list of what happened after beginning, I did not expect it to manifest itself in any way. So I don't have specific dates when these happened because I absolutely did not expect anything to happen — except I knew I would be healthier. But here's what did happen after I began:

1. Within two and one-half days I lost such a considerable amount of weight that it showed up in the mirror — I wasn't even looking for that — but it was so obvious! (I ended up losing four dress sizes in approximately four to five months!)

2. After several weeks my food addiction was gone! I used to work for a company that taught people how to stop addictions. I learned and I taught that an addiction never goes away. You can learn to control your addiction for the rest of your life, but it'll never be gone. Well, it definitely was gone! I had taught about two thousand people how to control their addiction — it cost $400.00 and it took 10 hours plus mental and emotional work after the class was over. I wish I could tell every one of

those people, "Save your $400, save 10 hours, save all the mental and emotional calisthenics, just eat 100% raw foods!"

3. I needed and was satisfied with far less raw food than prior. I have NO cravings. (At that point I didn't know why. Later, when I read Nature's First Law: The Raw-Food Diet I learned why it was so much easier to do it 100% than to try to do less — it has to do with addictions to cooked foods! Had I read the book before I actually experienced it, I never would've believed it!)

4. My memory returned to normal. (I was especially worried about that because my mother was in the advanced stages of Alzheimer's and she was in her mid-eighties! Here I was — only 57!

5. My physical energy zoomed! I was used to being tired all day, even falling asleep at my desk! I couldn't believe how much energy I had. I felt ALIVE physically!

6. My brain came alive as well! It seems at this point that I had been in a fog prior to changing my eating. My work showed such an improvement — I was now faster, more efficient, many, many less errors, and getting ahead of my work instead of being behind!

7. My attitude towards other people (strangers) changed. I feel a strong sense of goodwill toward all people.

8. A vein in my leg that had stuck out considerably all my adult life became flat!

9. My nose cleared up. I never realized it was stuffy every morning until it stopped!

10. Decisions are much easier. I used to go over and over and over things and still couldn't make a decision. Now it's easy!

11. My eyes no longer feel dry and sandy like they used to every night. Sometimes they were so dry I'd have to close them just to stop the irritation.

12. My vision changed. I now have a much deeper range of vision that is clear without my glasses.

13. My blood sugar went from 280 to 80!

14. I have zero big or little aches and pains.

15. I like the color yellow now — I never used to!?! (I don't know what that means, it's just another change that happened).

16. The skin on my heels is now smooth. It used to be dry and cracked.

17. The nutritionist I was seeing told me, "What you're doing is working for you. Everything is in order. Don't come back!"

18. That which took the longest was the arthritis. But after five and a half months it was all but gone. Now I can barely tell it's there. My left knee was so bad that I had a moderate limp. I couldn't bend my leg all the way back or straighten it out. All my fingers were the same. I also had arthritis in my right neck and jaw. I know I still have it very, very slightly, but it does not hamper any movements at all!

19. One more thing — I used to get leg and foot and toe cramps all the time as well as finger spasms. They did also go away, but sometimes they come back. But now I know exactly what they're from. Pesticides in food! I can always tell when I get an overload of pesticides because the cramps and spasms will come back. It does not happen when I eat organic food!

I didn't buy the book that David Wolfe was selling at the lecture. I thought I knew "enough" about the subject. But after five and a half months of eating raw foods, I decided that maybe I was going to stick with this for a while! So, I bought Nature's First Law: The Raw-Food Diet by Arlin, Dini, and Wolfe. Well! As much as I was affected by my own experiences doing raw food — I was even more affected by the information in the book! This is not just about reversal and prevention of disease for me! This is about how raw eating can affect the world in many, many different aspects. I now fully promote the idea of 100% raw eating.

What to eat? Wonderful raw fruits, vegetables, nuts, and seeds! The variety is endless! When to eat? Whenever you want! How much to eat? As much as you want!

My wisest suggestion to you is to try it! Give yourself 4 or 6 or 8 weeks of pleasure eating only raw food and then see how you are affected! You will be amazed!

With heartfelt thanks for letting me share..."

About David Wolfe's Eden Retreats:

Elaine Nigro, a raw-living-foods chef from Los Gatos, California, writes:
"Thank you for the Best Weekend Ever! I had a lot of fun and was really inspired. David and Sequoia, you two make a great team, and presented a wonderful workshop...I really look forward to seeing you again and being around your awesome energy!"

Richard Chisholm, an investor from San Diego, California, writes:
"Eden Hot Springs is incredible. What an incredible secret! An all-raw retreat center with so many pools — the place is breathtaking. The hiking, the yoga in the 100-year old hotel, the mud baths! Sheer joy!

David Wolfe has truly synthesized an incredible diet and brought it here to this retreat center. I very highly recommend your retreats to everyone."

Sandra of Mountain View, California writes:
"David, I think of the retreat weekend often. I am thinking about also attending your next retreat, because your weekend retreat earlier this month was just so cleansing and purifying. Your presence in this world makes a huge difference. Thank you again for touching my life in such a powerful and positive way."

About Nature's First Law: The Raw-Food Diet:

Doug Swenson of South Lake Tahoe, California (an author of 3 yoga books) writes:
"I have very much enjoyed your book Nature's First Law: The Raw-Food Diet. At this time I am also on a 100% raw-food diet, for many years I was a strict vegetarian and about 70% raw. Last year I did 100% raw for 6 months and really got superior results, then, not because I needed to, I started eating cooked food again. As of 2 months ago, I am once again on all raw food. This time I have not been eating any sprouted or dehydrated grain and feel much more clear. I know that Dr. Walker, who ate mostly raw his whole life, did not eat grain at all and recently died at age 117. At this time I eat about 50% fruit and 50% vegetables, sprouts, greens, soaked and

sprouted nuts and seeds. In the summer the nuts and seeds are less appealing. The Raw-Food Diet is not hard for me, I just sometimes get sidetracked by social outings then slowly slip back to bad habits. There is no question in my mind as to this being the best diet for all of us and the whole human race would benefit by this practice. Perhaps I can find the willpower to stick to my diet this time around, thanks to people like you guys, who write books."

John Asadourian of Tenafly, New Jersey writes:

"I very much liked the conclusions drawn in your book describing the existence of the true body and the false body. It was a very important lesson for me and I thank you for it. In my own theories I never was able to bring together the knowledge that exists which governs our universe: it seems that there is a spirit of death and one of life. When this knowledge is portrayed on the physical level, much light is shed on the truth of our existence. As the opener for the Essene Gospel Of Peace, Book 1 states, "The spirits of truth and falsehood struggle within the heart of man; Truth born out of the spring of light, Falsehood from the well of darkness. And according as man inherits the truth, so will he avoid darkness."

I believe there is enough evidence available through the study of Orgone energy to state the results in scientific terms: the ingestion of living plant cells enhances the energy fields of our cells, while the ingestion of devitalized (cooked) plant tissues, not to mention cooked animal tissue, detracts from the energy fields of our cells...

I am happy to know that your organization came into existence for I feel you represent the great libraries belonging to the Citadels of Truth."

C.R. of Sanford, Maine writes:

"Thank you for Nature's First Law: The Raw-Food Diet. Less than two months ago I was very ill and dying. I became a raw-foodist by the third chapter of your book. I am busy here in Maine trying to share the message with the many sick folks I am in contact with. No easy task. I am 38 years old and have never felt so well or joyful. My doctors are amazed. I am passing your book around although I don't like to part with it. Thank you again.

G.A. of Slovenia (Europe) writes:

"...I was attacked by rheumatoid arthritis after a case of pneumonia in 95/96. I couldn't walk or use my hands. I was in this state all thru 96 and it was accompanied by an inflammation of all the internal organs, eyes included...I escaped from the hospital. I left with the words — 'In 3 months your kidneys will fail!' — thrown in my back! This was a year and a half ago. I now run for 10 kilometers without even getting tired. I even gained my body weight, only this time my muscles grew up on raw food. Your book is a very brave work. I thank you for it from all my heart."

Raw-Food Restaurants

Arnold's Way
4438 Main St.
Philadelphia, PA 19127
215-483-2266
Arnold's Way offers raw-food meals and juices. A quaint, wonderful place located in the heart of Philadelphia.

Caravan Of Dreams
405 East 6th Street
New York, NY 10009
212-254-1613
Contact: Angel Moreno
Caravan offers organic vegan cuisine and raw-food dishes. Caravan hosts seminars and lectures.

Delights Of The Garden
2616 Georgia Ave. NW
Washington D.C. 20001
202-319-8747
Delights Of The Garden is a raw-food restaurant located in the heart of the nation's capital.

Enzyme Express
1330 East Huffman Road
Anchorage, Alaska 99515
907-345-1330
Even in Alaska you can be served raw vegetarian foods! Enzyme Express offers raw-food dishes and juices.

Garden Taste Restaurant
1237 Camino Del Mar
Del Mar, CA 92014
619-793-1500
Contact: Sheila or Nava Gabayson
Nestled in the author's hometown of Del Mar, Garden Taste provides organic vegan food along with raw-food dishes, juices and smoothies.

The Hygeia Center
18 East 23rd Street
New York, New York
212-353-5000
A part-time raw-food restaurant!

Karyn's Fresh Corner
3351 North Lincoln Ave.
Chicago, IL 60657
773-296-6990
Fax: 773-296-0583
Karyn's Fresh Corner is a raw-food restaurant
in Chicago, Illinois. Raw-food potlucks are held
on the 3rd Saturday of each month at 5 pm.

Living Community Center
330 East Seventh Street
Tucson, Arizona
520-623-0913
Contacts: Alan, Jason, Janice, & Wes
E-mail: alan@livingcommunitycenter.com, wes@livingcommunitycenter.com
Web-site: www.livingcommunitycenter.com
A raw-food restaurant is scheduled to open at the center in Spring 2001.

Organic Garden Restaurant & Juice Bar
294 Cabot St.
(near the Cabot Cinema — Rte. 62 off Rte. 128)
Beverly, Massachusetts 01915
978-922-0004
Contact: Robert Reid
The ultimate raw experience for everyone in the Boston area and the northeast United States. This restaurant was founded by two totally dedicated raw-foodists.

Quintessence
263 East 10th Street
New York City, NY 10009
(located between 1st Ave. and Avenue A)
646-654-1823
Fax: 646-654-1804
Contact: Tolentin
Quintessence is a 100% raw-organic restaurant servicing the needs of New York
City's exploding organic raw-food movement.

Raw

1849 West 1st Avenue
Vancouver, British Columbia
Canada V6J 5B8
www.rawhealthcafe.com
604-737-0420, Fax: 604-737-0430
Contact: Maureen Powers

A progressive health cafe in Vancouver, committed to supplying you with the freshest certified raw organic ingredients available.

Raw Energy: Organic Juice Cafe

2050 Addison (between Shattuck/Milvia)
Berkeley, CA
510-665-9464
Contact: Vicky Lee

The owner of this raw-food bar has been a long-time supporter of Nature's First Law. Her bar is a great place to eat for all those in the San Francisco Bay Area.

The Raw Truth Cafe, Healing Center, And Eco-Shop

3620 East Flamingo Road
Las Vegas, NV 89121
702-450-9007
Contacts: Bob Saladino

This is the prototype for the raw-food restaurant of the future!

Source Of Life Juice Bar

@Everlasting Life Health Food Supermarket
2928 Georgia Avenue, NW
Washington D.C. 20001
www.everlastinglife.net
202-232-1700
Contact: Ahuvyah

This is a vegan juice bar located within a vegan health food supermarket which strongly favors living foods. This health food complex provides educational seminars on living foods at their lecture hall next door to the juice bar.

Super Sprouts

205 Spadina Ave.
Toronto, Ontario
M5T 2C8
Canada
416-977-7796
Contact: Marie

Not truly a raw-food restaurant yet, Super Sprouts is a raw-food resource center located near the exotic fruit shops in Chinatown Toronto. Super Sprouts is becoming a raw-food lifestyle clearinghouse for all of Canada.

Tree Of Life
771 Harshaw Road
Patagonia, AZ 85624
520-394-2589

The Tree Of Life Rejuvenation Center has a raw-food restaurant open to the public. Fresh foods directly from the garden are served in a delightful outdoor setting connected with nature. Patagonia is approximately 1 hour south of Tucson.
Please call for more information and/or directions.

Well Springs Garden Cafe
2253 Highway 99
@Jackson Hot Springs
Ashland, OR 97520
541-488-6486
Contact: John Larsen

This is a small cafe servicing the nutritional needs of Jackson Hot Springs with raw-vegetarian food!

Organizations

Nature's First Law Inc.
P.O. Box 900202
San Diego, CA 92190
619-596-7979
888-729-3663 - orders
www.rawfood.com
E-mail: nature@rawfood.com
Contacts: David Wolfe & Stephen Arlin
Nature's First Law is The World's Premier Source of
Raw-Food Diet Books, Juicers, Bulk Organic Foods,
Raw Lifestyle Videos & Audio Tapes.
Nature's First Law conducts raw-food seminars and retreats worldwide.

Brian Tracy International
462 Stevens Avenue, Suite 202
Solana Beach, CA 92075
619-481-2977
Fax 619-481-2445
www.briantracy.com
E-mail: dfrench@briantracy.com
Brian Tracy is one of America's leading authorities on the
development of human potential and personal effectiveness.
He is the author/narrator of the book, **Maximum Achievement**,
and more than 200 hours of audio and video learning programs
covering the entire spectrum of personal development technology.

Civis
Via Leonardo da Vinci 26
I-20060 Vignate (Milan) - Italy
Tel/Fax: (0039) 02 95 36 06 28
E-mail: civitas@info-tel.com
This organization is dedicated to the complete abolition of vivisection (animal
experimentation). The founder, Hans Ruesch, author of **Naked Empress**, is absolutely
unwaivering in his inspiring commitment towards freeing all animals. **Civis** publishes
a highly recommended eye-opening newsletter.

Essene Church Of Christ
P.O. Box 1113
Creswell, OR 97426
541-895-2190
E-mail: esseneinfo@aol.com
www.essene.org
Contact: Abba Nazariah

One of the most ancient and yet progressive churches on the planet. The Essenes advocate a raw-food vegetarian diet and lifestyle. Each summer they hold a nationwide celebration/conference in Oregon. The church is currently headed by Abba Nazariah who has been a raw-foodist for 23+ years. Please write or call for more details.

European Vegetarian Union
Bluetschwitzerweg 5
CH-9443
Widnau, Switzerland
Tel/Fax +41 71 7226 445
E-mail: sdeleo@rheintal.ch or evu@openoffice.ch
Contact: Sigrid De Leo

EVU is a pan-European organization dedicated to promoting vegetarian, vegan, and raw-food lifestyles. Each year EVU hosts an international vegetarian congress. EVU also releases an excellent publication 4 times a year entitled: **EVU - News** which is distributed all over the world. Please contact Sigrid for subscription information

Excellence, Inc.
514 East 5th Street #10
New York, NY 10009
212-420-8270
Contacts: Annie & Dr. David Jubb

Excellence, Inc. has their emphasis on LifeFood Nutrition, languaging, and Whole Brain Functioning. Excellence, Inc. conducts events throughout the United States. Please write or call for information pertaining to retreats, trainings, and seminars.

Farm Sanctuary
PO Box 1065
Orland, CA 95963
530-865-4617, Fax: 530-865-4622
www.farmsanctuary.org

Farm Sanctuary is a national, nonprofit organization dedicated to rescuing and protecting farm animals. Farm Sanctuary helps prosecute farm animal abusers, helps pass landmark laws to outlaw animal cruelty, exposes the animal food industries, and operates coast-to-coast animal shelters.

The FRESH Network
P.O Box 71
Ely CB7 4GU
ENGLAND
Director: Karen Knowler
Tel + 44 (0) 870 800 7070
E-mail: karenk@easynet.co.uk
FRESH is a Fruitarian & Raw-Food Diet support organization
and network throughout the United Kingdom and Europe. FRESH works closely
with Nature's First Law. FRESH is directed by Karen Knowler, a truly amazing and
dedicated spirit. This organization receives the author's highest recommendation.

The Fruitarian Raw-Food Centre Of London
37 Grasvenor Avenue
Barnet, London
EN5 2BY
United Kingdom
+44 (0) 181 446 2960
+44 (0) 181 441 6252
Contact: Karen Noble
This organization offers weekend workshops and consultations on the raw energy
lifestyle, juicing, fasting, detoxification, wild foods (food for free), and preparation of
raw recipes. Guidance is offered for safe, reliable weight control, body-building,
strengthening the immune system, increasing longevity, and conscious breathing. This
group has made a study of the philosophy, antecedents, and ethics of raw veganism
with references in religion and ecology.

Gentle World
Two locations:
P.O. Box 44397
Kamuela, HI 96743
808-889-1133
Victoria Valley, RD 1
Kaitaia, New Zealand (09) 408-2188
E-mail: gentle@aloha.net
Contacts: Golden
Gentle World is a vegan community of mostly sunfoodists.
They publish books and host seminars on the vegan diet and lifestyle.

The Hygeia Center
18 East 23rd Street
New York, NY 10010
212-353-5000
Contact: Narda
This is a health-empowerment educational community center offering classes on
raw-foods and environmentally safe lifestyles.
A raw-food restaurant is scheduled to open upstairs.

The Institute For Vibrant Living
www.vibrantliving.org
E-mail: DanL@vibrantliving.org
650-961-9541
Contact: Larry Levine, Dan Ladermann

Every fall the Institute hosts the annual Raw-Living Foods Health Expo. The Institute is dedicated to developing raw-food support communities throughout the world. The Institute also plans to bring into being a string of raw-food juice bars and restaurants throughout North America.

Last Chance For Animals
8033 Sunset Blvd., suite 35
Los Angeles, CA 90046
Tel: 888-882-6462, Fax: 310-271-1890
E-mail: office@LCAnimal.org
Web-site: www.LCAnimal.org
Contact: Chris DeRose

This is a no-nonsense animal rights organization founded by former Hollywood star Chris DeRose.

Living Community Center
330 East Seventh Street
Tucson, Arizona
520-623-0913
E-mail: alan@livingcommunitycenter.com, wes@livingcommunitycenter.com
Web-site: www.livingcommunitycenter.com
Contacts: Alan, Jason, Janice, & Wes

The Living Community Center currently offers 2 incredible studios with sprung-wood floors, and an enclosed garden patio for communing while enjoying the Arizona sun. On any given day there may be a raw foods potluck, yoga, martial arts, international folk dance, or intensive weekend workshops and seminars given by internationally recognized speakers, artists, and spiritual teachers. On Friday and Saturday evenings, the Center opens the main studio for a smoke and alcohol free environment in which musicians and other artists have the opportunity of performing in a clean setting to be enjoyed by people of all ages. This group is highly recommended.

Living Light Culinary Arts Institute
800-484-6933, ext. 6256
Web-site: www.rawfoodchef.com
Contact: Cherie Soria

This institute offers certification courses in raw-live food cuisine. Instruction is hands-on for individuals, chefs, and teachers.

Living Light House
1457 12th Street
Santa Monica, CA 90401
310-395-6337
Fax 310-394-2858
Contacts: Landon, Don Kidson
The Living Light House hosts Tuesday and Thursday night gourmet raw-food
meals. Landon and Don invite ecological lecturers and
activists to present at the house. Owner, Don Kidson,
produces a long-running cable television program entitled:
The Hardware Humanitarian Show that focuses on
alternative healing and ecology issues.

Naturaliche Gesundheit
Muhlenberg 15
D-25782 Tellingstedt
GERMANY
Contact: Helmut Wandmaker
Helmut is one of the foremost promoters of The Raw-Food Diet
in Germany. He is the author of many wonderful German
books on raw foods. Helmut's books are carried as specialty
items by Nature's First Law. Contact Nature's First Law (800-205-2350)
if you would like to purchase one or more of Helmut's books.

Nature of Wellness
PO Box 10400
Glendale, CA 91209-3400
Contact: Javier Bourgos
High-integrity, no-compromise anti-vivisection (animal
experimentation) activism and information. Write or call
for free information. They produced the **Lethal Medicine** video.

People For The Ethical Treatment Of Animals (PETA)
501 Front St.
Norfolk, VA 23510
757-622-7382
Contact: Bruce Friedrich
With over 600,000 members worldwide, PETA is the
world's largest animal rights group. Write or call for free information.

Planet Health
319 East 9th Street
New York, NY 10003
800-398-6237
E-mail: helthbound@aol.com
Contacts: Ed Lieb
Planet Health promotes The Raw-Food Diet and Natural

Hygiene in New York City. Planet Health distributes books, informational products, and rebounders. Ed Lieb produces a television program entitled: **Accent On Wellness** which is aired on Manhattan Cable (Channel 16) on Saturdays at 7:30 am and on Brooklyn Cable (Channel 56) on Saturdays at 9:30 pm.

RAW
Ground Floor
33 Wilbury Avenue
Hove, East Sussex
BN3 6HS
ENGLAND
www.goraw.com
Telephone: 00 44 (0)1273 734454
Contact: Jonathon Cole

RAW offers support and information for people transitioning to the raw-food diet on whatever level is appropriate for them.

Raw Babe Inc.
16113 East Calder Drive
Loxahatchee, Florida 33470-4139
561-333-4013, Fax: 561-333-4014
Web-site: www.rawbabe.com
Contact: Brooke Peterson

Raw foods is a catalyst to consciousness. Brooke's vision is to see people being catalyzed into their highest potential through a T.E.A.M. approach (Transformational Evolutionary Alignment Members). Brooke's services include seminars, special events, and personal trainings in: Whole Life Coaching, Manifestation Magic, and Living Foods (which includes a culinary adventures academy). She encourages everyone to "Join the Raw Revolution."

Raw-Foods Foundation
HC 77, Box 41
Annapolis, MO 63620
E-mail: rawfoods@earthlink.net
314-725-6085
Contacts: Chris & Steve

This foundation is a raw-food educational organization providing services for the Midwest United States. The directors, Chris and Steve, provide potlucks, uncooking classes, retreats, and other fun adventures for raw-food enthusiasts.

Robbins Research International, Inc.
9191 Towne Centre Dr., suite 600
San Diego, CA 92122
800-445-8183
Web-site: www.tonyrobbins.com

Anthony Robbins is the most dynamic success speaker on

the planet Words alone would be inadequate to describe
the contributions this man has made towards a better planet
for all of us. Please contact his office and schedule you
and your family to attend an Anthony Robbins' seminar.

San Diego County Living Foods:
A Vegetarian Raw Foods Support Group
P.O. Box 3397
Vista, CA 92085-3397
619-360-6968
E-mail: troi2000@hotmail.com
Contacs: Safari Cass, Helene Idels
This support group meets at least once monthly for a
raw-food potluck. Each month the group participates and
hosts numerous ecological and self-empowering events. The
group's founder, Helene Idels, is extremely well-connected
in the raw-food, vegan, and vegetarian movements.

Self Empowerment Academy
P.O. Box 737
Kenmore
4069 Queensland
AUSTRALIA
www.selfempowermentacademy.com.au
Tel +61 7 3878 2446
Fax +61 7 3878 2564
E-mail: jasmuheen@selfempowermentacademy.com.au
Self Empowerment Academy represents the cutting edge
of the human potential movement. The Academy provides
resource tools and literature on the subjects of mind-mastery,
meditation, and living on light. The Academy is directed by
breatharian Jasmuheen and gets the author's highest recommendation.

The Temple of Health and Beauty
1530 Dekalb Ave., NE, Suite E
Atlanta, GA 30307
404-524-4488
Contact: Richard Byrd
The Temple is a living-foods center that offers a wide range of services to visitors.
The Temple is a first-class operation.

Vitalities Incorporated
Kauai, Hawaii
csilla@vitalities.org
www.vitalities.org
Contact: Csilla Jacobson
This company offers culinary showcases, a yearly calendar, a twice a year glossy magazine, and other services.

Wild Food Adventures
5036 SE Mitchell St.
Portland, OR 97206-4814
503-775-3828
Contact: John Kallas
This organization educates, informs, and serves as a forum for wild-food enthusiasts. Plants and events of interest are covered from anywhere in North America.

Healing Retreats

Eden Retreats
Nature's First Law
PO Box 900202
San Diego, CA 92190 USA
888-729-3663
E-mail: nature@rawfood.com
Web-site: www.rawfood.com

Nature's First Law conducts several raw-food retreats each year. At the moment, David Wolfe and Nature's First Law operate a raw-food rejuvenation retreat center in Eden, Arizona. Plans are currently underway to establish a full-time retreat center in San Diego. Please contact Nature's First Law to sign up for a retreat vacation.

The Annapurna Inn
538 Adams St.
Port Townsend, WA 98368
800-868-2662
annapurna@olympus.net
www.annapurnaretreat-spa.com
Contact: Robin

A raw-food bed and breakfast nestled in the Pacific Northwest.

Ann Wigmore Foundation
P.O. Box 399
San Sidel, NM 87049
505-552-0595

The Ann Wigmore Foundation is a retreat and healing center
that advocates enzyme-rich plant-foods to heal the body.
Educational classes are offered. Call or write for more information.

Ann Wigmore Institute
P.O. Box 429
Rincon, Puerto Rico 00677 USA
Tel: 787-868-6307, Fax: 787-868-2430
Web-site: www.annwigmore.org
E-mail: wigmorc@coqui.net
Contacts: Leola, Lalita

The Ann Wigmore Institute is a retreat and healing center. The Institute offers detoxification and healing programs using wheatgrass and enzyme-rich plant-foods to heal the body. Educational classes are also offered. The Institute is highly recommended by the author. Call or write for more information.

Creative Health Institute (CHI)
112 West Union City Rd.
Union City, MI 49094
Tel: 517-278-6260, Fax: 517-278-5837
E-mail: creative@coldwater.net
Web-site: www.creativealternatives.org
Contacts: Hiawatha Cromer, Don Haughey

CHI is a healing center offering an incredible 2-week cleansing and detoxification program as specified and fine-tuned by Dr. Ann Wigmore. This program uses wheatgrass to improve blood quality and raw plant foods to maintain a healthy diet. CHI is accessible from all areas of the northern midwest and is only a 3-hour drive from Chicago. CHI operates under a progressive philosophy and is highly recommended by the author.

East County Holistic Care
7303 Broadway
Lemon Grove, CA 91945
619-589-7546
Contact: Jenny

One of the best colon hydrotherapy, lymphatic drain, and massage offices in the nation! East County Holistic Care is nestled just two blocks from The Optimum Health Institute in San Diego County. The owner of East County Holistic Care, Jenny, can host up to six guests. She recognizes the relationship between the lymphatic system and vibrant health. Her therapy involves opening up the lymph ducts through massage and the use of The Lustre PC — a hand-held electrical device. The application of The Lustre PC to the body soothes and relaxes in the way that Sunshine stimulates the opening of a blossom. The Lustre PC gently brings electrical energy into the dark, contracted parts of the body encouraging those areas to let go of scar tissue, chronic tension, and backed-up lymph fluid. This device is *highly* recommended for anyone who works in the field of colon hydrotherapy, massage, and/or lymphatic drainage. (Compatible international Lustre PCI 120/240 V models are available).
Jenny and The Lustre PC receive the author's highest recommendation.
Please contact Jenny and let her know where you
discovered her and The Lustre PC!

Esser's Hygienic Rest Ranch
P.O. Box 161
Lake Worth, FL 33460
Tel. 561-965-4360
Contact: William Esser, Dr. Carlos Arguello, M.D.

Serving primarily as a raw-vegetarian, fasting, and sunshine healing center, this operation is supervised by long-term natural hygienist William Esser and Carlos Arguello, M.D. This ranch is located in the heart of sub-tropical Palm Beach county in Florida. The retreat is conveniently situated on 10 acres on Route 802 at 4005 Lake Worth Road. Spacious private rooms are available. If advised in advance, the ranch will send someone out to meet and pick up guests at the Palm Beach International Airport, or the major bus and railroad depots nearby.

Hippocrates Health Institute
1443 Palmdale Court
West Palm Beach, FL 33411
800-842-2125
Fax 561-471-9464

Hippocrates is a healing retreat run by Brian Clement emphasizing the use of raw plant foods. For more information write or call.

L.O.V.E.-I.N.G.
(Longevity from Organic Vegetarian Enzymatic Indigenous / Indoor Nutriceutical Garden)
P.O. Box 2853
Hot Springs, AR 71913
1-800-WHEAT-GRASS
www.naturalusa.com/viktor/sanctuary.html
Contacts: Viktoras Kulvinskas & Youkta

This resort/school is situated on 90 acres within Ouchita National Forest. Each year in the spring, LOVING hosts an "International Women Festival Of The Healing Arts." LOVING promotes the following themes:

1. Micro-agriculture and live-food preparation
2. Divine Life-Style Consultant & Self-Healing Training
3. Spiritualized Guidance Applied to the 21st Century (How to know, before the Earth changes visit your area, what to do, how to enjoy the now, and grow spiritually under all conditions)

Write for a detailed brochure.

Optimum Health Institute (OHI)
6970 Central Ave.
Lemon Grove, CA 91945
619-464-3346
Fax 619-589-4098

OHI is one of the best detoxification institutes in the United States. They have 1, 2, 3, and 4 week programs. 100% raw plant-foods are served on the premises. OHI offers very affordable rates. Write or call for a free brochure.

Optimum Health Institute (OHI)
Rural Route 1
Box 339-J
Cedar Creek, TX 98612
512-303-4817
Fax 512-303-1239

The new OHI in Texas operates a similar program to that found at OHI in San Diego. Write or call for a free brochure.

Rest Or Your Life Health Retreat
P.O. Box 102
Barksdale, TX 78828
830-234-3488
E-mail: vvvhaag@swtexas.net

Nestled on a crystal clear river in the Texas Hill Country away from the noise, smog, and maddening crowds, this Natural Hygiene center provides a peaceful, restful, and relaxing environment. This retreat is run by two medical doctors: Gregory and Tosca Haag. Tosca is Dr. Vivian Vetrano's daughter; Dr. Vetrano is Dr. Herbert Shelton's greatest student.

Tree Of Life Rejuvenation Center
P.O. Box 778
Patagonia, AZ 85624
520-394-2520

Tree Of Life was founded by raw-foodist, Dr. Gabriel Cousens. This center now features residential rooms for guests, a raw-food restaurant open to the public, beautiful gardens, trainings, and meditations. Tree Of Life is one of the best healing retreats in the world and receives a high recommendation.
Write or call for more information.

Resources

Bulk Organic Food
Nature's First Law
PO Box 900202
San Diego, CA 92190 USA
Toll-Free: 888-729-3663, International: +001-619-596-7979
E-mail: nature@rawfood.com
Web-site: www.rawfood.com
Nature's First Law now delivers bulk nuts (in the shell), raw-organic nut butters, dried fruit, cassia (a pod-fruit laxative), stone-crushed olive oil, olives by the jar or by the case, coconut oil from Fiji, and other foods. The world's best type of nutcracker is also available (no mess, no spray, cracks all nuts cleanly, easy to use). Order by e-mail, by standard mail, or by telephone.

Coconut Oil
Nature's First Law
PO Box 900202
San Diego, CA 92190 USA
Toll-Free: 888-729-3663, International: +001-619-596-7979
E-mail: nature@rawfood.com
Web-site: www.rawfood.com
In February of 2000, David Wolfe had the good fortune of visiting the Fijian islands where he met with a fourth-generation coconut grower who produces the finest cold-pressed coconut oil in the world. We have arranged to have barrels of this oil shipped to the United States. The oil is packaged at the Nature's First Law offices for world-wide distribution. This oil is 100% raw and sourced from wild coconuts on Fiji.

The Date People
P.O. Box 808
Niland, CA 92257
760-359-3211
Contact: Jamie & Angela Jones
Jamie & Angela grow and distribute the world's best
organic dates. Exotic varieties are available.

Eco-Organics
www.eco-organics.com
E-mail: Eco-organics@aol.com
201-333-8840
888-Eco-Organics
Contact: Nanda or Nick
Eco-Organics distributes organic fruits, vegetables, and
organic cotton and hemp accessories throughout North America. Anyone with a
mailbox can gain access to organic foods!

EJUVA
237 Miramar Dr.
Santa Cruz, CA 95060
831-457-1323
Contact: Steven Hurwitz
EJUVA offers herbal cleansing and rejuvenation products
designed to clear the intestines and restore balance to the
body. EJUVA's herbs are 100% raw, organic,
and of the highest quality available. EJUVA products are distributed by Nature's
First Law, call toll free 888-RAW-FOOD.

Exotica: Rare Fruit Nursery
Nursery location: 2508-B East Vista Way, Vista, CA 92084
Mailing address: PO Box 160, Vista, CA 92085
760-724-9093
Contacts: Chris Carter, Steve Spangler
Exotica is located in the San Diego/Southern California area. This nursery offers the
best exotic fruit trees and unique edible plants in North America.
Plants are available by mail order.

The Fire Within, Inc.
510-653-5050
Contact: Jon Cotton
E-mail: jon@thefirewithin.com
www.thefirewithin.com
The Fire Within specializes in: cleansing & detoxification
products, firewalks, workshops, educational vacations, and
counseling. Jon Cotton is a distributor for Arise & Shine Herbal Products —
an intestinal and full-body cleansing program. Call for a free newsletter.

First Choice Nutritionals
P.O. Box 2823
Sequim, WA 98382
www.1stchoicenutritionals.com
E-mail: 1stchoice@prodigy.net

Tel. 360-452-9523

Fax. 360-452-9292

Order line: 888-357-3456

This company distributes 100% enzymatic products, whole-food supplements, natural shampoos, and lotions. Also, this company is opening, in Spring 2001, Quiet Waters Retreat, located in Sunny Sequim on the Washington Peninsula. Quiet Waters is a holistic retreat providing nutritional fasting, internal cleansing, therapeutic body work, herbal wraps, stretching classes, meditation.

HealthForce Nutritionals

PMB 299

2240-D Encinitas Blvd.

Encinitas, CA 92024

1-800-357-2717

www.healthforce.net

Contacts: Jamey Dina, N.D., Kim Sproul N.D.

HealthForce researches and offers nutritional superfoods based on a unique understanding of raw foods, enzymes, lifeforce, Mother Nature and true science. A great company for the raw fooder (cleansing products, enzymes, superfoods, herbs, etc.). Jamey & Kim are the authors of **Uncooking With Jamie & Kim**!

High Vibe Health & Healing

85 East 3rd Street

New York, NY 10003

212-777-6645

www.lifefood9.com

Contact: Peter, Dagger

High Vibe Health & Healing supplies an incredible array of products to support your transition to a raw plant-food-based lifestyle including parasite flushes, herbs, specialized supplements, and much more. Call for info or a catalog.

The Living Temple

15123 Brookhurst St., #306

Westminster, CA 92683

714-531-8295

800-640-2670

Fax 714-531-8573

www.thelivingtemple.com

E-mail: rjonestlt@earthlink.net

Contact: Robin Jones

The Living Temple specializes in organic cotton clothing, hemp clothing, shower filters, and other vegan products and literature. The author gives The Living Temple his highest recommendation.

Loving Foods

P.O. Box 576

Paia, HI 96779

808-573-4207
E-mail: allraw@lovingfoods.com
Contact: Jeremy Safron
Loving Foods offers select raw-food products and conducts raw-food retreats. Jeremy is the co-author of **The Raw Truth: The Art Of Loving Foods**!

Dr. Robert Morse
God's Herbs
2404-A Tamiami Trail
Port Charlotte, FL 33952
888-863-4317 (toll free)
941-766-8068 (herb shop)
941-255-1979 (office)
Contacts: Dr. Morse or Theresa Bellmore
Dr. Morse specializes in healing cancer and in assisting with tissue/nerve regeneration, especially spinal injuries. His approach involves a total raw-plant-food diet and herbs. He believes strongly in empowering the individual spiritually, emotionally, mentally, and physically. Dr. Morse has been a raw-foodist for 30 years.

Native Seeds / SEARCH
526 North 4th Avenue
Tucson, AZ 85705
520-622-5561
Fax 520-622-5591
SEARCH (Southwestern Endangered Aridlands Resource
Clearing House) is a regional seed bank designed to preserve
ancient desert plants and heirloom farming practices. They
offer heirloom (non-hybridized) seeds and wild seeds.

Nature's First Food
Nature's First Law
PO Box 900202
San Diego, CA 92190 USA
Toll-Free: 888-729-3663, International: +001-619-596-7979
E-mail: nature@rawfood.com
Web-site: www.rawfood.com
Nature's First Food is the most nutrient dense superfood product ever created. It was designed to David Wolfe's specifications by Jamey Dina, N.D. Dr. Dina is the world's leading superfood authority and researcher. He has formulated Nature's First Food with a unique understanding of lifeforce energy, enyzmes, raw foods, Mother Nature, and true science. Designed to to be taken on a daily basis and especially during cleansing. Contains 100% raw, organic or wildcrafted superfoods, the best probiotic formulation ever put together (designed to implant good bacteria in the intestines), soil organisms, and a full digestive enzyme complex. Neutral tasting, easily dissolvable powder. Can be added to smoothies and juices. Contains no fillers. Currently available in a 10 ounce amber glass bottle with metal lid and oxygen absorber for optimum nutrient preservation.

Olives & Stone-Pressed Olive Oil
Nature's First Law
PO Box 900202
San Diego, CA 92190 USA
888-729-3663
E-mail: nature@rawfood.com
www.rawfood.com
Nature's First Law now has the best Olives and Stone-Pressed
Extra-Virgin Olive Oil available. Order by e-mail,
by standard mail, or by telephone.

Raw Health
2909 SE 77th Ave.
Portland, OR 97206
503-771-7096
kris@rawhealth.net
http://www.rawhealth.net
Contact: Kris Pletschke
Raw Health conducts raw-food events in the Portland area and offers an array of
excellent internal cleansing and anti-parasite products.

Rhio's Raw Energy Hotline
212-343-1152
Call Rhio's Hotline for the latest information on raw-food
events in the New York City area.

Seeds Of Change
P.O. Box 15700
Santa Fe, NM 87506-5700
505-438-8080
Fax: 505-438-7052
Contact Seeds Of Change to order heirloom
(non-hybridized) seeds for your garden!

Barbara Simonsohn
Holbeinstr. 26
27607 Hamburg
Germany
Tel. + 49 (0) 40 895 338
Fax. + 49 (0) 40 893 497
Barbara is the author of four German books on fruits and vegetables. She is one of
foremost proponents of raw-food and fruit-based diets in Germany. Barbara is cur-
rently assisting in the translation of this book into German. She is David Wolfe's pri-
mary liason in Germany. Barbara is fluent in English.

Soil Remineralization & Rock Dust
Earth Health Regeneration
P.O. Box 620478
Woodside, CA 94062-0478
Contact: Don Weaver

Don Weaver has been eating 100% raw plant foods for over 22 years. He is the world's foremost authority on soil remineralization and rock-dust gardening. For information on how to include powdered rocks in your garden, write to him at the address above.

Super Sprouts
205 Spadina Ave.
Toronto, Ontario
M5T 2C8
Canada
416-977-7796
Contact: Marie

Super Sprouts is the raw-food lifestyle clearinghouse for all of Canada. Nature's First Law and Super Sprouts work together to distribute books and food into Canada. Highly recommended.

Lenny Watson
P.O. Box 356, Suite 169
Maui, HI 96779
808-573-3590

Lenny Watson has been a raw-foodist since 1976. In the field of deep tissue massage and bodywork, Lenny Watson is at the top. His holistic practice on the island of Maui includes: massage therapy, nutritional counseling, fasting, cleansing, colon therapy, and astanga yoga.

Publications

Just Eat An Apple Magazine
(6 issues/year)
From the Nature's First Law head office: This is the world's
premier magazine on The Raw-Food Diet. An uncompromising approach to the
RAW lifestyle. Editor: Frederic Patenaude.
Regular Features: Interviews * Incredible Recipes * Fascinating Raw Philosophy *
What's Raw, What's Cooked * What's Happening In
The Raw-Food World * Networking Contacts * Personal Singles
Ads * Book Reviews * Letters Corner * Food & Sex
And much more! Excellent format, high quality, 28+ pages/issue.
$30/1-year subscription (US$40 Canada, US$45 foreign)
$50/2-year subscription (US$65 Canada, US$70 foreign)
To subscribe, write, call, or e-mail:
Nature's First Law, PO Box 900202, San Diego, CA 92190 USA
888-729-3663
E-mail: nature@rawfood.com

FRESH Network News
(5 issues/year)
FRESH is dedicated to promoting and supporting the raw food diet in the UK and
abroad. Catering for everyone, whatever their current lifestyle, in every issue you will
find: Readers' letters * personal stories * shopping reports * raw food
recipes * thought-provoking articles * raw-food parenting * permaculture *
raw communities * raw issues * lonely hearts * national/international contacts
and practitioners * coordinator's news * raw news from around the world * and
much more. Dedicated to personal and planetary health, FRESH assists and
supports you through these changes and beyond. FRESH is caring, fun,
friendly, informative, honest, comprehensive and packed full of information
every 40-page issue. $45.00/year (includes shipping charges from England)
To subscribe, write, call, or e-mail:
Nature's First Law, PO Box 900202, San Diego, CA 92190 USA
888-729-3663
E-mail: nature@rawfood.com

Fruitarian Network News
(4 issues/year)
Support for fruitarians world-wide.
Director: Rene Beresford
Regular Features: International Contacts * Fruit Poetry * Self-Help Information *
Interviews * Fruit Facts.

$41/year (worldwide).
To subscribe write, call, or e-mail:
Nature's First Law, P.O. Box 900202, San Diego, CA 92190 USA
888-729-3663
E-mail: nature@rawfood.com

Boletin Crudivegano
(4 issues/year)
Boletin Crudivegano is a Spanish magazine covering topics such as: vegetarianism, veganism, Natural Hygiene, fruitarianism, animal liberation, organic food, and agriculture. The magazinecontains excellent world-wide networking contacts are listed. 48+ pages. To subscribe, write or call:
Boletin Crudivegano, Apartado 29, 29100 Coin
Malaga, Spain
Tel: 95236 0930
Contact: Balta
The editor of this magazine, Balta, is founding a raw-food community called Eco-Aldea in Malaga, Spain. Please write him for more information.

Naturlich Leben
(6 issues/year)
A German magazine (written in the german language) dedicated to promoting vegetarianism, veganism, and the raw-food vegetarian lifestyle. Regular contributors: Franz Konz, Dr. K.J. Probst, Nicole Maurer, and others. **Naturlich Leben** is truly on the cutting edge of natural health, raw-food nutrition, and progressive thought. Very high-quality, large format, color cover, 50+ pages. To subscribe, write, call, or e-mail:
Bund Fur Gesundheit
Talstr. 36, D-52525 Heinsberg, Germany
Tel 02452-22678
Fax 02452-101078
E-mail: BFGeV@t-online.de

Wandmaker Aktuell
(6 issues/year)
A German magazine (written in the german language) dedicated to promoting fruitarianism, fasting, and the raw-food vegan lifestyle. Regular contributors: Helmut Wandmaker, Barbara Simonsohn
Very high-quality, large format, color cover, 36+ pages. To subscribe, write, call, or e-mail:
Helmut-Wandmaker-Stiftung
Hauptstrasse 4, D-25782 Tellingstedt, Germany
Tel: 04838-78047
Fax: 04838-7435
E-mail: Helmut.Wandmaker@t-online.de
Web-site: www.Helmut-Wandmaker.de

Permissions

The author and publisher wish to express thanks and appreciation to those listed below who granted permission to use the following material:

Avery Publishing Group for permission to quote from **Enzyme Nutrition** by Edward Howell, (c) 1985; published by Avery Publishing Group, Inc., Garden City Park, New York, (800) 548-5757.

Campbell Thomson & McLaughlin Ltd. for permission outside of the United States and Canada to quote from **Shattering The Myths Of Darwinism** by Richard Milton.

Chelsea Green Publishing Company for permission to quote from **Whole Foods Companion** by Diane Onstad.

Dell Books for permission to quote from **Illusions** by Richard Bach.

Essence Of Health for permission to quote from **Fruit The Food And Medicine For Man** and **Diet, Health, And Living On Air**.

Health Research for permission to quote from **Man's Higher Consciousness** by Professor Hilton Hotema.

Inner Traditions International for permission in the United States and Canada to quote from **Shattering The Myths Of Darwinism** by Richard Milton.

The University Of Chicago Press for permission in the United States and Canada to quote from **Year Of The Gorilla** by Dr. George Schaller.

Art Today: http://www.arttoday.com for their use of copyrighted images throughout the text. Maul Brothers Publishing contracted with Ken Seaney (Ground Zero Graphic Design) who helped design the text layout. Ken Seaney (Ground Zero Graphic Design) is a member of Art Today.

Sapoty Brook for permission to reprint and discuss his CaPNaK mineral balancing chart which may be found in his book **Eco Eating**.

The author and publisher made all reasonable efforts to contact all other literature sources quoted in the text.

Recommended Reading

The Raw-Food Diet

*Blatant Raw-Foodist Propaganda** by Joe Alexander

*Conscious Eating** by Dr. Gabriel Cousens

*Eating For Beauty** by David Wolfe

*Eco-Eating** by Sapoty Brook

L'Homme, Le Singe, Et Le Paradis** (French) by Albert Mosseri

*Nature's First Law: The Raw-Food Diet** by Arlin, Dini, and Wolfe

*Raw Power!** by Stephen Arlin

*Rohkost Statt Feuerkost** (German) by Helmut Wandmaker

*Spiritual Nutrition And The Rainbow Diet** by Dr. Gabriel Cousens

*Survival Into The 21st Century** by Viktoras Kulvinskas

*The Essene Gospel Of Peace, Book I** translated by Edmond Bordeaux Szekely

*Think Before You Eat** by Diane Olive

Ur-Medizin** (German) by Franz Konz

*Willst Du Gesund Sein? Vergiss Den Kochtopf!** (German) by Helmut Wandmaker

Raw-Food Recipe Books

*Garden Of Eden Raw Fruit And Vegetable Recipes** by Phyllis Avery

*The High Energy Diet Recipe Guide** by Dr. Douglas Graham

*Living In The Raw** by Rose Lee Calabro

*The Raw Gourmet** by Nomi Shannon

*The Raw Truth: The Art Of Loving Foods** by Renee Underkoffler and Jeremy Safron

*RAW: The Uncook Book**

*Sunfood Cuisine** by Fred Patenaude

*Uncooking With Jamie & Kim** by Jamie Dina & Kim Sproul

Natural Hygiene
*Awakening Our Self-Healing Body** by Art Baker
Choose To Live Peacefully by Susan Smith Jones
*Superior Nutrition** by Herbert Shelton

Fruitarianism
*Biotrophic Protocol** by Joshua Rainbow
*Fruit: Best Of All Foods** by Klaus Wolfram
*Fruit The Food And Medicine For Man** by Morris Krok
*Fruitarian Diet And Physical Rejuvenation** by Dr. Abramowski
*Perfect Body** by Roe Gallo
*Physical Fitness** by Professor Arnold Ehret
*Raw Courage World** by R.C. Dini
*Spiritualizing Dietetics: Vitarianism** by Dr. Johnny Lovewisdom

Vegetarianism
*Beyond Beef** by Jeremy Rifkin
*Conscious Eating** by Dr. Gabriel Cousens
*Diet For A New America** by John Robbins
*Diet For All Reasons** (video) by Dr. Michael Klaper
*Mad Cowboy** by Howard Lyman
*The Sunfood Way To Health** by Dugald Semple

Food Combining
*Fit For Life** by Marilyn & Harvey Diamond
*Food Combining Made Easy** by Dr. Herbert Shelton

Juicing
*Fresh Vegetable & Fruit Juices** by Dr. Norman Walker
*The Wheatgrass Book** by Ann Wigmore
*The Juiceman's Power Of Juicing** by Jay Kordich

Cleansing And Healing
*Cleanse & Purify Thyself, Book 1.5** by Dr. Richard Anderson

***Colon Health** by Dr. Norman Walker
 Fats That Heal, Fats That Kill by Udo Erasmus
***Golden Path To Rejuvenation** by Morris Krok
***Juice Fasting & Detoxification** by Steve Meyerowitz
***Mucusless Diet Healing System** by Professor Arnold Ehret
***Sunlight** by Dr. Zane Kime
***Surgery Electives** by John McCabe
***The Golden Seven Plus One** by Dr. C. Samuel West
***The Great AIDS Hoax** by T.C. Fry
***Thus Speaketh The Stomach: The Tragedy Of Nutrition** by Professor Arnold Ehret

Fasting
***Fasting Can Save Your Life** by Dr. Herbert Shelton
***Rational Fasting** by Professor Arnold Ehret
***The Miracle Of Fasting** by Paul Bragg

Breatharianism
***Diet, Health, And Living On Air** by Morris Krok
***Living On Light** by Jasmuhcen
***Man's Higher Consciousness** by Professor Hilton Hotema

Natural Mothering
***The Continuum Concept** by Jean Liedloff
***Primal Mothering In A Modern World** by Hygeia Halfmoon

Gardening
***Gardening Without Digging** by A. Guest

Nature
***Edible Wild Plants: North American Field Guide** by Elias and Dykeman
 The Secret Life Of Plants by Peter Tompkins and Christopher Bird
 Year Of The Gorilla by Dr. George Schaller

Science

Biological Transmutations by Louis Kervran

Chaos by James Gleik

Cracking The Bible Code by Dr. Jeffrey Satinover

Darwin On Trial by Phillip Johnson

*****Jubb's Colloidal Biology & Secrets Of An Alkaline Body** by Annie & Dr. David Jubb

The Learning Revolution by Gordon Dryden and Jeannette Vos

*****On Form And Actuality: A Refutation Of The Theory Of Evolution And Adaptation** by David Wolfe

Shattering The Myths Of Darwinism by Richard Milton

*****The Survival Of Civilization** by John Hamaker and Don Weaver

Anti-Vivisection

*****Lethal Medicine** (video)

*****Naked Empress** by Hans Ruesch

Inspirational

The Aladdin Factor by Mark Victor Hansen and Jack Canfield

*****As You Think** by James Allen

*****Children Of The Sun** by Gordon Kennedy

*****The Healing Power Within** by Ann Wigmore

The Master Key To Riches by Napoleon Hill

Maximum Achievement by Brian Tracy

Peace Pilgrim compiled by Friends Of The Peace Pilgrim

Spirit Of Shaolin by David Carradine

Success Through A Positive Mental Attitude by Napoleon Hill and W. Clement Stone

The Treasury Of Quotes by Jim Rohn

Think And Grow Rich by Napoleon Hill

*****Unlimited Power** by Anthony Robbins

Ye Are Gods by Annalee Skarin

Philosophy

IS Philosophy by Stephen Arlin
Joyful Wisdom by Friedrich Nietzsche
*****Life In The 21st Century** by Viktoras Kulvinskas
*****Major Achievements Of The Cooked-Food Eater** by Stephen Arlin
Thus Spoke Zarathustra by Friedrich Nietzsche

Classics

*****Autobiography Of A Yogi** by Parmahansa Yogananda
Desert Solitaire by Edward Abbey
Journey To Ixtlan by Carlos Castaneda
Illusions by Richard Bach
Ramayana retold by William Buck
The Odyssey of Homer
Walden by Henry David Thoreau
*****Yoga Gave Me Superior Health** by Theos Bernard

*****Books now available from: Nature's First Law 1-800-205-2350**

Index

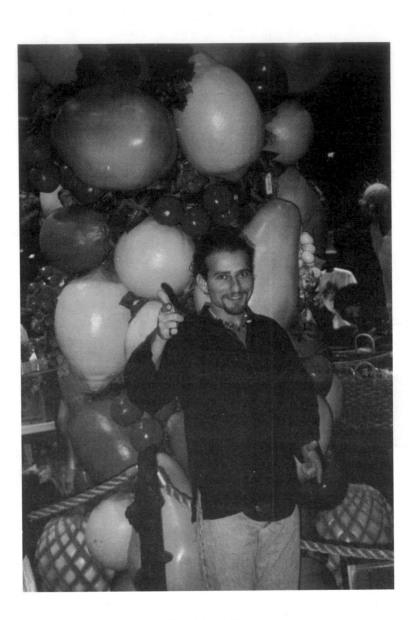

David Wolfe
"Radical Health Transformation"

About The Author

David Wolfe (b. August 6, 1970): David Wolfe is the middle son of two medical doctors. His father is an osteopath with over 35 years experience. His mother is an anesthesiologist.

David Wolfe has degrees in Mechanical and Environmental Engineering and Political Science. He has studied at many institutions including Oxford University. He concluded his formal education with a law degree from the University of San Diego.

In 1995, along with Stephen Arlin and R.C. Dini, David Wolfe founded Nature's First Law, the world's largest distributor of books, booklets, juicers, audiotapes, and videotapes to assist people in adopting, maintaining, and enjoying raw plant-food-based lifestyles. Along with his partners in health, Mr. Wolfe co-authored the book: **Nature's First Law: The Raw-Food Diet** in 1996 which has attracted world-wide notoriety.

At age 14, David Wolfe began reading and studying success and health books. At age 18, he read the book **Fit For Life** and adopted the diet lifestyle and food combining principles outlined there. Eventually he let go of all animal foods. In 1995, he adopted a 100% raw-food vegetarian diet. Through years of personal experimentation, research, nutritional counseling and problem solving, seminar speaking, and communications with thousands of individuals experimenting with raw-food vegetarian lifestyles, he eventually developed **The Sunfood Diet Success System** and his new book **Eating For Beauty**.

David Wolfe travels the world lecturing and speaking on raw-food nutrition, beauty, and success.

For the latest updates on David Wolfe, including current seminar tours and vacation retreat information, please visit:

www.davidwolfe.com

or

www.rawfood.com/events.html

Additional Copies Of
The Sunfood Diet Success System

Additional copies of **The Sunfood Diet Success System** may be ordered directly from Nature's First Law. One book is $24.95 plus $5.00 shipping and handling ($10.00 s&h if outside the United States or Canada). For each additional book please add $1.50 shipping and handling ($6.00 s&h if outside the United States or Canada). California residents add 7.75% sales tax. **Bulk discounts are available**.

If you have any questions or comments about any of the material contained in this book, feel free to write, call, or e-mail Nature's First Law. We seek correspondence with all like-minded individuals seeking to reach their maximum potential.

Also, check out the **Nature's First Law Catalog**. Each Catalog contains a listing of the highest-quality books, booklets, juicers, audiotapes, and videotapes to help assist, maintain, and enjoy a raw plant-food-based lifestyle. To receive a free copy of the **Nature's First Law Catalog** please write, call, or e-mail Nature's First Law.

To receive free exclusive e-mail bulletins (concerning upcoming events, David Wolfe's seminars, new products, exciting news, media coverage) from Nature's First Law and David Wolfe, simply send an e-mail to: nature@rawfood.com requesting to be added to the subscriber list.

Nature's First Law
Mailing Address: PO Box 900202, San Diego, CA 92190 U.S.A.
Store Location: 1475 N. Cuyamaca St., El Cajon, CA 92020
(888) 729-3663 - orders only
International: +001-619-596-7979
Fax: 619-596-7997
E-mail: nature@rawfood.com
Internet Homepage: www.rawfood.com

Found a family,
Plant a forest,
Rule your mind,
And laugh with the gods.